Second Edition

Building Better Caregivers

A Caregiver's Guide to Reducing Stress and Staying Healthy

Kate Lorig, DrPH • **Diana Laurent**, MPH
Maureen Gecht-Silver, OTD, MPH, OTR/L
Dolores Gallagher Thompson, PhD, ABPP
Marian Minor, RPT, PhD • **Virginia González**, MPH
David Sobel, MD, MPH • **Richard Reimer**, MD

Bull Publishing Company
Boulder, Colorado

Published by Bull Publishing Company
P.O. Box 1377
Boulder, CO, USA 80306
www.bullpub.com

Library of Congress Cataloging-in-Publication Data

Library of Congress Cataloging-in-Publication Data

Names: Lorig, Kate, author. | González, Virginia (Virginia M.) author. | Laurent, Diana, author. | Sobel, David S. (David Stuart), author. | Gecht-Silver, Maureen, author. | Gallagher-Thompson, Dolores, author. | Minor, Marian A. (Marian Adams), author.

Title: Building better caregivers : a caregiver's guide to reducing stress and staying healthy / by Kate Lorig, DrPH, Virginia González, MPH, Diana Laurent, MPH, David Sobel, MD, MPH, Maureen Gecht-Silver, OTD, MPH, OTR/L, Dolores Gallagher Thompson, PhD, ABPP, Marian Minor, RPT, PhD.

Description: 2nd edition. | Boulder, Colorado : Bull Publishing Company, [2025] | Includes index.

Identifiers: LCCN 2024061793 (print) | LCCN 2024061794 (ebook) | ISBN 9781945188572 (trade paperback) | ISBN 9781945188589 (adobe pdf)

Subjects: LCSH: Caregivers--Health and hygiene. | Caregivers--Psychology. | Long-term care of the sick.

Classification: LCC RA645.3 .L67 2025 (print) | LCC RA645.3 (ebook) | DDC 362/.0425--dc23/eng/20250218

LC record available at https://lccn.loc.gov/2024061793

LC ebook record available at https://lccn.loc.gov/2024061794

Printed in U.S.A.

30 29 28 27 26 25   10 9 8 7 6 5 4 3 2 1

Interior design and project management: Dovetail Publishing Services

Cover design and production: Shannon Bodie, BookwiseDesign.com

To Jim Bull and Erin Mulligan, who made this book possible

The Authors

Kate Lorig, DrPH, is professor emerita at Stanford University School of Medicine and a partner in the Self-Management Resource Center (SMRC). As director of the Stanford Patient Education Research Center she was a co-developer of the Building Better Caregivers educational program. For 20 years, Kate watched her mother care for her father, who was severely disabled by a stroke.

Diana Laurent, MPH, is a health educator and partner in the Self-Management Resource Center. During her over 30 years at Stanford School of Medicine, she co-developed the Building Better Caregivers program, as well as several other educational programs. Diana was and is a caregiver of her parents and in-laws; she also has experience in participating in the care of relatives who have dementia.

Maureen Gecht-Silver, OTD, MPH, OTR/L, is a retired assistant professor of clinical family and community medicine and occupational therapy at University of Illinois Chicago. Currently, an adjunct faculty member in the occupational therapy program at DePaul University in Chicago, Illinois, she has taught collaborative communication skills to health professionals in both clinical and academic settings. Her work has focused on improving self-management skills and quality of life of people with chronic conditions and disabilities as well as their caregivers. She, along with her sisters, was a caregiver for her father, who lived to age 98.

Dolores Gallagher Thompson, PhD, ABPP, is board-certified in clinical psychology and geropsychology and is professor emerita at Stanford University School of Medicine and co-director of the Optimal Aging Center in Los Altos, California. She has 30 years of experience in conducting funded intervention research with family caregivers and worked directly with caregivers in her clinical practice at Stanford. Dolores entered this field after being a long-distance caregiver for her mother who suffered multiple strokes before her death; at that time few resources for caregiving families were available and her experience shaped her subsequent career choices.

Marian Minor, PT, MSPH, PhD, is a professor emerita at the University of Missouri School of Health Professions where she taught and did research on exercise. She has contributed exercise information for self-management education for a variety of populations. Marian has been a caregiver herself and has supported other caregivers for many years.

Virginia González, MPH, is a health educator and partner in the Self-Management Resource Center (SMRC). She has over 15 years of experience working at the Stanford School of Medicine, where she was a co-developer of various self-management programs and was instrumental in the cultural adaptation and Spanish translation of these programs for Latino/Hispanic communities. After leaving Stanford and before becoming a partner in SMRC, Virginia was raising her children, while caring for her aging, chronically ill parents and in-laws. She also has personal experience with caring for extended family members with dementia and mental illness.

David Sobel, MD, MPH, is adjunct lecturer, Department of Medicine, Stanford University School of Medicine. As the medical director of Patient Education and Health Promotion for Kaiser Permanente Northern California he developed and evaluated programs to serve over 5 million members. In addition, he has served along with his brother as a caregiver for both parents in their 90's, and he is currently helping with the care of a neighbor with advanced dementia.

Richard Reimer, MD, is a Neurologist who is the Chief of the Neurology Service for the Veterans Administration Palo Alto Healthcare System and has been a Stanford University School of Medicine faculty member for over 20 years. He has assisted in the care for his parents as well as multiple other family members.

Acknowledgments

MANY PEOPLE HAVE HELPED US write this book. Among the most important are the first 200 participants of the Stanford University Building Better Caregiver studies. These have been followed by thousands of other online and small group workshop participants. These caregivers, along with our wonderful workshop leaders, have told us what information they needed and helped us make adjustments as we went along.

There are many professionals who have assisted us: We are especially thankful to the guidance and insights of Laural Traylor, MSW, and Theodore J. Hahn, MD, from the Veterans Administration, Bonnie Bruce, RD, DrPH, Cindy Tan, MPH, Chaplain Bruce Feldstein, MD, Catherine Regan, PhD, and Richard Seidel, PhD. To all of you, your help has been gratefully received.

There are also Fran Rice, Jean Thompson and many other friends, leaders and trainers who have given us wonderful advice and have added richness to our thinking.

A Special thanks to Canary Health and Katy Plant who have made this program available through the Veterans Administration.

We would also like to thank the publishers for permission to adapt sections from *The Healthy Mind, Healthy Body Handbook* (also published as *The Mind & Body Health Handbook*) by David Sobel, MD, and Robert Ornstein, PhD (published by DRx).

Finally, thanks to David Bull. David was our first publisher and had faith in this project that allowed us to proceed. Without him, there may never have been a book. His son Jim has continued the family tradition with support and encouragement.

If you would like to learn more about our continuing work, online internet programs, trainings, and materials see our website:

https://www.selfmanagementresource.com

If you would like to find workshops near you see:

https://selfmanagementresource.com
/license-locator/

We are continually revising and improving this book. If you have any suggestions or comments, please send them to:

smrc@selfmanagementresource.com

Contents

Disclaimer

This book is not intended to replace common sense, or professional medical or psychological advice. You should seek and get appropriate professional evaluation and treatment for problems—especially unusual, unexplained, severe, or persistent symptoms. Many symptoms and diseases require and benefit from specific medical or psychological evaluation and treatment. Don't deny yourself or your care partner proper professional care.

- If your or your care partner's symptoms or problems persist beyond a reasonable period despite using self-care recommendations, you should consult a health professional. What is a reasonable period will vary; if you're not sure and you're feeling anxious, consult a health care professional.
- If you receive professional advice in conflict with this book, you should rely upon the guidance provided by your or your care partner's health care professional. They are likely to be able to take your specific situation, history, and needs into consideration. If you are experiencing violence in your home, get out and seek help from health care professionals and/or law enforcement.
- If you are having thoughts of harming yourself in any way, please seek professional care immediately.

Medical treatment and knowledge are continually evolving. This book is as accurate as its publisher and authors can make it at the time of publication, but we cannot guarantee that it will work for you or your care partner in every case. The authors and publisher disclaim any and all liability for any claims or injuries that you may believe arose from following the recommendations set forth in this book. This book is only a guide; your common sense, good judgment, and partnership with health professionals are also needed.

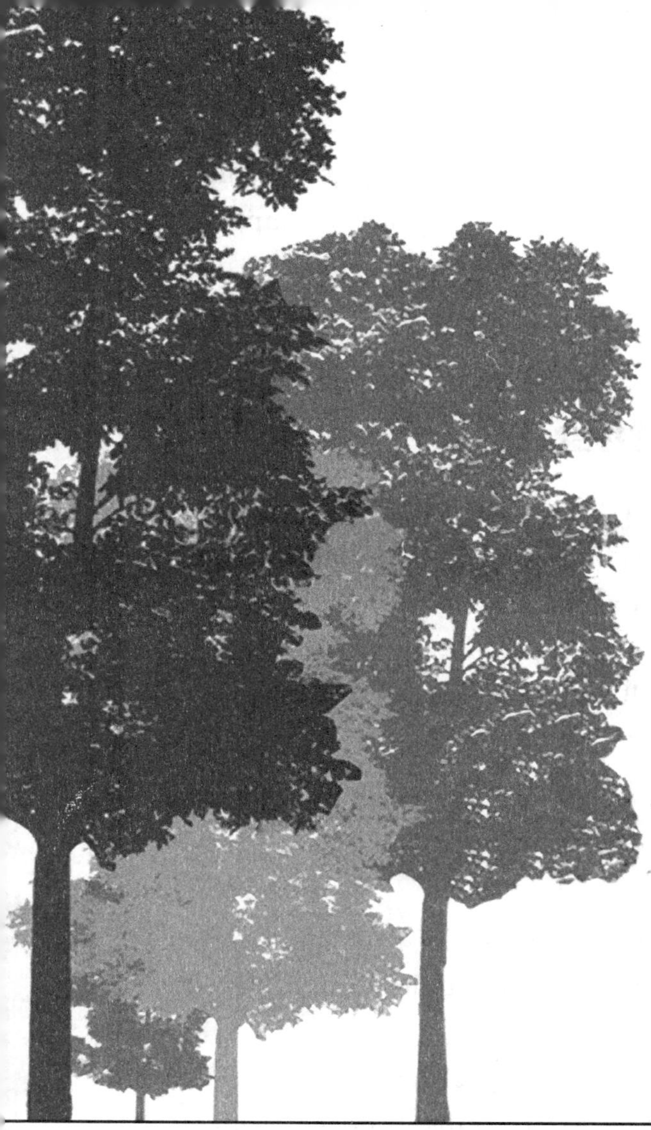

CHAPTER 1

Introduction: A Blueprint for Better Caregiving

AS PEOPLE PLAN THEIR LIVES, there are many things they prepare for and expect. People go to school, go to work, choose partners, have children, lose loved ones, become empty nesters, retire, etc. Caregiving is not usually part of anyone's expected life plan. Most people do not ask to be caregivers or prepare to be caregivers, and sometimes, people do not want to be caregivers. Nevertheless, people are caregivers and, more importantly, they have chosen to be caregivers.

That last statement may seem a little strange. You did not choose to have a relative, spouse, or friend become ill or injured and need care. What you did choose, however, was to care for them. Many people for one reason or another do not make this choice and do not provide care to others. So, congratulations for making that choice and being a caregiver! You are a very special person! As the authors of this book, we are here to share our expertise and the best in caregiving research. We also share what we have learned from thousands of people like you, as well as our own experiences as caregivers.

Together, we hope to help you gain skills to take care of yourself and your care partner(s). Probably the most important thing that these skills will give you is confidence to manage your life and reduce your stress. Our goal is to improve the quality of life for both you and your care partner.

What Is a Care Partner?

You may be wondering just what is a care partner? Your care partner is the person for whom you are caring. Your care partner may be Sally, or Jose, your sweetie, your mom, or your old man. No matter what you call the person, in this book, we refer to this person as a *care partner*. We do this because it is awkward to always say "the person you are caring for." A wonderful group of caregivers suggested this name and it works well for our purposes in this book.

Using This Book

Before we go any further, let's talk about this book and how to use it. Throughout, you will find information to help you learn and practice your caregiving skills. Some of these skills will help your care partner, but most of the skills are aimed at helping you both to care for someone else and to care for yourself. This is not a textbook. You do not need to read every word in every chapter. Instead, we suggest that you read the first two chapters and then use the table of contents to hunt out and find the information you need. Feel free to skip around. In this way, you will find and learn the skills you need to negotiate your individual path when you most need those skills.

What is in this book? This is your Caregiver's Toolbox. You will not find any miracles or cures. But you will find accurate and reliable information and hundreds of tips and ideas to make your life easier. The advice in this book comes from physicians and other health professionals, as well as caregivers like you. The content is supported by research studies, and it is as up-to-date as possible.

Caregiving is a great leveler. Everyone can learn the necessary skills. It does not matter if you went to school for five years or 25 years. Nor are caregiving skills related to race, age, gender, or genetics. The good news is that there is no test, not even pass or fail.

Our assumption is that most caregivers are doing a terrific job under conditions that are often difficult. In addition to being a challenging job, caregiving can also be isolating. You may be cut off from friends and even family. This makes learning from others difficult. To help you overcome this isolation, we have talked to hundreds of caregivers, as well as people who study caregiving. What we have learned, we have put into this book. Our hope is that by sharing this wisdom and knowledge from others, we can help you and others like you become better caregivers.

Stress and Caregiving

Caregiving is stressful. This is one of the things that we have been told by everyone who has experience with caregiving and caregivers. It is almost impossible to be a caregiver without experiencing increased stress. For some, this may be a little stress and for others, lots of stress. Figure 1.1 illustrates stressors—the things that can cause caregiver stress. In this book, we discuss each of these stressors in detail and give you some information on how to develop the skills needed to deal with these stressors. As you gain more confidence in your skills, our hope is that your stress decreases.

You probably hear a lot about stress in everyday conversations and in the media. But what is stress? In the 1950s, the physiologist Hans Selye described stress as "the nonspecific response of the body to any demand made upon it." Other researchers and doctors have expanded this definition to explain that the body adapts to demands, whether pleasant or unpleasant. In short, stress is how people react emotionally to a stressor. The stressor can be a dog barking, receiving bad or even good news, someone saying unkind words, or fear of the future. For caregivers, it is often the frustrating or difficult behaviors of our care partners (more about this later). When you are exposed to stressors, not only do you have an *emotional* reaction, such as anger, sadness, or crying, but your body also reacts *physically* with muscle tension, headaches, fatigue, or pain. Your heart may beat faster, and you might have problems breathing. Stress can cause people to shout, weep, go quiet, flee, or smile nervously.

If all this seems complex to you, you are right. Stress is complex. Thankfully, you do not have to understand how stress works to do something about it. Consider the following two people and their stories:

- John has been a caregiver for Julianna for many months. He has lost contact with

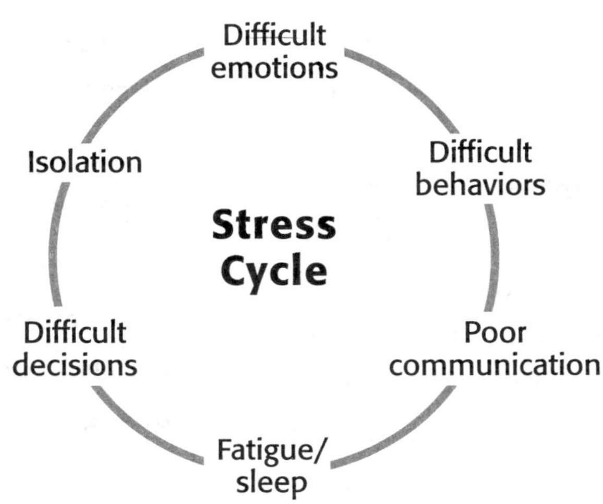

Figure 1.1 **The Stress Cycle**

most of their friends. Julianna has Alzheimer's disease, and it seems like every day she remembers less and less. John is worried about his ability to cope. One day Julianna cannot remember his name. John becomes angry, sits down, and cries. Julianna looks confused and frightened.

- Ellen has been the caregiver for Jose for many months. Jose has Alzheimer's disease, and it seems like every day his memory gets worse. Ellen is worried about her ability to cope, but she has found an online support group and she also talks to her friends about her concerns. One day, Jose cannot remember her name. Ellen is sad and mourns for all they both have lost. She takes a few minutes for herself and then gives Jose a dish of his favorite ice cream. He smiles.

These two examples are similar. The stressor—a care partner not remembering a caregiver's name—is the same. The immediate emotional reaction of the two caregivers is also similar. They both feel sadness. There are also differences. Ellen has some support. She has maintained contact with friends and joined an online support group. John does not seem to have any support. John's sadness is accompanied by anger which frightens his care partner. Ellen's sadness prompts her to try to show love to her care partner. Her reward is a smile.

In the chapters to follow, you will find many tools for dealing with stress. Chapter 2, Becoming a Better Caregiver: The Basics, gives you the basic tools discussed in this book and Chapter 3, Dealing with Stress and Difficult Care Partner Behavior, is a thorough introduction to the basics of stress.

Thinking About Caregiving

Just changing the way you think cannot cure stress. However, challenging negative thinking and certain caregiving skills can make caregiving easier. What you do about something is largely determined by how you think about it. For example, if you think that being a caregiver is like falling into a deep pit, you may have a hard time motivating yourself to crawl out, or you may think the task is impossible. The thoughts you have can greatly determine what happens to both you and your care partner. We talk more about this in Chapter 5, Using Your Mind to Manage Stress.

The following are some of the thoughts that caregivers have shared with us and some suggestions for ways to address the problems that these thoughts present:

"When things do not go right or my care partner behaves badly, it is my fault."

You are not to blame. You did not cause your care partner's condition. Your care partner's behavior is the result of trauma or genetic, biological, environmental, and/or psychological factors. We do not feel guilty when a young child has a tantrum or wets their pants. These behaviors are part of a developmental process. Similarly, your care partner's behaviors are caused by a disease, not by you. However, in both cases you are responsible for helping to manage these behaviors. We talk more about strategies to manage care partner behavior in Chapter 3, Dealing with Stress and Difficult Care Partner Behavior.

"I feel so guilty."

Guilt is a common caregiver feeling. You may feel guilty because you find caregiving difficult, you do not think you are doing enough, or you don't like all the tasks caretaking involves. You are probably doing the very best you can. You may also feel guilty because you want your old life back. Believe us when we say that almost every caregiver feels this way.

"I should have done that when I had the chance."

There are lots of "if only I had (fill in the blank with anything you wish you had done) when I had the chance" moments. Well, you have a chance now. We cannot remake or undo the past, but we can, to some extent, determine the present and the future.

"I am so isolated. I feel so alone. No one offers any help."

You don't have to do it alone. A common feeling for caregivers is isolation. As supportive as friends and family members may be, they often cannot understand what you are experiencing as you struggle to cope and survive daily. They do not know how to help and so they may stay away. You may have even told them that there is nothing they can do.

Connecting with other people with similar conditions can reduce your sense of isolation. A fellow caregiver's perspective can help you understand what to expect. Other people can offer practical tips on how to manage day-to-day, give you the opportunity to help others cope with their caregiving, help you appreciate your strengths, and realize that things could be worse. Your peers can inspire you to become a better caregiver. Support can come from reading a book or a newsletter about the experiences of other caregivers. It may come from regularly scheduled family meetings or from talking with others on the telephone, in support groups, or connecting online through computer and electronic support groups. Invite people to bring in a meal, connect on social media such as Facebook or Instagram, talk to someone on the phone, or use FaceTime or Zoom to video chat with distant friends and relatives. You will find more about getting support in Chapter 3, Dealing with Stress and Difficult Care Partner Behavior, and Chapter 7, Getting Help.

We know that caregivers do not have much time, but we also know that good caregivers do not do it alone. If you are not alone, then you or maybe someone else must manage caregiving. Your job can be made easier if you reach out to other caregivers, family, friends, health professionals, and social service agencies. Your job is to learn from and to manage these "consultants." You, as a caregiving manager, gather information, make decisions, and use consultants, such as health care professionals or caregiving help.

Succeeding as a Caregiver

In this book, we describe many skills and tools to help you succeed as a caregiver and address real problems such as caregiving stress. You may find that some skills and tools are more helpful than others. Some may not be helpful at all. We do not expect you to use them all. Pick and choose. Experiment. Set your own goals. All we ask is that you try something before you reject it. You might be surprised. It might work and then you will have a new caregiving tool. *What you do may not be as important as the sense of confidence and control that comes from doing something you want to do and succeeding at it.*

We have all noticed that some caregivers get on well and seem content with their task, while others have many daily problems and are miserable. The difference often lies in their caregiving skills and management style.

The keys to success in any undertaking are:

- defining the problem and exploring possible solutions (problem solving),
- deciding what you want to do and how you are going to do it (decision making), and
- learning the set of skills you need and practicing them until they have been mastered (action planning).

But knowing the skills is not enough. To succeed, you need a way of incorporating them into your daily life. Whenever you try a new skill, the first attempts may be clumsy or slow and might not work. It is easier to return to old ways than to continue trying to master new and sometimes difficult tasks. The best way to master new skills is through practice and evaluation of the results. In Chapter 2, Becoming a Better Caregiver: The Basics, we introduce and discuss three core caregiving skills: problem-solving, decision-making, and action-planning.

Being More than a Caregiver

When you are a caregiver, too often there can seem to be nothing in your life except caregiving. But you are more than a caregiver for your care partner. Grow areas of your life that you enjoy. Small daily pleasures can help balance uncomfortable and demanding tasks or emotions. Find ways to enjoy nature by growing a plant or watching a sunset; or indulge in the pleasure of human touch or a tasty meal; or celebrate companionship with family or friends. Finding ways to introduce moments of pleasure is vital.

Focus on your abilities and assets rather than disabilities and deficits. Celebrate small improvements—improvement in your caregiving, in your stress level, and in your care partner's emotions and behaviors. If caregiving teaches anything, it is to live each moment more fully. Within the true limits of whatever problems you and your care partner have, there are ways to enhance your sense of control and enjoyment of life.

Some of the most successful caregivers are people who think of caregiving as a path. This path, like any path, goes up and down. Sometimes it is flat and smooth. At other times, it is rough and frightening. To negotiate this path, one must use many strategies. Sometimes you can go fast, but other times you must slow down. There are obstacles to negotiate.

As we build better caregivers, we first must prepare to create an overall plan. In this chapter, we outlined some of the many challenges caregivers face and some basic ways you can approach those challenges. In the next chapter, we build the foundation and structure and walk you through building a personal action plan of your own. After that, you can read the chapters in whichever order you prefer and pick and choose the skills that will be most helpful to you. Just remember, this book is your Caregiver's Toolbox. You are the builder, and we are here to help.

For a complete list of suggested further readings, useful websites, and other helpful resources, please see: www.bullpub.com/resources.

Chapter 2

Becoming a Better Caregiver: The Basics

You know better than anyone that becoming a caregiver means making many changes in your life—changes in what you do and how you do it, and changes in how you socialize. It may mean giving up a paid job or working fewer paid hours. It also changes the dynamics of families and friendships. For some people, caregiving is full time, 24 hours a day every day. For other people, it takes up a few hours a week.

No matter how much time it takes or how complex the caregiving, as a caregiver, you have a major decision to make. Are you going to take it one day at a time and cope the best you can, or are you going to become a better caregiver by learning skills, problem-solving, and planning? Please note the word *decision*. There is no way to avoid deciding. If you choose to do nothing, that is a decision. If your decision is to become a better caregiver, then let's get started.

Like any skill, active caregiving must be learned and practiced. This chapter will start you on your way by presenting the three most important caregiving tools: problem-solving, decision-making, and action planning. Remember, as we mentioned in Chapter 1, Introduction: A Blueprint for Better Caregiving, you are the caregiving manager. Both at home and in the business world, managers direct the show. They don't do everything themselves; they work with others, including consultants, to get the job done. What makes them managers is that they are responsible for setting the agenda, solving problems, making decisions, and making sure that their decisions are carried out.

Like the manager of an organization or a household, you must do all the following things:

1. Identify problems and seek solutions (problem-solving).
2. Make decisions for both you and your care partner (decision-making).
3. Take action (action planning).

In the rest of this chapter, we explore each of these skills and discuss ways you can be a better manager and caregiver. One note: These skills are for you, the caregiver. Many care partners will not be able to master these tools.

Solving Problems: Identifying Problems and Seeking Solutions

Problems sometimes start with a feeling of general uneasiness. In order to think more about problem-solving, imagine yourself as the caregiver in the following story.

You may feel unhappy but you're not sure why. Upon closer examination, you find that you want some caregiving help from your family. Some of them live quite close, but except for an occasional phone call, they have all but disappeared from your life.

Your first thought is that they just don't want to be bothered and so you must do everything yourself. The more you think about this, this more you realize that this is not a solution. A solution would fix the problem, and you still have the problem. You also realize that you are not sure why they are staying away or exactly what help you need. You consider calling and telling them what you are thinking, but you are afraid your concerns will be made light of or be ignored. You think about getting help elsewhere but do not know how to start, and you worry that it may be too expensive. You talk about this with a good friend who suggests a family meeting. (We discuss family meetings in more detail in Chapter 7, Getting Help). You had never thought about this but decide to learn more.

The problem of getting help still seems overwhelming. This idea of gathering the family for a meeting is all so new and you are not sure you have the time or strength to face all that you must do. However, you decide to take the first step by finding out more about family meetings. You make this an action plan. (You will learn more about action planning later in this chapter).

To start your action plan, you promise yourself that this week you will gather more information about family meetings. You begin by looking at the content in this book about family meetings. You find this information helpful, but you need more. So, you search the topic on the internet. An internet search for family meetings leads to lots of links for families with young children, but that is not what you need. You decide to add the word *caregiver* and find lots of information that fits your needs. Now you know more than you did, but you think that you may need more help. You decide to call the local Alzheimer's Association (in Canada, Alzheimer Society of Canada) to see if they can help. You have just used the problem-solving tool in your Caregiver's Toolbox to achieve your goal of getting your family to help.

Let's review the specific steps you, as the caregiver in this situation, took to solve your problem:

1. **Identify the problem.** This is the first and biggest step in problem-solving—and usually the most difficult step as well. You may know that you are unhappy or stressed, but you may not know why until you think it over. With a little thought, you realize that you could use help and that your family has not been very helpful. In this example, the problem is needing help and feeling unhappy that family has not helped.
2. **List ideas to solve the problem.** Sometimes you may come up with a good list yourself. Other times, you may want to call on some of the "consultants" we mentioned in Chapter 1, Introduction: A Blueprint for Better Caregiving, to help you make that list. Consultants can be friends, family, members of a health care team, or community resources. Keep in mind that consultants cannot help you if you do not describe the problem well. For example, there is a big difference between just saying, "I am unhappy," and saying, "I need help and am disappointed that my family is not helping more."
3. **Choose an idea to try.** As you consider trying something new, remember that new activities are usually difficult. Feeling nervous or discouraged may be part of the process. Be sure to give your potential solution or problem-solving method a fair chance before deciding it doesn't work. Sometimes you have to try a couple of things. In our example, the first internet search was unsuccessful, but adding an extra search term helped uncover more helpful information. The thing to remember is to keep trying.
4. **Check the results.** After you've given your idea a fair trial, your problem may be solved. In this example, you still may not have found help, but two things have happened. First, you are working on a way of approaching your family for help. Second, you have reached out to a consultant, the Alzheimer's Association.
5. If you still have the problem, **pick another idea from your list and try again**. In our example, maybe you will decide not to have a family meeting, or the family meeting fails. You go to the list for another idea.
6. If your original list of ideas is not proving useful, **use other resources** (for example, other consultants) for more ideas. Then go back to step 3 with your new list of possible solutions.

Problem-Solving Steps

1. Identify the problem.
2. List ideas to solve the problem.
3. Choose one solution or method to try.
4. Check the results.
5. Pick another idea if the first didn't work.
6. Use other resources for a new list.
7. Accept that the problem might not be solvable now.

7. If you have gone through all the steps until all ideas have been exhausted and the problem is still unsolved, you may have to **accept that your problem might not be solvable right now**. This is sometimes hard to do. However, living with uncertainty is something we must all learn to do, and a caregiver's life contains more uncertainty than most. The fact that a problem can't be solved right now doesn't mean that it won't be solvable later or that other problems cannot be solved. Even if your path is blocked, there are probably alternative paths. Don't give up. Keep going.

Living with Uncertainty

In this chapter, we are sharing important tools for problem-solving, decision-making, and action planning. We know that sometimes it is hard to use these tools given the amount of uncertainty caregiving involves. Living with uncertainty is one of the hardest aspects of caregiving. It is something that most people cannot avoid. Uncertainty can be a stressor and one of the causes of emotional ups and downs. Facing the decline of someone important to you and becoming a caregiver takes away some of your sense of security and control. These processes can be frightening and introduce uncertainty into your life in a whole new way. You are following your life path, and suddenly, you are forced to detour onto a different, unwanted path. If you have been a caregiver for many months or even years, this uncertainty continues. Of course, everyone has an uncertain future, but most people are able to avoid thinking about it. When you become a caregiver, uncertainty becomes an unavoidable part of your life. We are uncertain about our care partner's health and function, and perhaps about our ability to continue as a caregiver. Often this uncertainty is the reason given for avoiding making decisions. Remember, no matter what you do, even if you do nothing, you are making a decision.

Making Decisions: Weighing the Pros and Cons

Like problem-solving, decision-making is another important skill in your Caregiver's Toolbox. The following are the steps for making a decision. They are a little like those for problem-solving.

1. **Identify the options.** For example, you may be feeling overwhelmed with housework and yard work. You have to make a decision about how to handle this problem. Your options include getting help in the house or continuing to do all the work yourself or maybe letting the yard work go. Sometimes your options are to change something and sometimes they are to *not* change something.
2. **Identify what you want.** What is important to you? Do you want to spend more time with your care partner or to take the time doing work in the house or yard to have a break from your care partner? Maybe what you really want to do is spend time alone shoveling the walkway, cutting the grass, or cleaning the house. Sometimes, identifying your deepest values helps you set priorities and increases your motivation to change.
3. **Write down pros and cons for each option.** List as many items as you can in two columns, one column for the pros and the other for the cons. Don't forget to list the emotional and social costs of each option.
4. **Rate each item on the pros and cons list** on a 5-point scale with 0 indicating "not at all important" and 5 indicating "extremely important."
5. **Add up the ratings for each column and compare them.** Noting which column has the highest total should help you identify the best decision for you. If the totals are close or you are still not sure, skip to the next step.
6. **Take the "gut test."** For example, does hiring someone to help you around the house feel right to you even if it means you might have to work more hours or make some financial sacrifices? If so, you have probably reached a decision. If not, the way you feel should probably win out over the math.

You may wonder, "If I am going to go with my gut, why do I have to do all the math?" This is a good question. The reason is that the thinking that goes on in steps 1–3 helps you to understand your gut decision and clarify issues.

Decision-Making Example

Should I get help in the house?

Pro	Rating	Con	Rating
I'll have more time	4	It's expensive	3
I'll be less tired	4	It's hard to find good help	1
I'll have a clean house	3	They won't do things my way	2
		I don't want a stranger in the house	1
Total	11		7

Add up the points for the pro and con lists. The decision in this example would be to get help because the pro score (11) is significantly higher than the con score (7). If this feels right in your gut, you have the answer.

Now it's your turn! Try making a decision using the following chart. It's OK to write in your book.

Decision to be made ______________________

Pro	Rating	Con	Rating
Total			

Note: The intent of this exercise is to help *you* make a decision. It is not for your care partner to make a decision. Many caregiving problems come from asking care partners to make choices that they may not be able to make. For example, you are going for a ride and ask your care partner, Maria, where she would like to go today. She says she'd like to visit her sister in St. Louis (this is 500 miles away). You say that this is not possible and your care partner is very unhappy. The problem is that the question was open-ended. It's better to ask, "Would you like to go to the grocery store or to the park?" We will talk much more about frustrating or problem care partner behaviors in Chapter 3, Dealing with Stress and Difficult Care Partner Behavior.

The key to successful problem-solving and decision-making is taking action. We talk about this next.

Taking Action

Simply knowing you want to do something is not enough. Once you have looked at a problem and made the difficult decision to take action, how can you begin? We suggest that you start by doing one thing at a time.

Setting Goals

Before you can take action, you must decide what you want to do first. Be realistic and specific when stating your goals. One caregiver wanted to have a few hours a week away from home. Another wanted to reduce anxiety and sleep better. Still another wanted to continue to ride their motorcycle but could no longer lift the 1,000-pound bike when it was lying on the ground. (Note that the tools in this chapter are not just for caregiving concerns but can be used for solving most problems, making decisions, and taking action.)

One of the problems with goals is that they often seem like dreams. They are so far off, big, or difficult that we are overwhelmed and don't even try to accomplish them. We'll tackle this problem next. For now, take a few minutes and write your goals below (add more lines if you need to). This should be something you *want* to do, not something you think you *should* do.

Goals

____

____

____

____

____

Put a star (☆) next to the goal you would like to work on first.

Don't reject a goal as unreachable until you have thought about all the possible alternatives. Sometimes people reject options without knowing much about them. In the earlier example, the caregiver looked for some ways to get the family to help and chose to learn more about family meetings. Although this was not a familiar option, it was not rejected without consideration.

Exploring Options

There are many ways to reach any specific goal. For example, a caregiver who wants to spend a few hours away from their caregiving responsibilities each week could ask a friend to stay with their care partner or might employ someone for a few hours. Maybe there is a high school student that could come in as part of a community service requirement. Or maybe they can ask for help in a church bulletin or email list. Maybe having their care partner spend two mornings a week at a local day health center would help. The caregiver who wants to be less anxious and get more sleep might look into relaxation exercises or yoga videos. They may make a list of the things interfering with sleep so they could start problem-solving how to change them. They might decide to talk to their health care provider about options. Our motorcycle rider could trade in their heavy motorcycle for a lighter one, use a sidecar, put training wheels on the bike, buy a three-wheeled motorcycle, or give up riding.

As you can see, there are many options for reaching each goal. The idea here is to list all the options you can think of and then choose one or two to try out.

Sometimes it is hard to think of all the options yourself. If you are having problems, use a consultant, just as you would in problem-solving. Share your goal with family, friends, and health professionals and ask them for suggestions. You can call community organizations such as Catholic or Jewish family services, a senior center, or the Area Agency on Aging. In Canada, you can reach out to the Service Canada call centre (1 800 O Canada) for programs and services for seniors or Dial 2-1-1. You can search the internet for almost anything.

Don't ask what you should do. Rather, ask for suggestions. It is always good to add to your list of options and to get a fresh perspective from a person who is new to the problem.

A note of caution: Many options are never seriously considered because people assume they don't exist or are unworkable. Never make this assumption until you have thoroughly investigated the option. One woman we know had lived in the same town all her life and felt she knew all about the community resources. When she was having problems with her health insurance, a friend from another city suggested contacting an insurance counselor. The woman dismissed this suggestion because she was certain that this service did not exist in her town.

It was only when, months later, the friend came to visit and called the Area Agency on Aging (which exists in most counties in the United States) that the woman learned that there were three insurance counseling services nearby. Our motorcycle rider thought that adding training wheels to a Harley was a crazy idea, but then explored the idea at a motorcycle shop. Using training wheels extended their riding life by 15 years. In short, never assume anything. Assumptions are major problem-solving and decision-making enemies.

Write the list of options for your main goal here.

Options

____

____

____

____

____

Put a star (☆) next to the two or three options you want to research further.

Action Planning: Making Short-Term Plans

For most of us, once we make a decision, we have a good idea of where we are going. However, some goals may seem overwhelming. How will you ever be able to move, how will you ever be able to make a life for yourself again, how will you ever be able to ____________________ (fill in the blank)? The secret to success is to ***not*** try to do everything at once. Instead, look at one thing that you can realistically expect to accomplish within ***the next week***.

This approach to moving forward is an *action plan*. An action plan is something that is short-term (usually a week), is doable, and sets you on the road toward your goal. Your action plan should be about something you want to do or accomplish. It should help you solve your problem and reach your goal. It is a tool to help you do what *you* wish. Do not make action plans to please your care partner, friends, family, or health care provider.

Action plans are probably your most used tool for success as a caregiver. Most caregivers can do things to make caregiving easier, but they fail to do them. Often, failing has more to do with not knowing how to make these new skills part of our daily routine than a lack of will or ability to master the skills. For example, most caregivers have the ability to practice the skills that will lessen their care partner's difficult or frustrating behaviors. However, few caregivers have a systematic plan for doing this. Think about your and your partner's activities of daily living (ADLs). ADLs are everyday things such as getting out of bed, bathing, dressing, preparing and eating meals, cleaning house, shopping, and paying bills. Can an action plan help you accomplish any of these tasks more efficiently? Can it help you find the energy to both accomplish your ADLs and be less stressed out?

An action plan helps you do the things you know you *should* do, but to create a successful action plan, it is best to start with something that you *want* to do. You can start with *anything*. In the following material, we go through the steps for making a realistic action plan.

Creating a Realistic Action Plan

First, decide what you will do this week. For someone seeking information, this might mean setting aside 15 minutes on each of three days this week to read, call community agencies, or look things up online. For the caregiver who wants to be less anxious and to sleep better, it may mean practicing a relaxation exercise at bedtime for four nights. The caregiver who wants to continue riding a motorcycle might spend half an hour over two days researching lighter motorcycles and motorcycle training wheels.

Make very sure that your plans are action specific. For example, rather than just deciding to lose weight (which is not an action but the result of an action), you plan to replace soda with tea (which is an action).

Next, make a specific plan. Deciding what you want to do is worthless without a plan to do it. The plan should answer all of the following questions:

- Exactly *what* are you going to do? Are you going to take a walk when you get stressed out or drink a big glass of cold water to avoid overeating when you feel anxious? Will you call someone when you start to feel stress build? What relaxation technique will you practice?

- *How much* will you do? This question is answered with something like time, distance, portions, or repetitions. Will you walk one block, walk for 15 minutes, eat half portions at lunch and dinner, or practice relaxation exercises for 15 minutes each evening?
- *When* will you do this? Again, this must be specific: in the late afternoon (when you know you are likely to be tired and more susceptible to stress and losing your temper), before lunch, at the evening meal, or before going to bed. Connecting a new activity with an old habit is a good way to make sure it gets done. Consider what comes right before your action plan that could trigger the new behavior. For example, you will do five minutes of relaxation breathing each afternoon right after you do the lunch dishes. Another trick is to incorporate your new activity into your routine right before an old favorite activity. For example, you could walk around the block before reading the paper or watching a favorite TV program.
- *How often* will you do the activity? This is a bit tricky. We would all like to engage in positive habits every day, but that is not always possible. It is usually best to decide to do an activity three or four times a week to give yourself wiggle room if something comes up. If you do it more often, so much the better. However, if you are like most people, you will feel less pressure if you can do your activity three or four times a week and still feel successful.

Here are some general guidelines for writing your action plan that may help. First, *start where you are*, start small, or start slowly. If you can walk for only one minute, start your walking program by walking one minute once every hour or two, not by trying to walk a block. If you have never done any exercise, start with a few minutes of warm-up. A total of five or ten minutes is enough. If you want to avoid stress overeating, set a goal based on your existing eat-

Success Improves Health

The benefits of change go beyond the payoffs of adopting healthier habits. Obviously, you will feel better and be a better caregiver when you are less stressed, communicate positively with your care partner, exercise, eat well, keep regular sleeping hours, stop smoking, and take time to relax. But regardless of the behavior that's changed, there's evidence that the feelings of self-confidence and control over your life that come from making any successful change improve your health.

Being a caregiver is sometimes not good for our self-image. For many people, it is discouraging to be faced by many problems and stressors each day and to find they do not possess all the coping skills they wish they did. By changing and improving one area of your life, whether it is approaching care partner problems differently, boosting your physical fitness, or learning a new skill, you regain a sense of optimism and vitality. By focusing on what you can do rather than what you wish you could do, you're more likely to lead a more positive and happier life. Taking steps to improve your self-confidence can make you feel better inside and out.

Elements of a Successful Action Plan

- The plan is something ***you*** want to do.
- The plan is achievable (something you can expect to be able to do that week).
- The plan is action specific.
- The plan answers the questions ***what, how much, when,*** and ***how often?***
- You are certain that you will complete your entire plan at a level of 7 or higher on a scale from 0 = not at all sure to 10 = absolutely sure.

ing behaviors. Don't state that you will never eat dessert gain. Instead, plan on serving yourself half portions for one meal a day.

For example, losing a pound this week is not an action plan because it does not involve a specific action; not eating after dinner for four days this week, by contrast, is a fine action plan.

Second, *give yourself some time off*. All people have days when they don't feel like doing anything. That is a good reason for saying that you will do something three times a week instead of every day.

Third, once you've made your action plan, *ask yourself* the following question: "On a scale of 0 to 10, with 0 being totally unsure and 10 being totally certain, how sure am I that I can complete this entire plan?"

If your answer is 7 or above, this is probably a realistic action plan. If your answer is below 7, you should look at your action plan again. Ask yourself why you are unsure. What problems do you foresee? Then, see if you can either solve the problems or change your plan to make yourself more confident of success. This is an opportunity to practice the problem-solving skills you learned earlier in this chapter.

Once you have made a plan you are happy with, *write it down* and post it where you will see it every day. Thinking through a weekly action plan is one thing. Writing it down makes it more likely you will take action. Keep track of how you are doing and the problems you encounter. (There is a blank action planning form at the end of this chapter. You may wish to make photocopies of it to use weekly.)

Carrying Out Your Action Plan

If your weekly action plan is well written and realistically achievable, completing it is generally not too difficult. There are a couple of strategies you can use to make it easier:

- Ask family or friends to check with you on how you are doing. Having to report your progress is good motivation.
- Keep track of your daily activities while carrying out your plan. Many caregivers make daily lists of what they want to accomplish.
- Check things off as they are completed. This will show you how realistic your planning is and that is useful for making plans. Plus, it is satisfying to make those check marks!
- Make daily notes, even of the things you don't understand at the time. Later, these notes may be useful in establishing a pattern to use for problem-solving.

How People Change

Thousands of studies have been done to learn how and why people change—or why they don't change. Here's what we have learned:

- Most people change by themselves, when they are ready. While health care providers, counselors, spouses, and self-help groups coax, persuade, nag, and otherwise try to assist people to change their lifestyles and habits, most people do so without much help from others.
- Change is not usually an all-or-nothing process. It happens in stages. Most of us change one small step at a time. Each step is an improvement over the one before it.
- In most cases, change resembles a spiral more than a straight line, with people going back to previous stages before advancing (two steps forward, one step back). Relapses are not failures but setbacks, which are a key part of change. Relapses provide feedback and help us figure out what doesn't work.
- Confidence in your ability to change is the key ingredient for success. Your belief in your own ability to succeed predicts whether you will attempt change in the first place, whether you will persist if you relapse, and whether you will ultimately be successful in making the change.

Checking the Results

At the end of each week, see if you completed your action plan and if you are any nearer to accomplishing your goal. Are you able to walk farther? Do you have more energy in the evenings after you walk? Are you less anxious? Taking stock is key. You might not see daily progress, but you should see a little progress each week. At the end of each week, check how well you have fulfilled your action plan. If you are having problems, this is the time to use your problem-solving tool.

For example, the sleep-deprived person we mentioned was not able to get more sleep during the first week they put their action plan to use. Each day, a different problem popped up: One night, their care partner got up and needed help; the next night, they woke to use the bathroom at three in the morning and could not go back to sleep; the next, the cats jumped on the bed; and so on. When looking back at the notes, the real problem became clear. They were afraid to sleep so deeply that they would not hear their care partner if anything happened. Putting a baby monitor in their care partner's room solved the problem.

Making Midcourse Corrections (Back to Problem-Solving)

When you are trying to overcome obstacles to make real changes, the first plan is not always the most workable plan. If something doesn't work, don't give up. Try something else. Modify your short-term plans so that your steps are easier. Give yourself more time to accomplish difficult tasks. Explore new options for reaching your goal. Check with your consultants for advice and assistance.

Not all goals are achievable. All caregivers know that caregiving means giving up some options. If this is true for you, don't dwell too much on what you can't do. Rather, start working on another goal you would like to accomplish. One caregiver we know talks about the 50 percent of things accomplished and the new skills learned. They don't dwell on the things they cannot do but the things they can.

Rewarding Yourself

The best part of managing caregiving is the reward that comes from accomplishing your goals and living a fuller and more comfortable life. However, there are other special ways to reward yourself on your path to improvement. Don't wait until your goal is reached. Reward yourself frequently for your short-term successes. For example, decide that you won't read the paper until after you exercise. Reading the paper then becomes your reward. One caregiver put a dollar in a jar each time they got through a half day without an upset. When there was enough money, they went out for ice cream. To begin with, this was only once every ten days or so, but as time went on, they were having ice cream more and more often. In fact, the caregiver had to change the reward to a dollar each day. The reward doesn't have to be ice cream. It can be a trip to the park or a cup of herbal tea in an outdoor cafe. There are many healthy pleasures that can add enjoyment to your life.

Use the form on page 22 to start your own action plan.

For a complete list of suggested further readings, useful websites, and other helpful resources, please see: **www.bullpub.com/resources.**

My Action Plan

When writing an action plan, be sure it includes all of the following:

1. What I am going to do (a specific action).
2. How much I am going to do (time, distance, portions, repetitions, etc.).
3. When I am going to do it (time of the day, day of the week).
4. How often or how many days a week I am going to do it.

Example: This week, I will walk (what) around the block (how much) before lunch (when) three times (how many).

This week I will ______________________________ (what)

______________________________ (how much)

______________________________ (when)

______________________________ (how often)

How sure am I that I can do this?
(0 = not at all sure; 10 = absolutely sure) ______

Comments

Monday ______________________________

Tuesday ______________________________

Wednesday ______________________________

Thursday ______________________________

Friday ______________________________

Saturday ______________________________

Sunday ______________________________

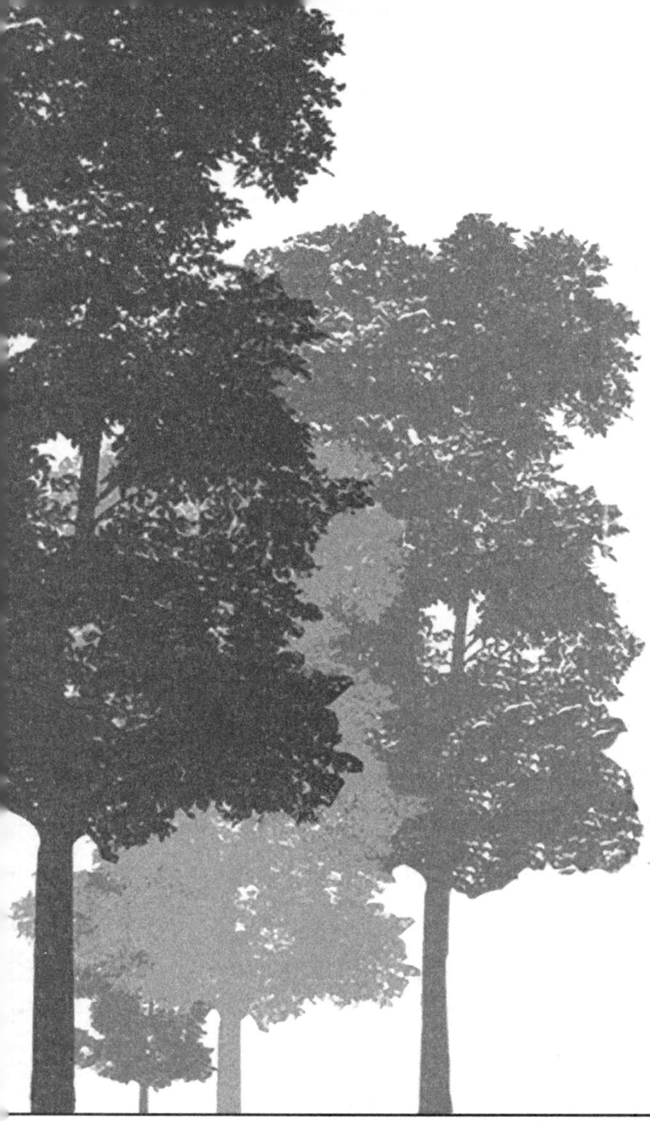

Chapter 3

Dealing with Stress and Difficult Care Partner Behavior

In Chapter 1, Introduction: A Blueprint for Better Caregiving, you learned that when you have a stressor, both your body and mind react. Stress can result in anger, frustration, slow thinking, tight muscles, and stomach upset—in fact, stress can affect almost any part of our minds or bodies.

Let's explore this idea a bit more. Imagine that you are on an elevator and feel someone or something poke you from behind. Your first reaction may be to feel startled. You may feel fear. What's going to happen? Are you going to be robbed? What is going on?! You tense up. You may start to breathe faster. You are stressed. You turn around and see a woman who is blind with a cane who didn't judge distance well. You are relieved. You no longer feel threatened and breathe with a sigh of relief. Your body relaxes. This example shows that stress comes from how you *interpret* the event, not the event itself.

Identifying Stress

When we ask caregivers what their biggest problem is, the reply is usually, "Stress." Then we ask what causes this stress and often hear things like:

- *"My care partner found the car keys and went for a drive. He got lost."*
- *"My care partner refuses to take a shower."*
- *"My care partner wants to be with me all the time."*
- *"My care partner refuses to get in the car to go to medical appointments."*

All of these are annoying or difficult care partner behaviors. Take a moment and think of one or two of your care partner's annoying or difficult behaviors. Write them down here:

1. ______________________________

2. ______________________________

Check your body for signs of stress like tightening muscles. Our guess is that just thinking about these behaviors has caused some stress.

Let's look at your stress level. Circle the number in the diagram below that describes your stress level right now. Then, you can do the same thing after you tried a stress breaker.

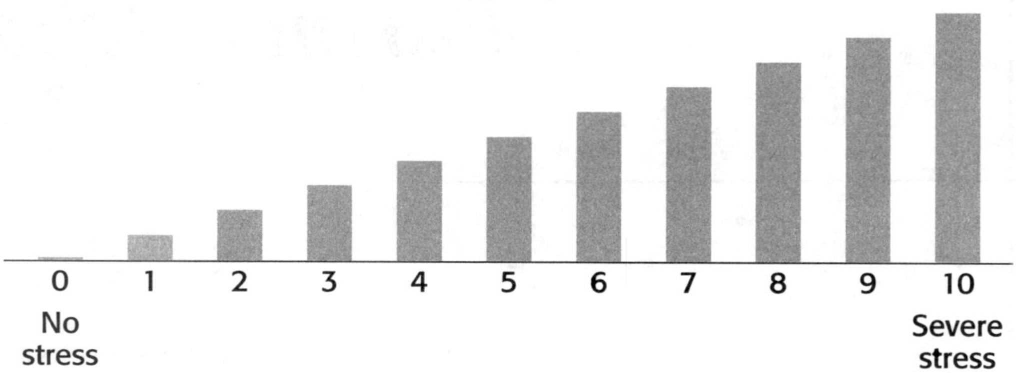

Before you can do anything about stress, you must notice the signs of stress. Your body may get tense, your voice may get louder, and you may feel it in your gut. Each of us reacts to stress a little differently. Your job is to know when this is happening. Pay attention to your body. You do not have to wait until you have a headache or a gut ache, or until you lose your temper or start crying. As soon as you notice stress starting to build, you can use thoughtful breathing as a quick stress breaker.

Breaking the Stress Cycle with Thoughtful Breathing

Thoughtful breathing is simple. We do not usually think about breathing. When you practice thoughtful breathing, you think about your breathing. This can help you relax. In other words, you breath with a purpose. It is like a time out. To begin thoughtful breathing, just take three or four deep breaths. You are taking deep breaths if your stomach moves more than your chest. Check this by putting one hand on your chest and one on your stomach. Take three or four deep breaths. If your lower hand is moving more than your upper hand, you are on target. If this does not happen right away, do not worry. It will with time. Right now, check with yourself. Are you feeling a little less stress?

You can also use thoughtful breathing during a stressful situation. Maybe your care partner is refusing to get out of bed. Somehow, this has escalated into a struggle. You can use thoughtful breathing to break the cycle. Take a moment to literally catch your breath. Sometimes all it takes is a small thing like thoughtful breathing to de-escalate.

While thoughtful breathing is a good way to deal with stress, it is even better if you can keep stress from escalating in the first place. One way of doing this is to identify and learn more about annoying or difficult care partner behaviors. Often people do not want to discuss these behaviors. Just the same, we know that many (if not most) care partners do have behaviors that their caregivers finding annoying, difficult, or just plain maddening. These behaviors are a major cause of caregiver stress. We also know that these behaviors usually happen for a reason and, as a caregiver, you can change at least some of these behaviors. The starting point is to break this problem into smaller parts.

Addressing Difficult Care Partner Behaviors

The following are eight steps you can use to deal with difficult care partner behaviors. After we list the steps, we explain each one in detail.

Step 1. Name the difficult behavior.

Step 2. If possible, determine the cause of the difficult behavior.

Step 3. Identify what happened before the behavior. This is the "trigger."

Step 4. Identify what you did during and after the behavior.

Step 5. Identify what your care partner did after the behavior.

Step 6. Determine how this made you feel.

Step 7. Evaluate your progress. Is the behavior changing? Are you feeling less stressed?

Step 8. Try something different.

Step 1: Name the Difficult Behavior

It is not always easy to define frustrating or difficult care partner behaviors, but most people tell us that they know it when it happens. It may be that you ask your care partner what they want for dinner, and they answer, "Ice cream." It may be that your care partner follows you around all the time. It may be that your care partner gets very angry any time you go out and leave them with someone else. It may be that your formerly clean and neat care partner now refuses to take a shower. If the behaviors cause either you or your care partner problems or stress, then they are probably difficult behaviors. You wrote down some difficult behaviors of your care partner on page 24. Look at these again. If you want to add or change something, do it now. If you are having trouble thinking of behaviors, then observe yourself and your care partner for a few days. You may discover things you have not before been able to name.

Step 2: Determine the Cause of the Difficult Behavior

Ask yourself, what are the reasons for difficult behaviors? There are several reasons for difficult care partner behaviors. The reasons may include the following:

- Your care partner wants attention.
- Your care partner wants or needs something: They are hungry, uncomfortable, or in pain.
- Your care partner needs stimulation or is bored.
- Your care partner wants to escape or avoid something unpleasant.
- Your care partner needs to go to the bathroom.
- Your care partner feels frightened or anxious.

This list can go on and on, and if your care partner cannot communicate well, then you may have to guess. After a while, the clues may become more obvious.

Notice that being angry or trying to annoy you (or "get your goat") is not listed as a reason for a difficult behavior. Trying to annoy or bug you are things someone does on purpose. This is usually not possible for someone with dementia or other brain injuries. Typically, what care partners are trying to do when they engage in difficult behavior is to express themselves. They are hoping you will understand their needs. Since people who need caregiving often don't communicate well verbally, caregivers must observe care partner behavior and try to figure out what it *could* mean and then act accordingly. While it is easy to take your care partner's behavior personally and then to feel guilty, in fact, most care partner behavior is not personally aimed at you or anyone else. Difficult behavior is caused by the condition that does not allow your care partner to communicate as they did in the past.

Consider this example. Myra does not communicate much and usually does not know where she is. Her husband, Richard, often sits her in front of the TV so he can get some work done. In just a few minutes, she is at his desk, calling out his name. This occurs many times a day. While we do not know the exact cause of this behavior, we can guess that Myra may be bored and may want attention. Guessing this, Richard decides to spend short time periods with Myra every hour and change her activities once or twice an hour. He discovers that the behavior disappears once he makes these changes. He also knows that he cannot spend every minute with Myra and decides that taking her to a senior day health program for a half day a few times a week may be a good solution for keeping her from getting too bored.

But then a new difficult behavior happens. Myra refuses to go to the day health center. She becomes angry every time it is suggested and won't get dressed or get in the car. Change is difficult for most people and even more so for someone with dementia. Myra may be frightened or feel abandoned. She is missing the stability of her familiar surroundings and her husband. This is a little like a toddler first going to day care. Myra would probably resist any new surroundings or unfamiliar people. Change must be handled slowly and more with actions than words. It might help if Richard and Myra stop by the senior day health center several times before Richard leaves Myra there alone. Or maybe Richard could go there for lunch with Myra. All these positive actions may help with the transition.

Here is another example. See if you can spot the cause. Several times during the day, Keenan follows Barbara around. He won't let her out of his sight, and he even wants to be there when she takes a shower. This drives Barbara up the wall and stresses her out. Barbara also notices that Keenan often soils himself during or after this behavior. What could be the cause of Keenan's behavior?

Boredom may be causing Keenan's behavior. As you just saw in the example with Myra, this is often a cause for difficult behaviors. Acting out (soiling himself) provides some excitement. Alternatively, Keenan may be trying to avoid soiling himself. However, he does not know how to express this or what to do about it. He may be following Barbara around to get her attention and seek her help in using the bathroom. There are a few things Barbara can try. She could structure several activities for Keenan during the day. He might fold the clothing, work on a hooked rug, watch a baseball game, or the two of them can go for a daily walk. Activity relieves boredom. She may also try leading Keenan to the bathroom every time the following behavior starts to occur. With a little trial and error and some keen observation, Barbara may stop the behavior or make it less frequent.

Once you think you know a little about what is causing difficult behaviors, it can be easier to find a solution. Your care partner may have difficult emotions such as anger or depression. However, they may not be able to express these. You may only know about these emotions by observing your care partner and by considering that emotions may be the cause of some difficult behaviors.

Many conditions impair cognition (memory) such as stroke, traumatic brain injury (TBI), Alzheimer's, post-traumatic stress disorder (PTSD), or Parkinson's. These same conditions can also change emotions.

People who have had strokes may cry or become very angry for what appears to you to be no reason at all or inappropriate reasons. A care partner may lash out. They might experience rapid mood changes, and their mood may not correspond to what is happening around them. In addition, someone who has had a stroke may be frustrated, angry, or depressed. The American Stroke Association has the following tips for caregivers:

- Always treat your care partner with respect.
- Give praise when your care partner is acting appropriately.
- When giving choices, let the person choose between two safe and appropriate alternatives.
- When necessary, set limits.

Someone with Alzheimer's might become more confused and agitated as the day goes on. This "sundowning" effect often accompanies the disease. It is especially common during the middle stages of Alzheimer's, as well as for people with some other types of dementia. Sundowning behavior tends to lessen as dementia increases. The Alzheimer's Association recommends the following suggestions for dealing with sundowning:

- As frustrating as this may be for you, always approach your care partner in a calm way and reassure them that they are in a safe place.
- Check triggers. Your care partner might need something or there may be a specific trigger.
- Sometimes it is helpful to remind your care partner of today's date and time.
- Don't argue or ask for an explanation.
- Do not take your care partner's actions or emotions personally.

People with Parkinson's-related dementia might hallucinate or become paranoid or depressed. The recommendations just listed for Alzheimer's symptoms may be helpful in dealing with these situations. In addition, sometimes antidepressants or antipsychotic medications can be helpful. Check with your care partner's primary health care provider.

People with post-traumatic stress disorder (PTSD) commonly experience three primary difficult emotions:

1. Hyperarousal, such as a very strong reaction to a common noise like the backfiring of a car. Having trouble sleeping, being easily startled, anger, problems concentrating, panic, and always being alert to danger are signs of hyperarousal.
2. Re-experiencing or going over an experience repeatedly, such as a battle or other traumatic experience. *Flashbacks* are a more common name for *re-experiencing*. These can include bad memories, nightmares, or exaggerated reactions.
3. Numbing, not having much emotion about anything. Numbing is a bit like depression. The person does not feel much of anything and may not be interested in anything. Numbing usually is accompanied by withdrawal. At the same time, the person might focus on avoiding any trauma or feelings that might be a reminder of trauma.

PTSD is usually treated by psychotherapy. As a caregiver, urge your care partner to get mental health treatment and be supportive should they choose to do so. If possible, ask to be part of the treatment. If your care partner talks of suicide, take it seriously and seek immediate help. Remember, you are not the cause of the problem.

People with traumatic brain injury (TBI) may feel many of the emotions discussed in this section. Just like people who have had a stroke, they may experience mood swings. For example, people who have TBI might break out laughing or become angry for no obvious reason. These periods usually last a very short time. Someone with TBI may also be anxious or depressed or have outbursts of anger.

Here is a list of things that you as a caregiver can do to help your care partner with TBI:

- Do not take the actions and words of your care partner personally. The TBI is the cause of the difficult emotions, not you.
- Remain calm. Work hard at not overreacting or becoming emotional.

- When possible, take your care partner to a quiet place to calm down.
- Tell your care partner that TBIs can cause difficult emotions and give your care partner a chance to talk about their emotions.
- If a topic is a trigger, when appropriate, gently redirect the discussion or activity to another topic. For example, if talking about the news is a trigger for difficult emotions, change the conversation to talk about hobbies or the family.
- Let your care partner know that some behaviors, such as yelling or threatening, are not acceptable. If these occur, refuse to engage. You may even leave the room.

  Learn more about TBI at

  http://braininjuryeducation.org/

  or

  https://braininjurycanada.ca/.

Depression is common for people who have these conditions.

Step 3: Identify What Happened Before the Behavior

What are the triggers for difficult behaviors? Often something happens before the difficult behavior that triggers the behavior. Here are some examples.

John asks Julianna what she wants for dinner. Julianna answers, "Ice cream." John does not think that ice cream is an appropriate dinner and sees this as a difficult behavior. The trigger was the open-ended question. What John really wanted to know was if Julianna wanted chicken or pasta. By using an open-ended question instead of giving a choice of two things, he inadvertently triggered the behavior. It is likely that Julianna thought of the food she liked best or the first thing that came into her mind.

In this example, it is clear that John does not like the idea of Julianna having ice cream for dinner. He might think that she is trying to annoy him. There are two things to consider with this example. First, why did John ask an open-ended question? The answer is often that John is trying to maintain Julianna's dignity by giving her choices. Unfortunately, sometimes he achieves the opposite result. Julianna's dignity is not maintained when she is frustrated at not being able to make a choice or her choice is unacceptable to John.

Another way of looking at this is that sometimes there is no good reason why Julianna should not have ice cream for dinner. John does not have to eat it. Perfect nutrition may not be important all the time. Maybe she will eat some pasta after the ice cream. Is this a behavior John should be concerned about? There is no right or wrong answer, but it is good to remember that a behavior is difficult only if it hurts the care partner or the caregiver sees it as difficult.

Let's look at another example. Rose is a full-time caregiver for her father Marcos. She has arranged to have someone from church come in and sit with Marcos for a couple of hours three times a week so she can shop and have lunch with a friend. When she comes home, Marcos shouts at her and says she does not care about him and that she is no good. Rose ends up in tears.

The trigger is easy to spot. It is Rose's leaving Marcos. The cause may not be so clear. It may be that Marcos shouting has to do with fear. However, taking a break is necessary and healthy for Rose and for all caregivers. The difficult behavior needs to be addressed, but not by

Rose giving up her outings. Instead the cause of the trigger needs to be dealt with.

When difficult behavior happens, you have two choices. You can change or avoid the trigger. Or you can change your reaction to the behavior. Here are some ideas for dealing with triggers.

- **Eliminate the trigger**. If the dog jumping up on your care partner's lap makes them angry or agitated, then the dog's jumping must be stopped. The dog can be trained, you can place the dog in a new home, or make sure that the dog and your care partner are never together. These are not easy decisions or choices, but the dog's behavior must be addressed in order to address your care partner's difficult behavior.
- **Arrange life so the trigger does not bother your care partner**. If a 3:00 a.m. train always wakes you or your care partner, you cannot get rid of the train. Earplugs, a soundtrack of white noise (recordings of the ocean or wind, for example), or double-paned windows may help.
- **Avoid the trigger**. If bright light is a trigger, offer your care partner dark glasses and help choose seats that face away from windows. If loud noises are a trigger, avoid places where these noises are likely to occur or try earplugs.
- **Distract your care partner**. Camille told Sally that it was time to take a shower. Sally hated showers and threw a fit. Camille realized that this was a familiar personality trait and an old trigger because Sally has never liked being told what to do. She suggested that they could go for a ride or work on a new puzzle after Sally's shower. In this situation Camille linked a reward (taking a ride or a puzzle) with taking a shower. There is a difference between being told, "Take a shower," and "Let's go for a ride after your shower."
- **Tolerate the behavior or think about it in a different way**. Consider the example of Marcos shouting at Rose whenever she returned from a short time away from the house. It may not be possible or healthy to change the trigger (Rose's leaving), but it is possible for Rose to react differently or to think differently about the behavior. She can remind herself that it is not her beloved father speaking but rather his illness.
- **Talk with your doctor or mental health professional about the trigger**. Professionals have techniques to help people become less sensitive to triggers. Sometimes consulting with a professional and learning new techniques is worth the effort, especially if the triggers cause very disruptive behavior.

Step 4: Identify What You Did During and After the Behavior

Often we cannot change difficult behavior, but we can almost always change how we react. To do this, we have to decide if the behavior really makes any difference. If the behavior does make a difference, then changing your reaction may break the cycle. Let us return to Rose and Marcos. When Rose returns home, Marcos gets mad and says things that hurt Rose. What does this accomplish? Marcos gets Rose's attention and establishes an emotional connection even if it is a negative one. Rose feels hurt and guilty. She ends up crying.

In this situation, Rose can do several things. She can tell Marcos how much she loves him before leaving while also making sure that he knows she is leaving. When she returns, she can immediately reassure him that she is now back, and she still cares for him. She can point out to him that she did not leave permanently but was gone only for a short while. She can tell him how much she missed him and maybe bring him a small treat. Before she leaves, Rose could set a timer for however long she will be gone and share it with Marcos. These will reassure Marcos that she is coming back.

If Marcos still responds angrily to her absence, Rose can sit quietly, not doing anything, until Marcos calms down. Or Rose can excuse herself and leave the situation for a few minutes. The important thing is that Marcos does not earn attention by behaving negatively.

Step 5: Identify What Your Care Partner Did During and After the Behavior

Rose was always so upset with Marcos's reactions that she never really thought about what he did after the blow up. When she thought about it, she realized that he was always very quiet and almost reserved after he was done shouting. It took them several hours or a day to get back to "normal."

Once she realized this, Rose thought that at some level he might be sorry or at least uncomfortable about his actions. She decided that if the behavior happened again, she would leave the room for a few minutes, and when she returned, she would say to Marcos that she realized that this was hard for him. She would explain that it was also hard for her and tell him that they could work together to figure out how to get through the difficulty.

Step 6: Determine How This Made You Feel

John was unhappy because Julianna wanted ice cream. After he stopped to think for a moment, he realized that there was no reason not to give her ice cream for dinner occasionally. He also knew her well enough to know that if she saw him eating pasta, she might want some as well. This is a win-win. Julianna gets what she wants, and John gets his pasta. Of course, if Julianna insisted on only eating ice cream over several days, other solutions would be needed.

By looking at the consequences for both parties, it is easier to determine what to do or sometimes not do. For Rose and Marcos, the consequence is lose-lose if Marcos gets angry and makes Rose cry. Both Rose and Marcos are unhappy. If Rose doesn't cry and instead leaves the room, it is a win for her even though it is a loss for Marcos. If she is able to reassure Marcos before and after she leaves that she is still going to be his caregiver and he does not lose his temper, it is a win-win. If Sally throws a fit about taking a shower, Camille must decide if Sally really needs a shower now. If the answer is no and Camille decides it is not worth the effort to fight, the situation is a win for both. If Camille decides that Sally needs a shower and convinces Sally to take a shower before they enjoy a ride, it is also a win-win.

Behavior Diary

Remember, you have two ways you can act to change a difficult behavior:

1. You can change or avoid the trigger.
2. You can change your reaction to the behavior.

Date:	
Behavior:	
Trigger:	
What, if anything, I did to change the trigger:	
What I did after the behavior:	
What my care partner did after the behavior:	
Results:	
Stress level: (circle number)	No stress 0 1 2 3 4 5 6 7 8 9 10 Extreme stress

Step 7. Evaluate Your Progress

There are many ways to deal with difficult care partner behaviors. To do so successfully means to step back a little and figure out how things are going and how you are feeling. After following the first six steps, is the behavior getting better? How do you feel? Are you feeling less stressed? If so, you may be on the right path. If not, it may be time to move on to step 8 and try something different. One of the best ways to track your efforts is by starting a behavior diary like the one included above.

Feel free to copy this diary and use it often. It is one of your most useful caregiver tools.

Step 8. Try Something Different

Don't be discouraged if difficult behaviors don't go away immediately. Not all your attempts will work, and sometimes it will take more than one try. If something doesn't work, try something else, and always evaluate if the behavior reduced your stress. Things change and something that worked once may not work all the time. It may take a few different approaches to change the triggers or change your reactions. Experimenting with new solutions is a worthwhile way to spend your time. As you experiment, you will become a better caregiver. Both you and your care partner will benefit.

Getting Help: Dangerous Care Partner Behaviors

So far, we have reviewed difficult, frustrating, or annoying care partner behaviors. Unfortunately, some care partner behaviors can be more than just annoyances, they can be dangerous for the care partner or for others. These include drug and/or alcohol abuse, hitting, biting, and kicking. You should know that you usually cannot change these behaviors. In fact, the harder you try to change a behavior, the worse it may get. What you can do is put safety first. Protect yourself and others who might be hurt. Get help.

Seeking Safety

We will start with the most difficult advice. If **you feel that you or others in your household are in danger, get out.** You may need to have an escape plan ready. If you think you might need to leave, have some clothing and your medications packed, money saved in a safe place, and gas in the car. You also need to think about where you would go. Maybe you can go to the home of a friend or relative. If you do not know where to go, call your local law enforcement or the Salvation Army. We know that this may sound drastic, but you cannot help your care partner if you or others in your family are in danger or are injured. If you do leave, and you fear for your care partner, call Adult Protective Services. You can also call 911 and ask them to call Adult Protective Services or send an officer who has special mental health training. In Canada, you can contact Canadian Network for the Prevention of Elder Abuse or Women's Shelters Canada.

Seeking the Help of Others

If you need to talk to a health care professional about dangerous behaviors, you can start by making an appointment with your care partner's health care provider. Go to the appointment without your care partner. This is something you may be able to discuss on a telephone or video call or even in a letter, email, or fax. When you talk with the provider, be as specific as possible. Focus on reporting the dangerous behavior with factual statements, like "My care partner drinks a six pack of beer every afternoon," "My care partner got so angry, they put a hole in the wall with their fist," or "My care partner insists on keeping a loaded gun in the house."

You can also add your own concerns, like "After about three beers, they become very angry. They yell and shout. I am afraid they will hit me or one of the children." Or "My care partner has never hit me, but I am afraid that someday they will. I am also afraid that they will hurt themselves." Or "Having a loaded gun around frightens me. I am afraid that my care partner will shoot me or commit suicide. They might even go and use it in public."

Finally, ask the provider for advice. Listen carefully. What you hear may not be something you want to hear, such as the need for you to get out of the house or call law enforcement. Maybe the behavior can be stopped, but it might be that the behavior will continue.

Never put yourself or your family at risk. Your primary responsibility is to protect yourself and your family.

When talking to the provider there are a couple of things you need to know. The provider can listen to you and make suggestions to you about what you can do but may not be able to tell you anything about your care partner. The provider cannot tell you anything about your care partner unless your care partner has previously given permission to do so or you have conservatorship. (We explain more about conservatorship in Chapter 13, Planning for the Future: Fears and Reality.) U.S. and Canadian laws protect patient-provider relationships and discussions.

Sometimes your partner's provider may not know how to help or is not approachable. If this is the case, you need to find other support. You can start at the Alzheimer's Association (in Canada, Alzheimer Society of Canada) or contact a social worker at your local senior center. You and your care partner do not need to be seniors, and your care partner does not have to have Alzheimer's to use these services. Try the caregiver support person at the local Veterans Administration (VA) Hospital or clinic or Veterans Affairs Canada, Carers Canada. If your care partner ever served in the armed services (even 60 years ago and even if they never before received services from the VA), you can still get great help from the VA caregiver support services. You can usually call these organizations and tell them your problem. They may not be able to help, but they often can refer you to some place that can. You will find helpful organizations, phone numbers, and websites in the online resources for this book.

Finally, remember that if you feel like you or those around you are in danger, get out. Do not wait.

For a complete list of suggested further readings, useful websites, and other helpful resources, please see www.bullpub.com/resources.

CHAPTER 4

Dealing with Difficult Emotions

DIFFICULT EMOTIONS AND CAREGIVING OFTEN GO TOGETHER. Having these emotions is perfectly normal. Many caregivers experience feelings of sadness, irritability, anxiety, grief, and/or guilt. Having such feelings is understandable. Caregiving is often stressful and for most people, negative emotions are part of the stress response.

These feelings tend to ebb and flow over time. Often, in the early stages, caregivers are angry about the changes that their loved one is experiencing and are not sure what to do to improve things. They often ask why did this happen? My partner did everything "right" and still is very ill. They may also feel anger because their lives have also changed. Caregivers in the earlier stages also tend to be anxious about the future and wonder: When will the next decline happen? Questions like this are common. How bad will it be? What can I do to cope?

As diseases progress and your care partner is less able to function, anger and anxiety can change to sadness. Many caregivers become depressed. Some feel as if they have done all they can do and ask why their loved one doesn't improve. Is there nothing more that can be done? Others feel guilty and think they haven't done enough and think if only they had done X or Y, their care partner would have improved, or at least not declined as rapidly. Growing awareness of the losses that have occurred (and the future losses ahead) can result in feelings of grief.

In the final stages of illness, some caregivers report feeling more "at peace"—they have reconciled themselves to what is next and have come to terms with what they did (and didn't) do for their care partner. But this is not always the case: Other caregivers become very depressed at the coming loss and do all that they can to prolong their care partner's life.

Depression

Caregivers often find depression to be the most difficult emotion. Several studies have reported that up to 50 percent of caregivers (particularly those caring for a relative with Alzheimer's disease or other forms of dementia) report symptoms of depression sometime during their caregiving. Depression is not the same as stress. Stress is something one experiences in response to specific situations (like your loved one repeatedly asking, "What's for lunch?" within an hour after having lunch). Stress is something that comes and goes over the course of a day, while depression often hangs over your head like a black cloud for days or weeks at a time. You know you have a problem with depression when your usual ways of coping, of feeling better, don't work anymore. Or they work for just a short time and then you're downhearted and blue again.

Sometimes caregivers do not realize they are depressed or think that they are feeling down because of all the things that are going on around them. And often they do not want to admit to being depressed. Like other symptoms, the symptoms of depression can be treated with self-management techniques, with counseling, and with medication. The best treatment is specific to each person and is usually a combination of these.

Feeling sad sometimes is common. Typically, sadness is a temporary feeling, often linked to a specific event or loss. People sometimes mistakenly use the word *depressed* to describe feeling sad or disappointed. A person might say, "I'm really depressed about missing out on visiting with my friends." In these circumstances people feel sad, but they can still relate to others and find joy in other areas of their lives.

Sometimes sadness affects people more deeply or lasts longer, as when you lose a loved one or you or someone near to you is diagnosed with a serious illness. If, however, your sad feelings are especially severe, long-lasting, and recurrent, you may be experiencing clinical depression. Clinical depression drains the pleasure out of life, leaving you feeling hopeless, helpless, and worthless.

Am I Depressed?

Here is a quick test for depression: Ask yourself what you do to have fun. If you do not have a quick answer, consider your mood over the past two weeks. Have you had any of the following symptoms?

- **Little interest or pleasure in doing things.** An inability to enjoy life or other people may be a sign of depression. Symptoms include not wanting to talk to anyone, go out, or answer the phone or doorbell.
- **Feeling down, sad, or hopeless.** Feeling persistently blue can be a symptom of depression.
- **Trouble falling or staying asleep, or sleeping too much.** Awakening and being unable to return to sleep or sleeping too much and not wanting to get out of bed can signal a problem.
- **Feeling tired or having little energy.** Fatigue—feeling tired all the time—can be a symptom of depression.
- **Poor appetite or overeating.** This may range from a loss of interest in food to unusually erratic or excessive eating.
- **Feeling bad about yourself.** Have you felt that you are a failure or have let yourself or your care partner down? Do you doubt your self-worth or have a negative image of your body?
- **Trouble concentrating.** Have you found it hard to do such things as read the newspaper or a magazine, listen to a podcast, or watch television?
- **Sluggishness or restlessness.** Have you been moving or speaking so slowly that other people have noticed? Or the opposite—have you been much more fidgety or restless than usual? Either can be a sign of depression.
- **Wishing yourself harm or worse.** Thoughts that you would be better off dead or of hurting yourself in some way are often a strong sign of clinical depression.

Depressed people may also gain or lose weight, lose interest in sex or intimacy, lose interest in personal care and grooming, struggle to make decisions, and have more frequent accidents.

If several of these symptoms seem to apply to you, please seek help from someone you trust—your health care provider, a member of the clergy, a psychologist, or a social worker. Do not wait for these feelings to pass. If you are thinking about harming yourself or others, get help now. Don't let a tragedy happen to you and your loved ones. In the United States, the national suicide prevention lifeline is 1-800-273-8255. In Canada, the national suicide crisis helpline is 9-8-8.

Fortunately, treatments for depression, including antidepressant medications, counseling, and self-management techniques, are highly effective in decreasing its frequency, length, and severity. Depression, like other symptoms, can be managed.

If you are experiencing clinical depression, you may become numb. Even crying brings no relief. Depression affects everything: the way you think, the way you behave, the way you interact with your care partner and others, and even the way your body functions.

Depression is not caused by personal weakness, laziness, or lack of willpower. Heredity, chronic conditions, medications, even the weather can all play a role in depression. The way you think, especially negative thoughts, can also produce and sustain a depressed mood. Negative thoughts associated with depression can be automatic, recur endlessly, and often are not linked to any event or triggering cause.

Feelings and emotions also contribute to depression. They include:

- **Fear, anxiety, or uncertainty about the future.** Worries about finances, your family, or your abilities as a caregiver can lead to depression. If you address these issues as soon as possible, you, your care partner, and your family will spend less time worrying and have more time for life's small joys. This can have a healing effect.
- **Frustration.** Frustration can have many causes. You may find yourself thinking, "I just can't do this any longer," "I feel so helpless," "I used to have a life of my own but now all I have is caregiving," or "Why doesn't anyone understand me?" The longer you entertain and accept these feelings, the more alone and isolated you are likely to feel.
- **Worry about loss of control over your life.** When you are a caregiver, many things can make you feel like you are losing control. These include having to be on call many hours each day and night, getting your care partner the help they need, and having to count on others to help you do things you or your care partner used to do yourselves. Feeling like you have lost control can make you lose faith in yourself and your abilities. Even though you may not be able to do everything yourself, you can still be in charge.

Depression can lead to withdrawal, isolation, and inactivity. These behaviors can create more depressed feelings. One of the major problems of depression is that the more you isolate yourself (and often your care partner as well), the more you drive away the people who can support and comfort you. Friends and family want to help you feel better, but often they don't know what to do. Sometimes unrealistic cheeriness masks what a person is really feeling, and only the most sensitive observer recognizes the brittleness or phoniness of the mood. Refusal to accept offers of help, even in the face of obvious need for it, is a frequent symptom of unrecognized depression. As you reject efforts to comfort and reassure you, others may become frustrated and eventually quit trying. The result is that a depressed person can end up saying, "See, I was right. Nobody cares."

Treating Depression

As we mentioned earlier, the most effective treatments for depression are antidepressant medications, counseling, and self-management techniques. We discuss each of these here.

Medication and Depression

Antidepressant medications help balance brain chemistry and are highly effective. These medications can be prescribed by health professionals with prescribing privileges, who are generally physicians, nurse practitioners, or physician associates. In addition to treating depression, antidepressants can also help relieve pain (if pain is a problem), lessen anxiety, and improve sleep. It can take several days to several weeks for most antidepressant medications to begin to work. Don't be discouraged if you are prescribed antidepressants and you don't feel better immediately. Stick with it. To get the most benefit, you may need to take medications for six months or more.

Most people experience side effects of antidepressant medication in the first few weeks. Side effects then lessen or go away. If you have side effects and they are not especially severe, continue to take your medication. As your body gets used to the medication, you will usually begin to feel better. Remember to take antidepressant medication every day. If you stop because you're feeling better (or worse), you may relapse. Antidepressant medications are not addictive. If you have significant side effects or if the medication is not helping, talk with your health care provider before stopping or changing your dose.

Counseling and Depression

Several types of psychotherapy, particularly cognitive behavioral therapy (CBT), can be highly effective in treating depression. Psychotherapy or counseling is often referred to as "talk therapy." Cognitive behavioral therapy is a form of counseling that focuses on challenging and changing unhelpful thought patterns. CBT aims to help people regulate their emotions and behaviors and learn coping strategies. CBT can help people think more realistically by encouraging them to change their thoughts, feelings, and behavior, including their stress responses. See more about this in Chapter 5: Using Your Mind to Manage Stress.

As with medications, counseling rarely has an immediate effect. You may see a counselor for weeks (or longer) before you see improvement. The time of therapy appointments can be brief, usually under an hour. Typically, people attend one to two sessions a week for several months. Counseling can be a good investment of your energy and time. By teaching you new skills and ways to think and relate, psychotherapy can help reduce your risk of recurrent depression.

We understand that as a caregiver you may not have the time or resources for counseling and dismiss this idea. Before you dismiss counseling, talk with your health care provider. Counseling can often be done via video sessions on your computer or tablet. Sometimes it is even done by phone. Health plans and employers are paying more attention to the needs of caregivers. You may have mental health coverage in your current plan.

Tools for Depression Self-Management

Depression self-management techniques can be surprisingly effective. You can learn many psychotherapy techniques on your own. For mild to moderate depression, or just to lift your mood, the self-management strategies discussed here can be very productive. One study showed that reading and practicing self-help advice improved depression in nearly 70 percent of patients.

These skills and strategies can be used alone or with medications and counseling.

- **Eliminate drugs that are downers.** Using alcohol or other drugs usually leaves you feeling worse. Prescription tranquilizers or narcotic painkillers such as Valium®, Librium®, Restoril®, Vicodin®, codeine, sleeping medications, or other "downers" intensify depression or may cause depression as a side effect. If you have been prescribed one of these medicines, do not stop taking it before first talking with your health care provider. There may be reasons for continuing its use, or you may have withdrawal reactions if you quit without tapering.

  Alcohol is a depressant or downer. One of its key effects is making you feel more discouraged. For most people, one or two drinks in the early evening are not a problem. However, if you can't stop thinking about alcohol during your day, or if alcohol is interfering in your caregiving or life in general, you are having trouble with this drug. Talk about your alcohol use with your health care provider or seek help from a twelve-step program such as Alcoholics Anonymous.

  Marijuana is now widely available legally. People with depression may turn to marijuana to help with their depression or other negative emotions. While marijuana does not seem to cause depression and may even seem to help in the short run, it is not an approved treatment for depression and may lead to other problems such as increased depression, an unwillingness to seek other help, and lower motivation.

- **Plan for pleasure.** If you don't feel much emotion and the world seems colorless, make an effort to put some living back into your life. When you are feeling blue or depressed, the tendency is to withdraw, isolate yourself, and restrict activities. That is the opposite of what you need to do. Maintaining or increasing activities is one of the best antidotes for depression. We know that this is especially hard when you are a caregiver. Don't leave good things to chance. You may have to plan pleasurable activities. Consider making a list of what you'd like to do with your free time during the week. (We know that it can seem like there is no free time, but if you look carefully, you can probably find a few minutes or more here and there). Schedule your fun each week. Even if you don't feel like doing it, try to stick to your activity schedule. Sometimes having fun isn't such an easy prescription. You might think having fun means attending a big event. You may find enjoyment in small events. We call these small joys. That nature walk, cup of tea, or half hour of listening to music may improve your mood. Surprisingly it might improve the mood of your care partner too. You will never know if you do not do it.

  Here are some ideas that you might try.

  - Go for a short walk either alone or with your care partner.
  - Sign up for a free exercise course at a local center.
  - Call or video chat with a friend.
  - Look at a sunset.
  - Watch a funny movie.

- Follow along to a yoga video.
- Join a caregiver's group. Some of these even meet online. Go to a bookstore or library and look through your favorite section.
- Listen or dance to some upbeat music.
- Exercise or schedule a massage so you can reconnect with your body.
- Eat your favorite spicy food.
- Treat yourself to a fragrant herbal bath, or try a cold shower.
- Go to a garden center and smell all the flowers.
- Plant some young trees.
- Make plans and carry them out.
- Look to the future. Look forward to your grandchildren's graduation from college even if they are now just toddlers.
- If you know that one time of the year is especially difficult, such as Christmas or a birthday, make specific plans to be active during that period. Invite a couple or friends who understand your situation for lunch and ask them to bring the lunch and cake.

Activities like these can keep your spirits up and prevent or lessen depression. Don't wait to see what happens. Be prepared to enjoy something every day.

- **Take action.** Continue your daily activities. Get dressed every day and take pride in your appearance. Make your bed, get out of the house, go shopping, or walk your dog. Plan and cook meals. Force yourself to do these things even if you don't always feel like it. If time is the problem, do these things but simplify them. A meal can be eggs or fresh fruit with yogurt and granola.

  Taking action to solve your most immediate problems provides the surest relief from negative feelings. You might decide to clean or organize a room or just a desk drawer. Even a single simple action can boost your mood. Search websites you trust to learn more about a current events topic you are interested in. Call or write to an old friend or distant relative.

  When you are feeling emotionally vulnerable, do not set major or difficult goals for yourself. As a caregiver, you have a big responsibility and it may be time to share the load. Consider getting help. (See Chapter 7: Getting Help.) Break large tasks into small ones, set some priorities, and do what you can as best you can. It is best not to make big life decisions when you are feeling depressed although you may have to make big decisions for your care partner. For example, don't sell your house because your care partner has problems with stairs. Think about how you can move to the first floor. Moving can be a sign of withdrawal. If you have to make plans for alternative care for your care partner, get help from family, friends, or professionals, such as social workers. If family members urge you to move closer to them, get help with the decision. Moving may be a good idea if you will get more support and you have ties in the area to which you will move. On the other hand, depression often intensifies when you are in a location away from your current friends and acquaintances.

Besides, many troubles may move with you, and you may have left behind the support you may need to cope.

- **Socialize.** Don't isolate yourself. Seek out positive, optimistic people who can lighten your heavy feelings. Make an effort to see family and friends. Stay involved with church groups, book clubs, etc. Your friends will understand if your care partner cannot fully participate or has changed. If you can't get out, consider video chatting with friends, starting an online book club with people you know, or joining a group on the internet. If you join a public online group, be sure it is moderated and that someone enforces the rules of the group.
- **Move your body to change your mood.** Physical activity lifts depression and negative moods. Depressed people often complain that they feel too tired to exercise. But the feelings of fatigue associated with depression are not due to physical exhaustion. Try to get 20 to 30 minutes of some type of exercise every day. It can be walking, yoga, yard work, chair dancing—anything. You may find that you have more energy once you start moving regularly. Movement may also be good for your care partner, and by moving yourself, you are setting a positive example. For more information on how to safely start moving and keep moving, see Chapter 9, Exercising for Health and Wellness.
- **Think positive.** Many people tend to be excessively critical of themselves, especially when they're depressed. You may find yourself thinking untrue things about yourself. Challenge automatic negative thoughts by changing the negative stories you tell yourself. For example, you may say to yourself, "Unless I do everything perfectly, I'm a failure." Try changing this belief to, "Success is doing the best that I can in any situation. I do not always need to earn an A grade. Earning a C is often good enough." To learn more about use of adaptive thinking to challenge negative self-talk, see pages xxx–xxx.

Don't be discouraged if it takes some time to feel better even once you start using these techniques. If, however, these self-management strategies are not improving things for you and your depression becomes more severe, seek help from your health care provider or a mental health professional. Counseling or antidepressant medication (or both) can go a long way toward relieving depression. Seeking professional help and taking medications are not signs of weakness. They are signs of strength.

Embarrassment

Like depression, embarrassment is another feeling commonly reported by caregivers. Maybe your care partner eats with their hands. People often lose social skills when they lose some of their cognitive ability (their brains do not function as well as they did before). Most people are taught that what other people think is important. Embarrassment is really our concern about what other people will think. Sometimes, as a caregiver, you have to put your old beliefs behind you and learn new techniques for interacting with the world.

You can also take active steps to deal with your own embarrassment. You can ask to sit in a corner with your partner facing the wall so others will be less like to notice their behaviors. Or the Alzheimer's Association has business-type cards you can get that say something like, "This person has Alzheimer's or dementia; their brain doesn't work like yours or mine. Thank you for understanding." You can also make cards like this yourself. The idea is that you can slip this to a server in a restaurant, to someone next to you in church, or to a clerk/salesperson, etc. This can help lessen your embarrassment and helps the other person know what's going on. You will most likely find that folks are kind and that they have probably faced similar situations or know of someone who has.

Grief and Guilt

We often think of grief as something that happens when someone dies. When someone you care about, be it a family member or friend, changes or becomes ill, you also may grieve. You may grieve for the lives you used to have together and grieve for the future you could have had together. The reality of the present is not what you wanted or expected. Folks that are grieving sometimes deny what is happening. Instead of facing a care partner's decline or realizing their behavior is resulting from an illness, you may say things like, "Cherise is just having a bad day and will get better" or "She is acting that way because I am not a good enough caregiver, and she is angry."

Sometimes grief is expressed as anger. A caregiver may say, "It's not fair that our lives were disrupted" or "It is all the hospital's fault for not catching this sooner." Bargaining is yet another way of expressing grief. "If you will just let us have a few good days, I will be happy."

Many caregivers feel guilty that they feel this sense of loss and grief. You may think you are betraying your partner, or it's a sign you don't love them anymore. This is not the case. A sense of loss and feelings of grief are common, particularly as symptoms such as dementia progress and there is "less of a person" left in your loved one. After a time, most grief works itself out and you gain acceptance and peace. But this does not happen all at once, and the path can be difficult and painful.

Dealing with Difficult Emotions

It is often difficult to put a name on a difficult emotion. The name does not matter. What does matter is that you are feeling them and that there are things you can do about them. We will start with some things you can do for all difficult emotions, and then we will explain a few specific emotions.

Step 1: Acknowledge What You Are Feeling

Many people go through life acting as though nothing is bothering them. But all people have feelings. When you don't own your feelings, sometimes they bubble up and show themselves at inopportune times. For example, you may be angry with your care partner or worried about your own health. You may not even realize you are angry or worried. What happens is that you yell at the dog or become angry with a salesclerk. If things like this are happening to you, stop a moment. Think about what is happening and acknowledge to yourself that you are worried, angry, embarrassed or feeling guilty. Once you name your feelings and look at the causes, you may be able to do some problem solving. Just saying I feel sad, I feel angry, I feel embarrassed, or I feel guilty can help.

Step 2: Give the Feelings a Name, Such as Anger or Guilt

Do not worry about giving your feelings the "right" names. There is no right or wrong. Naming an emotion and acknowledging you feel it does not make you a bad person. It makes you a strong and thoughtful person. For example, it is alright to say that you are angry about your condition, about having to be a caregiver, and having your life disrupted. Almost all caregivers tell us that they feel this way at one time or another.

Step 3: Try to Identify What Is Causing the Feeling

See if you can state how you feel in a sentence. For example, you could say, "I feel resentment that my sister does not help more" or "I worry that my care partner will get worse and I will not be able to cope."

Sometimes there is more than one cause for a feeling. When it comes to guilt, there may be many reasons. You might feel guilty for not being kinder to your care partner before you understood their problems. You might feel guilty because you think that your care is not good enough. You may feel guilty because you feel trapped. It is also common for caregivers to feel guilty because they want more time for themselves or because they hope that the caregiving will soon end.

Step 4: Take Action

So far, we have been naming and explaining difficult emotions. Now it is time to do something about them. The following ideas are things you may want to try. You do not need to do all of them. Look over the list and decide where you want to start.

- **Talk with someone.** Talking to someone about what you are feeling often softens the feelings. You can talk to a professional, such as a social worker, counselor, psychologist, health care provider, or leader of your religious community. You can also talk with your family and friends. You can talk to more than one person. Depending on whom you talk with, you can expect different outcomes. A professional may be very good at giving you suggestions, and friends and family may offer love and sympathy. By talking with people honestly, you may get some help you did not expect.

  You might want to talk to a group of peers—other people who are caregivers. They will know exactly what you are talking about and understand your situation. You can find such groups online, through organizations such as the Alzheimer's Association, or groups at your local senior center. Many people shy away from such groups because they think that a group meeting is just a "pity party." This is not the case at all. At meetings like these, people share experiences as well as what has worked and what has not worked.

- **Write in a journal.** Thanks to good science, we now know that sometimes just writing down your feelings helps you to feel better. You do not need to show what you write to anyone—just write. You do not even have to think much about your writing. Sit down with paper and pen, or at a computer, and start a journal. Write down the date and then any feelings that come into your head and anything else you want to express. Five minutes is enough, but if you want to write longer, fine. Try to do this every day, even if you write only a line or two.

  Several things happen when people write like this. First, they feel better just expressing their emotions in writing. Second, over time, they are surprised and learn things when they look back. Your journal acts like a road map to help you see where you have been. It may also offer insights into the future. For example, you might begin to see patterns. You might read about how you feel very sad every time your care partner gets a little worse. You may also note that after a day or two, you adjust, and life goes on. This may help the "downs" not to be so deep in the future. We cannot tell you what you will learn or how you will feel. We do know that keeping a journal has provided numerous benefits to many people.

  Writing is powerful, so we want to offer a word of caution. Journaling might stir up some thoughts and emotions that make you more feel depressed, stressed, or frightened. If this occurs, it can be a sign that you need help. Seek out an expert such as a psychologist or social worker if this is the case.

Adaptive Thinking

Earlier, we talked about changing negative thoughts. The way to do this is with adaptive thinking. This means changing the way you look at things to include thoughts that are more helpful to you. When you think adaptively, you still see the negatives, but you don't dwell on them. These negative thoughts can get you down, but if you take a broader view that lets you look at things in different ways, you can think about things in different ways. Adaptive thoughts help to reduce your stress. You feel better and can go on more easily day to day. Sometimes we cannot change things, but we can change the way we think about things.

Some adaptive thinking hints are especially helpful for caregivers. Focus on being the best caregiver you can be today. Do not reflect on what might have been or what the future might hold. Face the facts of the current situation and work within it.

Unfortunately, there might be very little that you can do as a caregiver to make your care partner better, but you can make each day the best it can be for both of you. To do this, you may need to rethink about what caregiving means to you. Take a minute and complete the following sentence. For me caregiving is: ______________

____

____.

Now, look at what you wrote. Is it largely negative? If so, how could you change your statement to be more positive? Can you think of any small joys you have gotten from caregiving? You do not want to be a Pollyanna or false in your definition. What you want to do is to think about caregiving in the most positive, neutral, or least negative way possible. For example, instead of, "Caregiving is ruining my life, and nothing will ever be the same," you might think, "Caregiving is really hard, and I am doing the best I can." Here is another example: "For me, caregiving is so frustrating. He can't do anything. All he does is shout and whine. He does not appreciate anything I do." You might change this to: "For me, caregiving is a challenge. His condition is hard for both of us. I will do what I can to make him comfortable. I know he would thank me if he could."

Adaptive thinking takes practice. It does not come easily. However, it is worth the effort. The following four steps will help you adapt your thoughts:

1. Identify your frequent reoccurring negative thoughts.
2. Write these thoughts down.
3. Think how you might change each thought.
4. Every time you catch yourself having a negative thought, change it to your less negative or more positive choice.

With practice, your thinking will adapt, and, as this happens, you may well find yourself with fewer difficult emotions.

Sometimes it takes more than just adapting our thinking. It takes action, especially setting priorities and not trying to do it all.

Establishing Priorities

We often hear from caregivers that they are overwhelmed. There is too much to do. You may feel like what you do is never good enough. The work is never-ending. It is not surprising that you may be angry, depressed, and stressed. Caregiving is never-ending work, but so is life.

An important caregiver tool is establishing priorities. A good way to start is to write down all the things that *have to be done* and then add to this a list of all the things *you would like to do.*

Go through your list and mark everything that is important to your care partner's health and safety. See if there are items that are nice but not necessary. Do not cross out things that you would like to do. Try to find a few things that you do not need to do or that you can do less often. Are there some things that could be done more easily? Can some of the things (housework or yard work) be done by someone else? If so, then come up with an action plan to make that happen.

Now, look again at the things you would like to do. Mark the three or four things that you would like to do most. Choose at least one and see if there is any way that you can make

We have included an example form here:

Priorities Worksheet

Things That Have to Be Done	Things I Would Like to Do

this happen. Sometimes this means changing your thinking. For example, a caregiver visits her husband in a nursing home for three hours every day. She would like to take a short trip to see her grandchildren but thinks she can't because she would miss her regular visits to her husband for a few days. The visits are her duty. Her visits do not add to the health or safety of her care partner. To try to figure out a way to make the trip to her grandchildren's, she might try some adaptive thinking. "If I visit my grandchildren, I will have more to talk about with my husband. He will enjoy hearing about them and looking at the photos I will take. Maybe I can get someone at the nursing home to help him with Zoom or FaceTime, and we can all be together for a short time."

With so much to do, it is hard to establish priorities. However, you are doing this every day. This exercise makes you really think about your priorities. You might decide not to change a thing. That is OK, but until you look at what you are doing, it is hard to make the decision to change or not change.

Facing the Facts

No matter how much you set priorities or adapt your thinking, life is not always as you would like it to be. This is especially true when you are a caregiver. Sometimes people put a rosy glow on reality (this is another way of saying they are in denial). "There is nothing much wrong. He cannot find the bathroom at night, has frequent falls, and eats with his hands, but these are little things. We do not need any extra help. He will get better, and I can handle everything."

When you deny the facts, you can pretend that nothing has changed and that life will return to the "way it used to be." You also can preserve your pride in being the perfect family member and caregiver. Pretending, however, can come at a high price. In reality, you may be unhappy or depressed, but because you are so busy pretending everything is perfect, you can't talk to anyone about your problems. And on top of this isolation, you and your care partner might both be in physical or emotional danger. Your care partner's falls may result in injury. Your attempts to pretend everything is fine may put your care partner in more danger. It also puts you in danger. You may hurt yourself trying to help your partner.

Emotionally, your care partner might be very willing to admit that life has changed and find relief in giving up some of the pretenses of the "old normal." For the care partner, it can become more and more of a burden to pretend. Finally, there will come a time when this is no longer possible.

Unfortunately, not facing the facts often leads to a crisis. You or your care partner may break a hip. Your care partner may leave the house and the police find them the next day. You may alienate family members and friends because they clearly see the facts and probably are willing to help, but they become angry with your constant denials. Not knowing what to do or how to help, they stop coming around.

The big benefit to facing the facts is that it gives you control. No longer scrambling to hide from reality, you can have time to plan, to get help, and to find small joys with your care partner. Facing the facts allows you to explore a new phase of life.

Sometimes it is difficult to know where to start in facing the facts. Friends, family members, and your health care providers can help. Ask them what they see when they look at your care partner. Ask how you can be a good caregiver in the real-world situation you are in. The hard part is that you must listen carefully, not interrupt or try to tell them they are wrong, and, most importantly, not get angry or defensive. You may not like what you hear. Denial is very powerful. You can overcome it. The good news is that facing the facts usually leads to a better quality of life for both the caregiver and care partner.

Dealing with Peer Pressure

Although your own feelings and thoughts can get in the way of facing the facts, peer pressure can be troubling and difficult to deal with too. You might know people who fall into the following types:

- **The happy warriors.** Sometimes, well-meaning friends will tell you how they took care of their mothers for 15 years and that every day was a blessing and a joy. You may find caregiving difficult and not very joyful. Hearing this from a friend can make you feel guilty because you are not enjoying caregiving as she did. Worse, you might feel you are a bad person because sometimes you do not much like being a caregiver.
- **The "experts."** There are also "helpful friends." They have never been caregivers, but they tell you exactly what you should and should not do. Sometimes these experts are family members. "Experts" can cause stress because they do not know what they are talking about or because you do not want to offend them. They can also make you feel guilty because their advice on how to do things differently implies that you are not the best possible caregiver.
- **The doomsayers.** These people have been caregivers and it was a terrible experience for them. Doomsayers are more than happy to tell you all the gruesome details and to end every conversation by saying, "Just wait! It will get worse." Doomsayers give voice to your anxiety and uncertainty and cause stress, anger, and fear.

These are just a few of the "helpful" people you may meet. They usually mean well but, in fact, cause you extra stress and problems.

One technique for dealing with not-so-helpful people is called a broken record. Find a phrase such as, "Thank you for your input," "Let me think about this," or "I would rather talk about something else." No matter what they say, repeat your phrase. You don't engage in a conversation or an argument about these topics with them. It is best to keep your phrase neutral. Just keep repeating your phrase. Usually what happens is that, after hearing this phrase three or four times, the other person gives up.

You will find more ideas about how to communicate with not-so-helpful people as well as those from whom you need or want something in Chapter 6, Communicating Effectively.

Letting Go of What You Cannot Control

There are many things that, as a caregiver, you cannot control. This lack of control can make you feel guilty, sad, frightened, and angry. Recognizing and accepting what you cannot control is a great caregiver skill. Some caregivers find the serenity prayer used by Alcoholics Anonymous helpful:

God, grant me the serenity to accept the things I cannot change,

The courage to change the things I can,

And wisdom to know the difference.

Often in this book, we encourage you to recognize things you can change and offer various tools so that you can make changes. But we realize that not all things can be changed or improved. It is important that you know this too. When you encounter things you cannot change, you need to accept them and then let them go. Each person only has so much energy and emotional capacity. You are certainly not alone in your feelings. If the tools in this book are not enough to help you with acceptance, talk with a counselor or spiritual leader. This is especially important if you are so frustrated that you feel you might lash out at your care partner.

In this chapter, we have talked about some common caregiver stressors and given you some specific tools for dealing with these. We will continue with this theme in the next chapter.

For a complete list of suggested further readings, useful websites, and other helpful resources, please see: www.bullpub.com/resources.

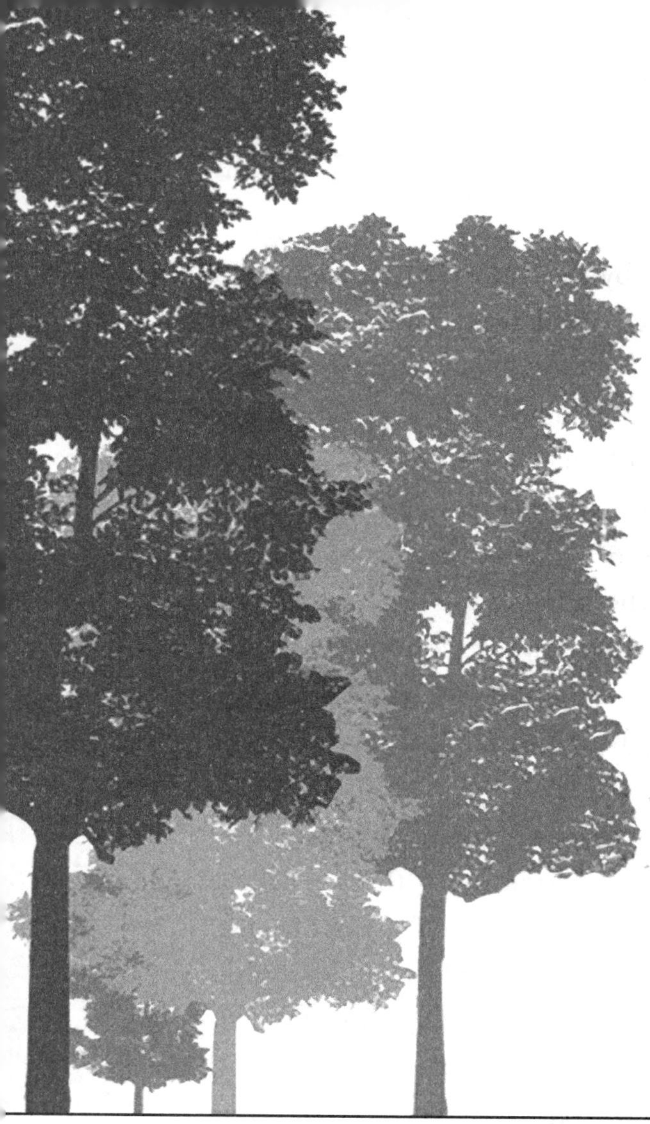

Chapter 5

Using Your Mind to Manage Stress

BEFORE WE SAY ANYTHING ELSE, WE WANT TO BE CLEAR—caregiving is stressful. Your caregiving stress is not all in your head, nor is the stress your fault. The goal of this chapter, like the last one, is to provide you with stress-managing tools. We know that no one can manage the stress of caregiving with just happy thinking. But we also know that there are many effective ways your mind can help you deal with stress. In this chapter, we introduce you to some of these mental tools.

Stress, the Mind, and the Body

There is a strong link between thoughts, attitudes, and emotions and mental and physical health. As one of the caregivers we work with so truly said, "It's not always mind over matter, but mind matters." Although thoughts and emotions do not always cause stress, thoughts and emotions have a big influence on how people handle and respond to stressors. Research has shown that thoughts and emotions trigger certain hormones and other chemicals that send messages throughout the body. These messages affect how the body functions. Thoughts and emotions can affect heart rate, blood pressure, breathing, blood sugar levels, muscle responses, concentration, and the ability to fight off illness.

All of us, at one time or another, have experienced the power of the mind and its effects on the body. Both pleasant and unpleasant thoughts and emotions can cause the body to react in different ways. For example, your heart rate and breathing increase or slow down or you experience sensations such as sweating (warm or cold), blushing, tears, and so on. Sometimes just a memory or an image can trigger these responses.

Try this simple exercise. Imagine that you are holding a big, bright yellow lemon slice. You hold it close to your nose and smell its strong citrus aroma. Now you bite into the lemon slice. It's juicy! The juice fills your mouth and dribbles down your chin. You begin to suck on the lemon and its tart juice. What happens? Even though you are not actually biting into a lemon slice, the body responds. Your mouth puckers and starts to water. You might even smell the scent of the lemon. All of these reactions are triggered by the mind and its memory of your experience with a real lemon.

This example shows the power the mind has over the body. It also gives you a good reason to work to develop your mental abilities to help you manage your symptoms. With training and practice, you can learn to use the mind to relax the body, to reduce stress and anxiety, and to reduce the discomfort or unpleasantness caused by physical and emotional symptoms. In this chapter, we describe several ways in which you can begin to use your mind to manage stress and other symptoms. These are sometimes referred to as "thinking" or "cognitive" techniques because they involve the use of thinking abilities to make changes in the body.

As you read, keep the following key principles in mind:

- Stress can have many causes. Because it can be caused by so many things, there are many ways to manage stress. If you understand the nature and causes of your stress or other symptoms, you will be able to manage them better.
- Not all management techniques work for everyone. It is up to you to experiment and find out what works best for you. Be flexible. This includes trying different techniques and checking your results to decide which management tool is most helpful under which circumstances.
- Learning new skills and gaining control of the situation take time. Give yourself several weeks to practice before you decide if a new tool is working for you.

- Don't give up too easily. Like exercise and other new skills, using your mind to manage stress requires both practice and time before you notice the benefits. So even if you feel you are not accomplishing anything, don't give up. Be patient and keep on trying.
- Stress reduction techniques should not have negative effects. If you become frightened, angry, or depressed when using one of these tools, do not continue to use it. Try another tool instead.
- Stress is not all bad. In fact, we need stress to help us prepare for challenging situations. Stress can make us tougher and more resilient. Learning new things and overcoming challenges often involves some positive stress.

Relaxation Techniques

You may have heard and read about relaxation, yet still be confused about what relaxation is, its benefits, and how to do it. Relaxation involves using thinking and behavioral techniques to reduce or eliminate tension from both the body and the mind. Relaxation usually results in less stress and frustration and improved sleep. It can also help with pain and shortness of breath. Relaxation is not a cure-all, but it can be a beneficial life skill.

The goal of relaxation is to turn off the outside world so that the mind and body are at rest. This allows you to reduce the tensions that can increase the intensity or severity of stress. Here are different types of relaxation techniques. Each has specific guidelines and uses. Some techniques are used mostly to achieve muscle relaxation. Others are aimed at reducing anxiety and emotional stress or diverting attention.

Getting Started: Ideas for Relaxation

Some of these suggestions require advance planning or setting aside enough time to make them worthwhile (for example, starting a small garden). Others are quick and easy, like curling up to read or listen to a good book, or stroking or playing with your pet. Review the list and star the ones you can do often, without too much fuss or bother. Start with these. In the meantime, you can be thinking about the others we list here that take more time and possibly some advanced planning. There is no better time than the present to think about how and when you can begin to do them as well.

Some types of relaxation are so easy, natural, and effective that people do not think of them as "relaxation techniques." They include the following:

- Take a nap or a warm, soothing bath.
- Curl up and read or listen to a good book.
- Watch a funny movie or a favorite TV show.
- Make a paper airplane and sail it across the room.
- Get a massage.
- Enjoy an occasional glass of wine or beer.
- Start a small garden or grow a beautiful plant indoors.

- Do crafts such as knitting, pottery, or woodworking.
- Read a poem or an inspirational saying.
- Go for a walk.
- Start a collection (for example, coins, folk art, shells, or something in miniature) and add to it.
- Listen to your favorite music.
- Sing around the house.
- Crumble paper into a ball and use a wastebasket as a basketball hoop.
- Look at water (for example, ocean waves, a lake, or a fountain).
- Watch the clouds in the sky.
- Put your head down on your table and close your eyes for five minutes.
- Rub your hands together until they're warm, and then cup them over your closed eyes.
- Vigorously shake your hands and arms for 10 seconds.
- Call a friend or family member to chat.
- Smile and introduce yourself to someone new.
- Do something nice and unexpected for someone else.
- Stroke or play with a pet.
- Go to a vacation spot in your mind.

Relaxation Tools That Take Five to 20 Minutes

The techniques we discuss in this section, the body scan and relaxation response, may take a bit more effort and time to learn, but they are quite effective. The following are some guidelines to help you get the most out of the relaxation tools:

- Pick a quiet place and time when you will not be disturbed for at least 15 to 20 minutes. (If this seems too long, start with five minutes. Also, in some homes the only quiet place is the bathroom. That is just fine.)
- Try to practice the technique once or twice daily and not less than four times a week.
- Don't expect instant success. Your mind way wander. This is common. Most of these techniques take practice. Sometimes it takes three to four weeks of consistent practice before you start to notice benefits.
- Relaxation should be helpful. At worst, you may find it boring, but if it is an unpleasant experience or makes you more nervous or anxious, switch to a different stress management tool described in this chapter.

Body Scan

To relax your muscles, it is helpful to know how to scan your body and recognize where you are tense. If you know where you are tense, then you can release the tension. The first step is to become familiar with the difference between the feeling of tension and the feeling of relaxation. This exercise allows you to compare those feelings. With practice, you can learn to spot and release tension anywhere in your body. It is best done lying down on your back, but any comfortable position can work. A body-scan script can be found on page 55.

Relaxation Response

In the early 1970s, physician Herbert Benson studied what he calls the "relaxation response." According to Benson, our bodies have several natural states. One example is the fight or flight

Body-Scan Script

As you get into a comfortable position, allowing yourself to begin to sink comfortably into the surface below you, you may perhaps begin to allow your eyes gradually to close. . . . From there, turn your attention to your breath. . . . Breathing in, allowing the breath gradually to go all the way down to your belly and then breathing out . . . and again, breathing in . . . and out . . . noticing the natural rhythm of your breathing. . . .

Now, allowing your attention to focus on your feet. Starting with your toes, notice whatever sensations are there—warmth, coolness, whatever's there . . . simply feel it. Using your mind's eye, imagine that as you breathe in, the breath goes all the way down into your toes, bringing with it new refreshing air. . . . And now noticing the sensations elsewhere in your feet, not judging or thinking about what you're feeling, but simply becoming aware of the experience of your feet as you allow yourself to be fully supported by the surface below you. . . .

Next focus on your lower legs and knees. These muscles and joints do a lot of work for us, but often we don't give them the attention they deserve. So now breathe down into the knees, calves, and ankles, noticing whatever sensations appear. . . . See if you can simply stay with the sensations . . . breathing in new, fresh air, and, as you exhale, releasing tension and stress and allowing the muscles to relax and soften. . . .

Now move your attention to the muscles, bones, and joints of the thighs, buttocks, and hips . . . breathing down into the upper legs, noticing whatever sensations you experience. It may be warmth, coolness, a heaviness or lightness. You may become aware of the contact with the surface beneath you, or perhaps the pulsing of your blood. Whatever's there . . . what matters is that you are taking time to learn to relax . . . deeper and deeper, as you breathe . . . in . . . and out.

Move your attention now to your back and chest. Feeling the breath fill the abdomen and chest. . . . Noticing whatever sensations are there . . . not judging or thinking, but simply observing what is right here right now, allowing the fresh air to nourish the muscles, bones, and joints as you breathe in, and then exhaling any tension and stress.

Now focus on the neck, shoulders, arms, and hands. Inhaling down through the neck and shoulders, all the way down to the fingertips. Not trying too hard to relax, but simply becoming aware of your experience of these parts of your body in the present moment. . . .

Turning now to your face and head, notice the sensations beginning at the back of your head, up along your scalp, and down into your forehead. . . . Then become aware of the sensations in and around your eyes and down into your cheeks and jaw. . . . Continue to allow your muscles to release and soften as you breathe in nourishing, fresh air, and allow tension and stress to leave as you breathe out. . . .

As you drink in fresh air, allow it to spread throughout your body, from the soles of your feet all the way up through the top of your head. . . . and then exhale any remaining stress and tension. . . . And now take a few moments to enjoy the stillness as you breathe in . . . and out . . . Awake, relaxed, and still . . .

Now as the body scan comes to a close, coming back into the room, bringing with you whatever sensations of relaxation . . . comfort . . . peace, whatever's there . . . knowing that you can repeat this exercise at any appropriate time and place of your choosing. . . . And when you're ready, open your eyes.

▶ To order the *Relaxation for Mind & Body Audio Program*, go to: www.bullpub.com/tfhcd-g.html

response experienced by people who are faced with a great danger. During the *fight or flight response*, the body becomes tense as it prepares to "fight" or to "flee." This tension is eventually followed by the body's natural tendency to relax. This is the relaxation response. As our lives become more and more hectic, our bodies tend to stay tense for longer and longer periods. We lose our ability to relax. Practicing the relaxation response helps change this pattern.

To elicit the relaxation response, take the following steps:

1. Find a quiet place where there are few or no distractions. Get in a comfortable position. You should be comfortable enough to remain in the same position for 20 minutes.
2. Choose a word, object, or pleasant feeling. For example, repeat a word or sound (such as the word *one*), gaze at an object or symbol (perhaps a flower), or concentrate on a feeling (such as peace).
3. Adopt a passive attitude. A passive attitude is very important for this exercise. Empty all thoughts and distractions from your mind. You might become aware of thoughts, images, and feelings, but don't concentrate on them. Just allow them to pass on.

Focused/Mindful Breathing Techniques

If you don't like doing the body scan, or don't have the time to do the whole exercise, don't worry. There are options! Many people use focused or mindful breathing techniques to promote relaxation, and even though it seems very simple (after all, we all breathe all day long, don't we?), it's a very worthwhile practice to learn and to use when you are stressed. Below we explain how taking the time to do some deep, focused, slow breathing can bring you relaxation.

To begin focused or mindful breathing techniques, take the following steps:

1. Sit quietly in a comfortable position.
2. Close your eyes.
3. Relax all your muscles, beginning at your feet and progressing up to your face. Keep them relaxed.
4. Breathe in through your nose. Become aware of your breathing. As you breathe out through your mouth, if you chose a word, say it silently to yourself. Try to empty all thoughts from your mind. Concentrate on your word, sound, or symbol. When your mind wanders—as it certainly will—just gently guide your attention back to your chosen word, sound, or symbol.
5. Continue this for five minutes. You can do it for longer if you wish. It is OK to open your eyes to check the time, but do not use an alarm. When you finish, sit quietly for several minutes, at first with your eyes closed. Do not stand up for a few minutes.
6. Maintain a passive attitude, and let relaxation occur at its own pace. When distracting thoughts occur, ignore them by not dwelling on them and return to repeating the word you chose. Do not worry about whether you are successful in achieving a deep level of relaxation.

Practice this once or twice daily. If you don't have time to take all the steps just discussed, here is an even quicker mindful breathing technique. Spread out the fingers of one hand as you hold it in front of your body. With a finger from the other hand start at the bottom outside of the thumb and take a breath in as you move your finger to the tip of the thumb. Breathe out as you slowly move your finger down the inside of your thumb and breathe in as you move it up the next finger. Continue for all five fingers—five slow breaths in all. If you have time, you can come back in the opposite direction for ten breaths.

Note that if you have a smartwatch, it may have a one-minute meditation setting. There is nothing to download; the watch comes with this setting. Try using this feature. Even just one minute can help address your stress!

Distraction

Our minds have trouble focusing on more than one thing at a time. We can make our stress symptoms less intense by training our minds to focus attention on something other than our bodies and their sensations. This technique, called distraction or attention refocusing, is particularly helpful for those people who feel that their stress symptoms are painful or overwhelming. It is important to mention that with distraction you are not ignoring the stress. You are choosing not to dwell on it.

Distraction works best for short activities or times in which stress is anticipated. For example, if you know a certain caregiving job will cause discomfort or that falling asleep at night is difficult, you might try one of the following distraction techniques:

- Make plans for exactly what you will do after the unpleasant activity passes. For example, if getting your care partner to take a shower is a challenge, think about what you can do after the shower is over. If you have trouble falling asleep, try making plans for some future event, being as detailed as possible.
- Think of a person's name, a bird, a flower, or whatever, for every letter of the alphabet. If you get stuck on one letter, go on to the next. (This can be a good distraction for pain and for sleep problems.)
- Challenge yourself to count backward from 100 by threes (100, 97, 94, . . .).
- To get through unpleasant daily chores (such as sweeping, mopping, or vacuuming), imagine your floor as a map of a country or continent. Try naming all the states, provinces, or countries, moving east to west or north to south. If geography does not appeal to you, imagine your favorite store and where each department is located.
- Try to remember words to favorite songs or the events in an old story.
- Redirect your attention to a pleasurable experience.
- Picture something outside, such as your garden or the seashore.
- Remember positive experiences from the past, especially those you shared with your care partner.
- Think about how you felt when your team won the Super Bowl, the World Series, or the World Cup.

- Picture your children or grandchildren when they were babies.
- Remember a time when your pet did something funny.

There are, of course, many variations to these examples, all of which help you refocus attention away from your problem.

So far, we have discussed short-term refocusing strategies that involve using only the mind for distraction. Distraction also works well for long-term projects or stress symptoms that tend to last longer, such as depression.

In these cases, the mind is focused not inward but outward on some type of activity. If you are depressed or have continuous unpleasant feelings, find an activity that interests you and distract yourself from the problem. The activity can be almost anything, from gardening to cooking to reading or going to a movie. One of the marks of successful caregivers is that they develop a variety of interests and take time to restore themselves.

Positive (Helpful) Thinking and Self-Talk

We talk to ourselves all the time. For example, when waking up in the morning, you may think, "I really don't want to get out of bed. I'm tired and I don't think I can be a caregiver one more day." Or at the end of an enjoyable evening, you think, "Gee, that was fun. I had forgotten that my care partner and I could still have fun." What you think or say to yourself is called self-talk. The way you talk to yourself reflects how and what you think about yourself. Thoughts can be positive (helpful) or negative (unhelpful), and so is self-talk. Self-talk can be an effective self-management tool if it encourages positive and helpful thinking. Or it can be a weapon that hurts or defeats us if it leads to habitually negative or unhelpful thinking.

Self-talk is usually learned from others and becomes a part of people as they grow up. It comes in many forms. Unfortunately, these forms are often not helpful. Negative self-statements usually take the form of phrases that begin with something like, "I just can't do . . . ," "If only I could . . . ," "If only I didn't . . . ," "I just don't have the energy . . . ," or "How could I be so stupid?" This type of unhelpful thinking represents the doubts and fears people have about themselves in general. You may have thoughts like these about your abilities to deal with your role as a caregiver and your care partner's condition and its symptoms. Negative thinking damages self-esteem, attitude, and mood. Negative self-talk is unhelpful as it makes you feel bad and undermines your ability to deal with stressful challenges.

What you say to yourself plays a major role in determining your success or failure in becoming effective caregivers. Negative thinking tends to limit your abilities and actions. If you tell yourself "I'm not very smart" or "I can't" all the time, you probably won't try to learn new skills because this just doesn't fit with what you think about yourself. Soon you become prisoner of your own negative beliefs.

Fortunately, self-talk is not something fixed in your biological makeup, and therefore it is in your control. You can learn new, healthier ways to think about yourself so that your self-talk can work for you instead of against you. We suggest developing encouraging things to say to yourself, such as "I've handled worse situations" or "I am doing my best" or "This is challenging but if I take it one step at a time. I can manage and I'll get through it." You can develop a set of these kinds of statements and type them into a note on your phone or write them down on a notepad or on Post-its throughout your living space. These daily reminders can help defuse negative caregiver self-talk. By changing the unhelpful, self-defeating statements to helpful ones, you can manage stress and other symptoms more effectively. This change, like any habit, requires practice and includes the following steps:

1. **Listen carefully to what you say to or about yourself, both out loud and silently.** If you find yourself feeling anxious, depressed, or angry, try to identify some of the thoughts you were having just before these feelings started. Then write down all the negative self-talk statements. Pay special attention to the things you say during times that are particularly difficult for you. For example, what do you say to yourself when you start to get annoyed with your care partner or when you do not think you are doing enough? Challenge these negative thoughts by asking yourself questions to identify what about the statement is really true or not true. When you get annoyed because your care partner is being difficult tell yourself: "I can manage this situation better if I don't express my anger. I'm going to count to 10 and then deal with the situation." Or perhaps you are worrying too much about the future? It's true that things will likely get more challenging as memory loss or other symptoms progress, but focusing on that is not helpful and will just increase your anxiety. It's more helpful to tell yourself: "I don't know exactly what the future holds. Everyone progresses at a different rate. What will I accomplish by worrying? It's better to do some advance planning, to anticipate situations that *are* likely to happen—like my care partner needing more personal care—and think through my options. How can I prepare now, so that when that time comes, I'm able to handle it?"
2. **Work on changing each unhelpful statement to a more helpful one, or think up a positive statement to replace the negative one.** Write the helpful statements down so you can get in the habit of repeating them instead of the negative statements. For example, negative statements such as "I don't want to get up," "I'm too tired and it will just be another awful day," "I can't do anything that pleases my care partner, so why bother?" or "I'm good for nothing" become positive messages such as "I'm feeling pretty good today and I'm going to do something I enjoy," "I might not be able to do everything but I know that my care partner appreciates the effort even if they cannot express appreciation," or "My care partner needs and depends on me, so what I do is worthwhile and important." Making a written or audio "set" of such statements that you can review during the day is very helpful to making this a new habit.

3. **Read and rehearse these positive statements, silently to yourself or with another person.** This conscious repetition or memorization of the positive self-talk will help you replace those old, habitual negative statements.
4. **Practice these new statements in real situations.** This practice, along with time and patience, will help the new patterns of thinking become automatic.
5. **Rehearse success.** When you aren't happy with the way you handled a particular situation, try this exercise:
   - Write down three ways that it could have gone better.
   - Write down three ways it could have gone worse.
   - If you can't think of alternatives to the way you handled it, imagine what someone whom you greatly respect would have done.
   - Think what advice you would give to someone else facing a similar situation.

Remember that mistakes aren't failures. They're opportunities to learn. Mistakes give you the chance to rehearse other ways of handling things. This is great practice for future crises.

As you first do this, you may find it hard to adopt a positive attitude, to develop encouraging self-talk, and to change unhelpful statements into more helpful ones.

The following are some ideas to help you replace unhelpful thinking with more helpful thinking.

- **Use a shortcut.** A shortcut is to use either a thought stopper or a positive affirmation. A thought stopper can be anything that is meaningful to you (for example, a puppy, a polar bear, a rose, or an oak tree). When you have a negative thought, replace it with your thought stopper. It might sound silly, but try it. It works for many people and you may be one of them.

  A positive affirmation is a positive phrase that you can use over and over. It's ready to use when you need it. For example, "I am getting better every day," "I can do this," "This won't go on forever," or "God loves me." Like the positive statements, use this to replace negative thoughts.
- **Try to be realistic and set realistic standards for yourself.** Are you exaggerating the situation, generalizing, worrying too much, or assuming the worst? Are you thinking in terms of black and white? Could there be gray? Maybe you are making an unrealistic or unfair comparison, assuming too much responsibility, taking something too personally, or expecting perfection.

Many caregivers hold themselves to an impossibly high standard—expecting themselves to *always* make the right decision or *always* handle things in the most effective way. Thinking this way only sets you up for failure since no one is perfect. All caregivers regret things: things they did or said, and things they didn't do or say. Caregivers have to learn to forgive themselves for their human failings. That doesn't mean you don't strive to be the best caregiver possible. It does mean you "cut yourself some slack" when you are having a bad day. As a famous poet once said: "Yesterday is but a memory, tomorrow is a dream, today is all we have," so we try to make the best of each day.

Caregivers often feel frustrated with their care partner and then feel bad about themselves for being impatient or short with the person. Caregivers need to learn to develop and to practice self-compassion. The psychologist Kristen Neff has a number of exercises on her website (https://self-compassion.org/self-compassion-practices/#guided-practices) and has several YouTube videos on this topic. She says that self-compassion means giving the same kindness and sympathy to yourself as you would give to a good friend.

Here's an example to show you how this works. Your husband with moderately advanced dementia argues with you repeatedly about driving. He doesn't remember that he no longer has his license. One day you snap at him and yell loudly: "I've had it with you. You never listen to me and we argue all the time. I'm going to put you in a nursing home." Then you feel badly and start a chain of unhelpful thoughts, such as: "I'm no good at this anymore, I'm burned out, and I don't know how long I can take this," and you go into your bedroom and cry. Or maybe you scream out loud in the garage to get out some of the frustration you're feeling. What is the result of all of this? It's a negative spiral: You think negative thoughts about yourself as a caregiver, you feel badly about yourself, and you find it harder to get up and face the next hour or the next day. You're defeating yourself and making caregiving harder than it needs to be.

An alternative is to practice self-compassion. If a friend told you the exact same story, same circumstances, what would you likely say to them? Probably not, "What a bad caregiver you are!" but more likely, "Everyone has a bad day. That doesn't mean you're a bad caregiver! It means you need to find ways to take better care of yourself, here and now, so that you can continue." By putting yourself in your friend's place and talking to them as if you were talking to yourself, you will find that your stress eases and you are encouraged to face the next challenge with more of a sense of inner strength. Are you making assumptions about what other people think about you? What do you know for a fact? Look at the evidence so that you are better able to change these negative thoughts and statements.

- **Set intentions for helpful thinking.** Setting an intention in the morning is another good habit. Think about what kind of a day you intend today to be? Then think about how you can maximize your ability to make it a good day. What's likely to get in the way? How can you anticipate and potentially change negative things that might happen today?

  For example, if your care partner always struggles with getting dressed and ready to get out on time for appointments, you can set out necessary clothing, allow enough time, and be cheerful and encouraging, so that the desired outcome is more likely to occur. Starting the day with a positive attitude, and trying to problem solve in advance, will go a long way to reducing negative thoughts and feelings.

- **Change your perspective.** Sometimes you can relieve stress and break the cycle of negative thoughts by shifting your perspective. If you are upset, ask, "How important will this be in an hour, a day, a month, or a year?" Or you might consider how important this stress is compared to natural disasters or other calamities. This reframing often helps us sort out the things that are really important and need action versus the more minor annoyances that capture our attention.

Imagery

You may think that "imagination" is all in your mind. But the thoughts, words, and images that flow from your imagination can have very real effects on your body. Remember the lemon you imagined at the start of this chapter. Your brain often cannot distinguish whether you are imagining something or if it is really happening. Perhaps you've had a racing heartbeat, rapid breathing, or tension in your neck muscles while watching a movie thriller. These sensations were all produced by images and sounds on film. During a dream, maybe your body responded with fear, joy, anger, or sadness—all triggered by your imagination. If you close your eyes and vividly imagine yourself by a still, quiet pool or relaxing on a warm beach, your body responds to some degree as though you were actually there.

Guided imagery and visualization allow you to use your imagination to relieve stress symptoms. These techniques will help you focus your thoughts on healing images and suggestions.

Guided Imagery

This tool is like a guided daydream. It allows you to divert your attention. It can refocus your mind away from your symptoms and transports you to another time and place. It can help you achieve deep relaxation by picturing yourself in a peaceful environment.

With guided imagery, you focus your mind on a particular image. Imagery usually involves your sense of sight, focusing on visual images. Adding other senses—smells, tastes, and sounds—makes the guided imagery especially vivid and powerful.

Some people are highly visual and can see images with their "mind's eye." But if your images aren't as vivid as scenes from a great movie, don't worry. It's normal for the intensity of imagery to vary. The important thing is to focus on as much detail as you can and to strengthen the images by using all your senses. Adding background music can also increase the impact of guided imagery.

With guided imagery, you are always completely in control. You're the movie director. You can project whatever thought or feeling you want onto your mental screen. If you don't like a particular image, thought, or feeling, redirect your mind to something more comfortable, or open your eyes and stop the exercise and use a different script next time.

The guided imagery scripts presented on pages 64 and 65 can help take you on a mental stroll. Here are some tips for using imagery:

- Read the script over several times until it is familiar. Then sit or lie down in a quiet place and try to reconstruct the scene in your mind. The script should take 15 to 20 minutes to complete.

- Have a family member or friend read you the script slowly, pausing for about 10 seconds wherever there is a series of periods (. . .).
- Make a recording of the script and play it to yourself whenever convenient.
- Use a prerecorded tape, CD, or digital audio file that has a similar guided imagery script. For a complete list of suggested further readings, useful websites, and other helpful resources, please see www.bullpub.com/resources.

Visualization

This technique is similar to guided imagery. However, in guided imagery, the images are suggested to you. Visualization allows you to create your own images. Visualization is another way of using your imagination to create a picture of yourself doing the things you want to do. People use a form of visualization every day—when you dream, worry, read a book, or listen to a story. In all these activities, the mind creates images for you to see. You also use visualization intentionally when making plans for the day, considering the possible outcomes of a decision you have to make, or rehearsing for an event or activity. Visualization can be done in different ways and can be used for longer periods or while you are engaged in other activities.

One way to use visualization to manage stress is to remember pleasant scenes from your past or create new scenes. To practice visualization, try to remember every detail of a special holiday or party that made you happy. Who was there? What happened? What did you do or talk about? You can also try this by remembering a vacation or some other memorable and pleasant event.

During visualization you can plan the details of some future event or fill in the details of a fantasy. For example, how would you spend a million dollars? What would your ideal home or garden look like? Where would you go and what would you do on your dream vacation?

Another form of visualization involves using your mind to think of symbols that represent stress-related discomfort or pain felt in different parts of your body. For example, a stiff neck might be red, or a tight chest might have a constricting band around it. After forming these images, you can then try to change them. The red color might fade until there is no more color, or the constricting band will stretch and stretch until it falls off. These new images can change the way you think of your pain or discomfort.

Visualization helps build confidence and skill, and therefore is a useful technique to help you set and accomplish your personal goals (see Chapter 2, Becoming a Better Caregiver: The Basics). After you write your weekly action plan, take a few minutes to imagine yourself taking a walk, doing your exercises, or using a relaxation technique from this chapter. You are mentally rehearsing the steps you need to take in order to achieve your goals successfully.

Imagery for Different Conditions

You have the ability to create special imagery to help (though not cure) specific stress-related symptoms or feelings. Use any image that is strong and vivid for you—this often involves using all your senses to create the image—and one that is meaningful to you. The image does not have to be accurate for it to work. Just

Guided-Imagery Script: A Walk in the Country

Begin by getting into a comfortable position, whether you are seated or lying down. Loosen any tight clothing to allow yourself to be as comfortable as possible. Uncross your legs and allow your hands to fall by your sides or rest in your lap, and, if you are at all uncomfortable, shift to a more comfortable position.

You're giving yourself some time to quiet your mind and body. Allow yourself to settle comfortably, wherever you are right now. If you wish, you can close your eyes. Breathe in deeply, through your nose, expanding your abdomen and filling your lungs and, pursing your lips, exhale through your mouth slowly and completely, allowing your body to sink heavily into the surface beneath you. . . .

And once again breathe in through your nose and all the way down to your abdomen, and then breathe out slowly through pursed lips, letting go of tension, letting go of anything that's on your mind right now and just allowing yourself to be present in this moment. . . .

Imagine yourself walking along a peaceful old country road. The sun is gently warming your back . . . the birds are singing . . . the air is calm and fragrant. . . .

With no need to hurry, you notice your walking is relaxed and easy. As you walk along in this way, taking in your surroundings, you come across an old gate. It looks inviting and you decide to take the path through the gate. The gate creaks as you open it and go through.

You find yourself in an old, overgrown garden, flowers growing where they've seeded themselves, vines climbing over a fallen tree, soft green wild grasses, shade trees.

You notice yourself breathing deeply . . . smelling the flowers . . . listening to the birds and insects . . . feeling a gentle breeze cool against your skin. All of your senses are alive and responding with pleasure to this peaceful time and place. . . .

When you're ready to move on, you leisurely follow the path out behind the garden, eventually coming to a more wooded area. As you enter this area, your eyes find the trees and plant life restful. The sunlight is filtered through the leaves. The air feels mild and a little cooler. . . . You savor the fragrance of trees and earth . . . and gradually become aware of the sound of a nearby stream. Pausing, you allow yourself to take in the sights and sounds, breathing in the cool and fragrant air several times. . . . And with each breath, you notice how refreshed you are feeling. . . .

Continuing along the path for a while, you come to the stream. It's clear and clean as it flows and tumbles over the rocks and some fallen logs. You follow the path easily along the creek for a way, and after a while, you come out into a sunlit clearing, where you discover a small waterfall emptying into a quiet pool of water.

You find a comfortable place to sit for a while, a perfect niche where you can feel completely relaxed.

You feel good as you allow yourself to just enjoy the warmth and solitude of this peaceful place. . . .

After a while, you become aware that it is time to return. You arise and walk back down the path in a relaxed and comfortable way, through the cool and fragrant trees, out into the sun-drenched, overgrown garden. . . . One last smell of the flowers, and out the creaky gate.

You leave this country retreat for now and return down the road. You notice you feel calm and rested. You feel grateful and remind yourself that you can visit this special place whenever you wish to take some time to refresh yourself and renew your energy.

And now, preparing to bring this period of relaxation to a close, you may want to take a moment to picture yourself carrying this experience of calm and refreshment with you into the ordinary activities of your life. . . . And when you're ready, take a nice deep breath and open your eyes.

▶ To order the *Relaxation for Mind & Body Audio Program*, go to: www.bullpub.com/tfhcd-g.html

Guided-Imagery Script: A Walk on the Beach

Begin by getting into a comfortable position, whether you are seated or lying down. Loosen any tight clothing to allow yourself to be as comfortable as possible. Uncross your legs and allow your hands to fall by your sides or rest in your lap, and if you are at all uncomfortable, shift to a more comfortable position.

When you are ready, you allow your eyes gradually to close and turn your attention to your breathing. Allow your belly to expand as you breathe in, bringing in fresh new air to nourish your body. And then breathing out. Notice the rhythm of your breathing . . . in . . . and out . . . without trying to control it in any way at all. Simply attend to the natural rhythm of your breath. . . .

And now, in your mind's eye, imagine yourself standing on a beautiful beach. The sky is a brilliant blue, and as some fluffy white clouds float slowly by, you drink in the beautiful colors. . . . The temperature is not too hot and not too cold. The sun is shining, and you close your eyes, allowing the warmth of the sun to wash over you. . . . You notice a gentle breeze caressing your face, the perfect complement to the sunshine.

Then you find yourself turning and looking out over the vastness of the ocean . . . you become aware of the sound of the waves gently washing up on shore . . . You notice the firmness of the wet sand beneath your feet, or if you decide to take off your shoes, you may enjoy the feeling of standing, in the cool, wet sand. . . . Perhaps you allow the surf to roll up and gently wash across your feet, or perhaps you stay just out of its reach. . . .

In the distance, you hear some seagulls calling to one another and look out to see the birds gracefully gliding through the air. And as you stand there, notice how easy it is to be here, perhaps noticing some sensations of relaxation, comfort, or peace . . . whatever's there. . . .

Now take a walk along the shore. Turn and begin to stroll casually along the beach, enjoying the sounds of the surf, the warmth of the sun, and the gentle massage of the breeze. As you move along, taking your time, your stride becomes lighter, easier. . . . You notice the scent of the ocean. . . . You pause to take in the freshness of the air. . . . And then you continue on your way, enjoying the peacefulness of this place.

After a time, you decide to rest a while and find a comfortable place to sit or lie down . . . and simply allow yourself to take some time to enjoy this, your special place. . . .

And now, when you feel ready to return, you stand and begin walking back down the beach in a comfortable, leisurely way, taking with you any sensations of relaxation, comfort, peace, joy . . . whatever's there . . . noticing how easy it is to be here. Continue back until you reach the place where you began your walk. . . .

And now pausing to take one last long look around. Enjoying the vibrant colors of the sky and the sea . . . the gentle sound of the waves washing up on the shore, the warmth of the sun, the cool of the breeze. . . .

And as you prepare to leave this special place, taking with you any sensations of joy, relaxation, comfort, peace . . . whatever's there . . .knowing that you may return at any appropriate time and place of your choosing.

And now bringing your awareness back into the room, focusing on your breathing . . . in and out . . . taking a few more breaths . . . and when you're ready, opening your eyes.

▶ To order the *Relaxation for Mind & Body Audio Program*, go to: www.bullpub.com/tfhcd-g.html

use your imagination and trust yourself. Here are examples of images that some people have found useful:

For Tension and Stress

- A tight, twisted rope slowly untwists.
- Wax softens and melts.
- Tension swirls out of your body and down a drain.

For Fatigue

- A light bulb is plugged in and there is a sudden burst of energy.
- A puppy races around you with boundless energy and enthusiasm.
- You slowly take off a heavy winter coat, allowing you to feel lighter and more energetic.

For Pain

- The pain is washed away by a cool, calm river flowing through your entire body.
- All of the pain is placed in a large, strong metal box that is closed, sealed tightly, and locked with a huge, strong padlock.
- You grasp the TV remote control and slowly turn down the pain volume until you can barely hear it, and then it disappears entirely.

For Depression

- Your troubles and feelings of sadness are attached to big colorful helium balloons and are floating off into a clear blue sky.
- A strong, warm sun breaks through dark clouds.
- You feel a sense of detachment and lightness, enabling you to float easily through your day.

Use any of these images, or make up your own. Remember, the most effective images are vivid and have meaning to you. Use your imagination for health and healing.

Prayer and Spirituality

For many people, there is a relationship between spirituality and health. Spirituality is one way to find meaning, hope, comfort, and inner peace in your life. Many people find spirituality through religion. Some find it through music, art, or a connection with nature. Others find it in their values and principles.

Many people are religious and share their religion with others. Others do not have a specific religion but do have spiritual beliefs. Your religion and beliefs can bring a sense of meaning and purpose to your life, help you put things into perspective, and set priorities. Your beliefs may help you find comfort during difficult times. They can help you with acceptance and motivate you to make difficult changes. A spiritual or religious community can serve as a source of support when needed and give you the opportunity to help others.

Recent studies find that people who belong to a religious or spiritual community, or who regularly engage in religious activities, such as prayer or study, have improved health. There are many types of prayer. All types of prayer can contribute to improved health, including asking for help, direction, and forgiveness and offering words of gratitude, praise, and blessing, among others. In addition, many religions have a tradition of contemplation or meditation. Prayer does not need a scientific explanation. It is probably the oldest of all self-management tools.

Although religion cannot be "prescribed," we encourage you to explore your own beliefs. If you are religious, try practicing prayer more consistently. If you are not religious, consider adopting some form of reflection or meditative practice. If you and your care partner have a prayer tradition, continue it. Say prayers out loud. You might not think your care partner is listening or understanding. Hospital chaplains will tell you that when they pray with unconscious patients, the patterns on heart monitors tend to slow and become more regular.

If you or your care partner are religious, consider telling the caregivers who are part of the care team. Most won't ask. Help them understand the importance of religious beliefs in managing your and your care partner's health and life. Most hospitals have chaplains or pastoral counselors. Even if you are not in the hospital, these spiritual advisers will probably be willing to talk with you. Most respite and hospice services have chaplains. Ask for that person to visit at least once. You might find new support. If not, they do not have to come again. Their advice and counsel can supplement your medical and psychological care.

Other Techniques for Managing Stress

There are additional valuable techniques you can consider which can clear your mind, positively shift your emotional state, and reduce tension and stress.

Mindfulness

Mindfulness involves keeping your attention in the present moment, without judging what is happening as happy or sad, good or bad. It encourages living each moment—even painful ones—as fully and as mindfully as possible. *Mindfulness* is more than a relaxation technique; it is an attitude toward living. It is a way of calmly and consciously observing and accepting whatever is happening, moment to moment. Considerable research has demonstrated the benefits of mindfulness practice in relieving stress, easing pain, improving concentration, and relieving a variety of other symptoms.

Our restless, judging minds can make mindfulness surprisingly difficult. Just like a restless monkey jumps from branch to branch, our mind jumps from thought to thought.

Mindfulness practice is one form of meditation. In mindfulness, you focus the mind on the present moment. The goal of mindfulness is to observe without judgement—with no intention of changing or improving anything. People report being positively changed by the practice of mindfulness. Observing and accepting life just as it is, with all its pleasures, pains, frustrations, disappointments, and insecurities, often enables people to become calmer, more confident, and better able to cope with whatever comes along.

To develop your capacity for mindfulness, sit comfortably on the floor or on a chair with your back, neck, and head straight, but not stiff. When you are comfortable, begin the following practice:

- Concentrate on a single object, such as your breathing. Focus your attention on the feeling of the air as it passes in and out of your nostrils with each breath. Don't try to control your breathing by speeding it up or slowing it down. Just observe it as it is.
- Even when you resolve to keep your attention on your breathing, your mind will quickly wander off. When this occurs, observe where your mind went: perhaps to a memory, a worry about the future, a bodily ache, or a feeling of impatience. Then gently return your attention to your breathing.
- Use your breath as an anchor. Each time a thought or feeling arises, momentarily acknowledge it. Don't analyze it or judge it. Just observe it and return your attention to your breathing.
- Let go of all thoughts of getting somewhere or having anything special happen. Just keep stringing moments of mindfulness together, breath by breath.
- At first, practice this for just five minutes, or even one minute at a time. You may wish to gradually extend the time to 10, 20, or 30 minutes.

The practice of mindfulness is the practice of moment-to-moment awareness. You can apply it to anything: eating, showering, working, talking, running errands, or playing with your children or grandchildren. Mindfulness takes no extra time.

Quieting Reflex

The quieting reflex technique was developed by physician Charles Stroebel. It can help you deal with short-term stress events, such as the urge to overeat, yell at your care partner, or express road rage. This technique relieves muscle tightening, jaw clenching, and holding your breath by activating the sympathetic nervous system.

The quieting reflex technique should be practiced frequently throughout the day, whenever you start to feel stressed. It can be done with your eyes opened or closed.

1. Become aware of what is annoying you: a ringing phone, a rude comment, the urge to smoke, a worrisome thought—whatever.
2. Repeat the phrase "Alert mind, calm body" to yourself.
3. Smile inwardly with your eyes and your mouth. This stops facial muscles from making a fearful or angry expression. The inward smile is a feeling. It cannot be seen by others.
4. Inhale slowly to the count of three, imagining that the breath comes in through the bottom of your feet. Then exhale slowly. Feel your breath move back down your legs and out through your feet. Let your jaw, tongue, and shoulder muscles go limp.

With several months' practice, the quieting reflex becomes an automatic skill.

Nature Therapy

Many of us suffer from what has been called "nature deficit disorder." Thankfully, this disorder can be cured with regular doses of the outdoors. For thousands of years, exposure to natural environments has been recommended for healing. Taking a break from artificial lighting, excessive phone, computer, and TV screen time, and indoor environments can be restorative. A brief walk—even if only to the post box or to mail a letter at the corner—or a visit to a nearby park can restore the mind and body. Or bring nature indoors with plants, pets, and nature photography. Even a few minutes of playing with or stroking a pet can lower blood pressure and calm a restless mind. An added benefit of these examples is that even though you might be doing them for yourself, they can make your care partner feel better at the same time!

Worry Time

Worrisome negative thoughts feed anxiety. Ignored problems have a way of thrusting themselves back into our minds. You'll find it easier to set aside worries if you make time to deal with them.

Set aside 20 to 30 minutes a day as your "worry time." Whenever a worry pops into your mind, write it down and tell yourself that you'll deal with it during worry time. Jot down the little things (Will my care partner eat their dinner?) along with the big ones (What will I do if my care partner gets worse?). During your scheduled worry time, don't do anything except worry, brainstorm, and write down possible solutions. For each of your worries, ask yourself the following questions:

- What is the problem?
- How likely is it that the problem will occur?
- What's the worst that could happen?
- What's the best that could happen?
- How would I cope with the problem if it happens?
- What are possible solutions?
- What is my plan of action?

Be specific. Instead of worrying about what might happen if you cannot keep your job, ask yourself how likely it is that you will lose your job. And if you do, what will you do, with whom, and by when? Write a plan on how you might balance your job and caregiving or how you might take a leave of absence.

If you're anxious about possibly having to clean a care partner who cannot make it to the bathroom in time, imagine how you would manage the situation. Ask yourself if any of this is really unbearable. Remind yourself you might feel uncomfortable or embarrassed, but you'll survive.

Remember, if a new worry pops up during the rest of the day, jot it down and save it to address during worry time. After you jot it down, distract yourself by refocusing intently on whatever you were doing before the worry interrupted you.

Scheduling a definite worry time cuts the amount of time you spend worrying by at least a third. If you look at your list of worries later, you'll find that the vast majority of them never became realities. Or if they did really happen, they were not nearly as bad as you had anticipated.

Practice Gratitude

One of the most effective ways to improve your mood and overall happiness is by focusing your attention on what's going well in your life. What makes you feel grateful? Psychologists have done research to demonstrate that people can increase their happiness with gratitude exercises. We encourage you to try these three:

1. **Write a letter of thanks.** Write and then deliver a letter of gratitude to someone who was especially kind to you but has never been properly thanked. Perhaps it's a teacher, a mentor, a friend, or a family member. Express your appreciation for the person's help and kindness. The letter will have more impact if you include some specific examples of what the recipient has done for you. Describe how the actions made you feel. Ideally, read your letter out loud to the person and, if possible, face to face. Be aware of how you feel and watch the other person's reaction.
2. **Acknowledge at least three good things every day.** Each night before bed, write down at least three things that went well on that day. No event or feeling is too small to note. By putting your gratitude into words, you increase appreciation and memory of your blessings. Knowing that you will need to write each night changes your mental filters during the whole day. You will seek out, be more aware of, and specially note the good things that happen. If doing this daily is too much or it begins to seem like a routine chore, write your list once a week.
3. **Make a list of the things you take for granted.** Perhaps you can celebrate a day in which your care partner smiles or remembers your name. Counting your blessings can add up to a better mood and more happiness.

Compile a List of Strengths

Make a personal inventory of your talents, skills, achievements, and qualities, big and small. Celebrate your accomplishments. When something goes wrong, consult your list of strengths and put the problem in perspective. The something that went wrong then becomes just one specific experience, not an event that defines your whole life.

Practice Kindness

This world is plagued by acts of violence. When something bad happens, it's front-page news. As an antidote to this misery, despair, and cynicism, practice acts of kindness. Look for opportunities to give without expecting anything in return. Here are some examples of small acts that can make you and others feel better in a very real way:

- Hold the door open for the person behind you.
- Give an unexpected gift of movie or concert tickets.
- Send an anonymous gift to a friend who needs cheering up.
- Lend a hand to someone who is carrying a load.
- Tell positive stories you know of helping and kindness.
- Cultivate an attitude of gratefulness for the kindness you have received.
- Plant a flower or a tree.
- Smile and let people cut ahead of you in line or on the freeway.
- Pick up litter.
- Give another driver your parking space.

Be creative. Kindness is contagious and has a ripple effect. In one study, the people who were given an unexpected treat (cookies) were later more likely to help others.

Write Away Stress

It's hard work to keep deep negative feelings hidden. Over time, the cumulative stress of hiding emotions undermines the body's defenses and can weaken immunity. Confiding your feelings to others or writing them down puts them into words and helps you sort them out. Words help people understand and absorb a traumatic event and eventually put it behind them. Putting something in writing can give you a sense of release and control.

The psychologist Jamie Pennebaker in his books *Opening Up* and *Expressive Writing: Words That Heal* describes a series of studies that looked at the healing effects of confiding or writing. One group was asked to express their deepest thoughts and feelings about something bad that had happened to them. Another group wrote about ordinary matters such as their plans for the day. Both groups wrote for 15 to 20 minutes a day for three to five consecutive days. No one read what either group had written.

The results were striking. The writing "therapy" was surprisingly powerful. When compared with the people who wrote about ordinary events, the ones who wrote about their bad experiences reported fewer symptoms, fewer visits to the doctor, fewer days off from work, improved mood, and a more positive outlook. Their immune function was enhanced for at least six weeks after writing. This was especially true for those who expressed previously undisclosed painful feelings in their writing.

Try the "write" thing when something is bothering you. It can help when you find yourself thinking (or dreaming) too much about an experience, when you are avoiding thinking about something because it is too upsetting, or when there's something you would like to tell others but don't for fear of embarrassment or punishment.

Here are some guidelines for writing as a way to help you deal with any unpleasant or traumatic experience:

- Set a specific time aside for writing. For example, you might write 15 minutes a day for four consecutive days, or one day a week for four weeks.
- Write in a place where you won't be interrupted or distracted. This might have to be at night or early in the morning.
- Don't plan to share your writing—that could stop your honest expression. Save what you write or destroy it, as you wish.
- Explore your very deepest thoughts and feelings and analyze why you feel the way you do. Write about your negative feelings such as sadness, hurt, hate, anger, fear, guilt, or resentment.
- Write continuously. Don't worry about grammar, spelling, or making sense. If clarity and coherence come as you continue to write, so much the better. If you run out of things to say, just repeat what you have already written.
- Even if you find the writing awkward at first, keep going. It gets easier. If you cannot write, try talking into a tape recorder for 15 minutes about your deepest thoughts and feelings.

- Don't expect to feel better immediately. You may feel sad or depressed when your deepest feelings begin to surface. This usually fades within an hour or two or a day or two. The overwhelming majority of people report feelings of relief, happiness, and contentment after writing for a few consecutive days.
- Writing might help you clarify what actions you need to take, but don't use writing as a substitute for taking action or as a way of avoiding things.

Once established, relaxation, imagery, and positive thinking can be some of the most powerful tools you can add to your caregiver toolbox. They will help you manage symptoms as well as master the other skills discussed in this book.

As with exercise and other acquired skills, using your mind to manage your stress and other symptoms requires both practice and time before you begin to notice the benefits. So, if you feel you are not accomplishing anything, don't give up. Be patient and keep on trying.

For a complete list of suggested further readings, useful websites, and other helpful resources, please see: www.bullpub.com/resources

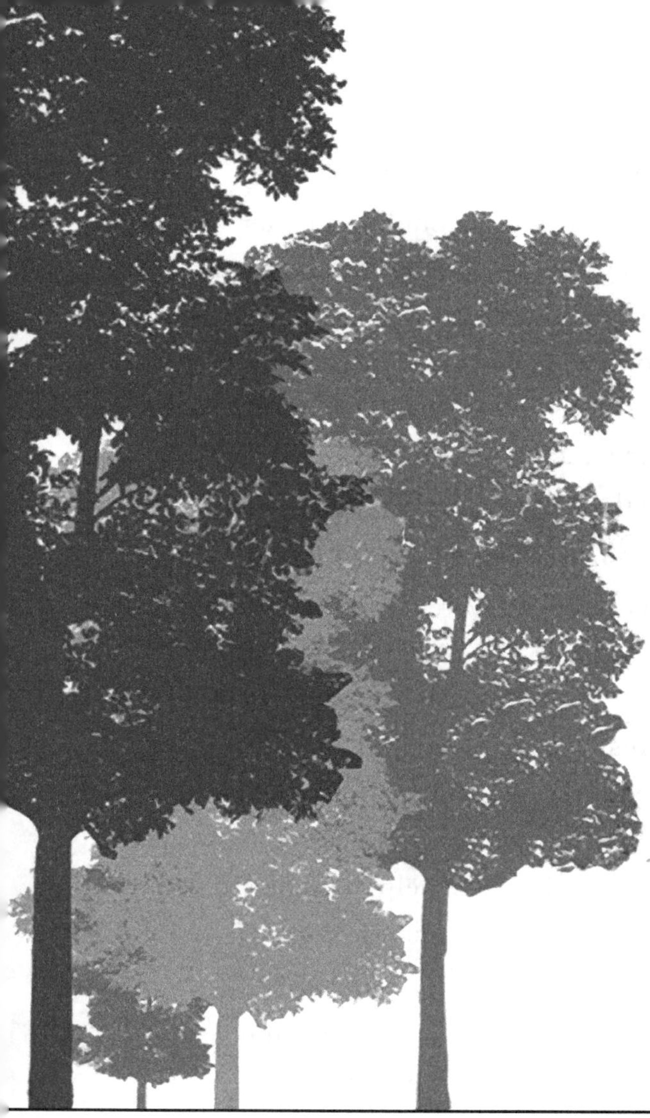

Chapter 6

Communicating Effectively

“I FEEL SO ALONE.” “No one understands what it is like to be a caregiver.” “My family and friends are no help.” “When I take my care partner to the clinic, no one seems to listen.” Being a caregiver is stressful and frustrating. Your world has changed. You must communicate and advocate not only for yourself but often also for your care partner. Notice we say both communicate and advocate. When we communicate, we want others to understand. When we advocate, we are trying to accomplish something specific. Good communication and advocacy can help with the frustration and stress of caregiving. Poor communication and advocacy can lead to anger, helplessness, isolation, and depression. It can also lead to not getting the best care for your care partner, which means more stress for you.

Healthy communication and advocacy are the lifeblood of relationships, and relationships are a lifeline to healthy coping. Poor communication is the biggest reason for strained relationships between spouses or partners. Poor communication also causes strain among other family members, friends, co-workers, or between you and members of your care partner's health care team. From our discussion about dealing with difficult care partner situations, you know that sometimes communicating is done through actions, not words, or by avoiding the situation. You also learned more about communication in Chapter 4, Dealing with Difficult Emotions, and Chapter 5, Using Your Mind to Manage Stress, when we discussed ways to manage difficult emotions and stress. In this chapter, we share some ideas for improving communication and advocacy for yourself and your care partner with family, friends, and members of the health care team.

Your family, friends, and your own health care providers and the health care team of your care partner should understand you. They also must know what you want. They should also be able to help you define what you want. Getting others to understand is communication. Getting others to act often takes advocacy. Advocacy does not need to be confrontational. It is usually just a matter of making what you want clear. Look at the difference in the following examples of an interaction between a caregiver and their care partner's health care provider. Here's an example:

Caregiver (at the end of a long visit with their care partners health care provider): "I think I could be a better caregiver. What should I do?"

Health care provider: "I want you to go home and keep doing what you are doing. You are doing a great job."

Now let's look at another example:

Caregiver: "I think I could be a better caregiver, but I am at the end of my rope. I am not getting any sleep. I worry constantly and wake often with my care partner. My partner shouts at me all the time. I am a wreck. Please tell me what to do or how to get help."

Health care provider: "I am sorry I did not ask how you were doing. You are doing a great job as a caregiver. This is a hard job. Thank you for asking for help. This takes real strength. I did not know about the shouting and not sleeping. It sounds as though you need some breaks and maybe some help at night. Do you have any ideas in mind?"

Caregiver: "Having some help would be great, but my care partner will not allow any strangers in the house."

Health care provider: "I am going to refer you to our social worker. Also, I suggest you look into the Senior Day Health program. Your care partner may be afraid of change, but remember, it is the disease talking. This is a common concern and can be overcome. To be able to continue caregiving, you need to think of both of you, not just your care partner. This is a hard transition time. Are you willing to seek some more advice and assistance?"

Caregiver: "Yes, I will follow through and thank you for not thinking of me as a complaining wimp."

In the first example, the caregiver:

- Said "I think I could be a better caregiver. What should I do?"
- The health care provider gave reassurance about the care that was being given.
- The caregiver did not get the needed help and the health care provider thought they had done a good job in giving reassurance.

The caregiver did not communicate their needs and the health care provider thought they understood what the caregiver was asking for without probing. Good communication was lacking on both sides.

In the second example, the caregiver:

- Started with the same statement about feeling they were a poor caregiver. But then they added that they were at the end of their rope. This was followed with some specific problems that made them feel this way.
- The provider gave reassurance and then made some suggestions.
- The caregiver said that the care partner would not like having someone else in the house.
- The provider reminded the caregiver that it was the disease that was talking and acknowledged that more help was needed. The provider acknowledged that asking for and accepting help is hard and that needing help is common. Then the provider suggested some resources for help and asked if the caregiver was willing to seek advice from a social worker.
- The caregiver was still not convinced that this would help but agreed to take the first step.

In this example, the needs of the caregiver were more clearly communicated. The concerns about the care partner's reactions to help were also discussed. While the problems were not immediately solved, the clear communication allowed both parties to understand and agree on first steps.

In this chapter, we are going to discuss several different communication skills and describe several example situations to illustrate how you can apply these skills.

Communicating: The Basics

The following are some basic tips for improving how you communicate:

- Be clear about the problem or what you want or need to communicate. This is very much like the first step in problem-solving. Remember that others cannot read your mind. Don't expect others to just know what you want. If you want to be sure they know, tell them.
- Become aware of your own assumptions and biases. Sometimes you may think you know the answer, think your situation is unique, or reject something out of hand. Be open to what others have to say.
- Listen carefully until the other person is finished talking. Sometimes it is hard not to just jump in and interrupt the other person. Good listeners seldom interrupt. Wait for a

few seconds after the other person has finished talking before responding. They may have more to say. If someone goes on too long, at least wait until the speaker takes a breath before you speak. (More about listening is on page xx.)

- Let the person know you heard them. This might be a simple "uh huh." Many times, the only thing the other person wants is acknowledgment, to know that they were heard. Sometimes all a person may need is a sympathetic listener.
- When needed, ask for more information. You will find more about this on page xx.
- Let the person know that you understand both the content and emotional impact of what they are saying. You can do this by restating the content. For example, "You are planning a trip." Or you can respond by acknowledging the emotions: "That must be difficult" or "How sad you must feel." When you respond on an emotional level, the results are often startling. These responses tend to open the gates for more expression of feelings and thoughts. Responding to either the content or emotion can help improve communication and discourage the other person from simply repeating what has been said.
- Avoid trying to talk people out of their feelings or telling them that they "shouldn't feel that way." Their feelings are real to them and telling them that they are wrong is insulting. Just listen and reflect.
- When offered suggestions from others, seriously consider them. Sometimes it is easy to become a victim. This happens when you are sure that nothing anyone suggests will work.
- Express gratitude. Thank others for listening and taking what you said seriously.

Listening

Good listening is a critical communication skill. Most of us are much better at talking than we are at listening. Sometimes, when others talk to us, we are only half listening because we are already preparing a response before they have even finished speaking. The following are suggestions for becoming a good listener.

Part of listening to what others are saying includes observing how they say it. Even when you say nothing, your body is talking. Sometimes it is even shouting. Research shows that body language is responsible for more than half of what people communicate. To improve your communication, you need to listen not only to the words of others but also to their tone of voice. Be sure to observe their body language and facial expressions. There might be times when the words don't tell the whole story. Is the voice wavering? Is the speaker struggling to find the right words? Do you notice body tension? Does the person seem distracted? Is the tone sarcastic? What is the facial expression? If you pick up on some of these signs, speakers may have more on their minds than the words alone express.

Body language should match what people say in words. If it does not, you may be sending mixed messages and creating misunderstandings. For example, if you want to make a firm statement, look at the other person and keep your expression friendly. Stand tall and confident. Relax your legs and arms and breathe. You might lean forward to show your interest. Try not to sneer or bite your lips. This might indicate discomfort or doubt. Don't move away or slouch. These actions can communicate disinterest and uncertainty.

When you notice that the body language and words of others do not match, gently point this out. Ask for clarification. For example, you might say, "I hear you saying that you would like to go with me to the family picnic, but you look tired and you're yawning as you speak. Would you rather stay home and rest while I go alone?"

In addition to reading people's body language, it is helpful to recognize and appreciate that everyone expresses themselves differently. Conversational style varies according to where people were born, how they were raised, their occupation, their cultural background, and, especially, their gender. For example, some people tend to ask questions that are personal. These show interest and help form relationships. Others are more likely to offer opinions or suggestions and state facts. These people may tend to discuss problems just to find solutions, not to share their feelings and experiences. No one style is better or worse. They are just different. By acknowledging and accepting these differences, you can reduce some of the misunderstanding, frustration, and resentment in your communications with others. Recognizing these differences is especially important when you are communicating with people from different cultures. Hand gestures, eye contact, and posture, for example, might have very different meanings in one culture than another. If you are confused, just ask.

Remember that you cannot change the communication of others. What you can do is change your communication to be sure you are understood.

Getting More Information: Asking Questions

Getting more information is a bit of an art. It can involve both simple and more complicated techniques.

Often people pretend to understand when they really do not. The simplest way to get more information when this happens is to ask: "I do not understand. Can you tell me more?" Or "Could you say that another way, so I might understand better?", "What do you mean?", "Could you expand on that?", and so on.

Be specific when you are asking for more information. If you want specific information, ask specific questions. For instance, "When you say sometime in the future, I do not understand what that means. Are you talking about days, months, or years?"

Let's look at the following examples of how specific questions can help in this encounter between a doctor and caregiver.

Doctor: "How has your care partner been feeling?"

Caregiver: "Not so good."

The provider has not gotten much information. The response from the caregiver is not very useful. Here's how the provider gets more information:

Making Sure Your Communication Is Clear

Good communication skills help make life easier for everyone, especially caregivers. Here are some words that can help or hinder communication.

Words That Help

Right now, at this time, at this point ("At this point, I do not need any help, but I might next week. Can I call you?")

Who, which, where, when ("What do you mean?", "Please explain," "Tell me more, I don't understand.")

Words That Hinder

Never, always, every time, constantly ("Every time I try to get out, it fails.")

You obviously ("You obviously have never been a caregiver.")

Why or why not ("Why did you, or didn't you, do that?")

Doctor: "Has your care partner been sleeping better?"

Caregiver: "Not really."

Doctor: "Could you tell me more?"

Caregiver: "Well, he goes to sleep but gets up four or five times a night and never goes back to sleep after 5:00 a.m.

Doctor: "What time does he go to sleep?

Caregiver: "About 7:30, and then I have a few hours to get things done."

Doctor: "Does he also take a nap?" . . . and so on.

Health care providers are trained to get specific information from patients, so they usually ask more specific questions, especially when a general question does not give them the information needed. Most people are not trained to do this, but you can learn to ask specific questions. Asking for specifics helps communication. Try clearly asking like this: "Can you be more specific?"

Avoid asking, "Why?", which is a general question. Rather, begin your question with "who," "what," "which," "when," or "where." These words usually get a more specific response.

Getting More Information: Paraphrasing

Another way to get more information is to paraphrase or repeat back what you heard in your own words. This is a useful tool if you want to make sure you understand what other people meant—not just what they said, but what they intended. Paraphrasing can either help or hinder effective communication. It depends on the way the paraphrase is worded. Remember to paraphrase in the form of a question, not a statement. Consider the following example:

Caregiver: "I don't know. My care partner is so messy when she eats, and she sometimes eats with her hands. I want to go to dinner with you, but I think everyone in the restaurant will be looking at us."

Paraphrasing as a statement: "Obviously, you're telling me you don't want to go to dinner."

This response might provoke an angry response such as, "No, I didn't say that! If you're going to be that way, we'll stay home for sure." Or the response might be no response—a total shutdown because of either anger or despair ("They just don't understand"). People don't like to be told what they mean.

Paraphrasing as a question: "Are you saying that you'd rather stay home than go to dinner?"

Response to the second paraphrase (the question): "That's not what I meant. I just think that we might do better at a restaurant where we would be less noticeable. How about that new Italian place? They have nice booths in the back that are more private."

As you can see, the second paraphrase helps communication. The questioner has discovered the real reason for expressing doubt about going to dinner. In short, you get more information when you paraphrase with questions.

Important Communication Skills for Different Situations

The following information is about different communication tools you can use for healthy communication and advocacy.

Using "I" Messages

Many people are uncomfortable expressing feelings, especially when it seems like you are being critical of someone else. When emotions are high, attempts to express frustration can be full of "you" messages. "You don't understand," "You make me so frustrated," "You never listen," and "You never call" are some examples of "you" messages. Using the word "you" can suggest blame, causing the other person to feel under attack. Suddenly, the other person is on the defensive and barriers go up. Situations can just escalate from there, leading to anger, frustration, and bad feelings.

"I" statements are clear and confident ways to share your thoughts and feelings, while "you" statements can sound like you are blaming or accusing someone. For example, it is better to use the I statement, "I try very hard to do the best work I can," instead of saying, "You always criticize me." Or "I appreciate it when you turn down the television while I talk," not, "You never pay attention."

Here are some more examples:

"*You*" message: "Why are you always late? We never get anywhere on time."

"*I*" message: "I get upset when I'm late. It's important to me to be on time."

"*You*" message: "There's no way you can understand how hard it is to be alone with Raj all day."

"*I*" message: "Being alone with Raj all day is hard. I could use a little help."

Watch out for hidden "you" messages. These are "you" messages with "I feel . . ." stuck in front of them. Here's an example:

"*You*" message: "You always walk too fast."

Hidden "*You*" message: "I feel angry when you walk so fast."

"*I*" message: "I have a hard time walking fast."

Exercise: "I" Messages

Try changing the following statement into "I" messages. (Watch out for hidden "you" messages!)

- "You expect me to wait on you hand and foot!"
- "Doctor, you never have enough time for me and my care partner. You're always in a hurry."
- "You hardly ever touch me anymore. You don't pay any attention to me anymore."
- "Doctor, you didn't tell me the side effects of all these drugs or why my care partners must take them."

"I feel that you are not treating me fairly" is a "you" statement disguised as an "I" statement. A true "I" statement is "I feel angry and hurt."

The trick to "I" messages is to avoid the use of the word "you" and, instead, report your personal feelings using the word "I." Of course, like any new skill, using "I" messages takes practice. Start by listening carefully to yourself and to others. (Grocery stores are a good place to hear lots of "you" messages as parents talk to their children.) In your head take some of these "you" messages and turn them into "I" messages (see the text box "Exercise: 'I' Messages"). You'll be surprised at how fast "I" messages become a habit. If using "I" statements seems difficult, try this format:

- I observe (state just the facts).
- I think (state your opinions).
- I feel (say what your feelings are).
- I want (state exactly what you'd like the other person to do).

Imagine that because you cannot go to a birthday party, you made a cake for a friend to take along. One of your kids comes into the kitchen, sees it on the counter, and cuts out a large slice. You're upset because, with a piece missing, the gift is ruined. You might say, "You ate the cake. You should have asked me about it first (opinion). I'm really upset and disappointed because I can't give it as a gift now (feeling). I'd like an apology and for you to ask me first next time (want)."

Also, there is another thing to learn from this example. The cakemaker assumed that a cake with one missing piece would not be appreciated. Telling the story about what happened to that slice could be fun to hear.

Here are some "I" message cautions. First, "I" messages are not a cure-all. Sometimes the listener needs time to really hear them. This is especially true if listeners are used to hearing "you" messages from you. If "I" messages do not work at first, continue to use them. Things will change as you gain skill and old patterns of communication are broken.

Second, some people use "I" messages as a means of manipulation. They may often express that they are sad, angry, or frustrated to gain sympathy from others. If used in this way, problems can escalate. Effective "I" messages must report honest feelings.

One last note: "I" messages are an excellent way to express positive feelings and compliments! "I really appreciate that you sent the cake. Everyone loved it and the story about the missing piece made everyone laugh."

Minimizing Conflict

In addition to using "I" messages, there are other ways to reduce conflict. Consider the following examples.

- **Refocus the discussion.** If you get off topic and emotions are running high, shift the focus of the conversation. Refocus and bring the discussion back to the agreed topic. For example, you might say, "We're both getting upset now and drifting away from the topic we agreed to discuss." Or "I feel like we are bringing up things other than what we agreed to talk about. I'm getting upset. Can we discuss these other things later and just talk about what we originally agreed to discuss?"
- **Ask for more time.** For example, you might say, "I think I understand your concerns, but I need more time to think about it before I can respond." Or "I hear what you are saying, but I am too frustrated to respond now. Let me find out more and then we can talk again."
- **Make sure you understand the other person's viewpoint.** Do this by summarizing what you heard and asking for more clarification. You can also switch roles. Try arguing the other person's position the best you can. This will help you to understand all sides of an issue. It also shows that you respect and value the other person's point of view.
- **Look for compromise.** You might not always find the perfect solution to a problem or reach total agreement. However, it may be possible to find something on which you can both agree. For example, you can do it your way this time and the other person's way the next time. Agree to part of what you want and part of what the other person wants. Or decide what you'll do and what the other person will do. These are all forms of compromise that can help you through some difficult times.
- **Say you're sorry and forgive others.** We'll address this in the next section.

Apologizing and Forgiving

We have all said or done things that have, on purpose or accidently, hurt others. Many relationships are damaged—sometimes for years—because people have not learned the powerful social skill of apologizing. Often all it takes to restore a relationship is a simple, sincere apology. Rather than a sign of weakness, an apology shows great strength. For an apology to be effective, follow these tips:

- **Admit the specific mistake and accept responsibility for it.** Name the offense. Don't gloss over it by saying something general like, "I'm sorry for what I did." Be specific. For example, you might say, "I'm very sorry that I was angry and hung up on you. I was at my wits' end." Explain what led you to do what you did. Don't offer excuses or sidestep responsibility.
- **Express your feelings.** A genuine, heartfelt apology involves some suffering. Sadness shows that the relationship matters to you.
- **Acknowledge the impact of the wrongdoing.** You might say, "I know that I hurt you and that my behavior cost you a lot. For that, I am very sorry."
- **Offer to make amends.** Ask what you can do to make the situation better or volunteer specific suggestions.

Making an apology can be difficult, but it is an act of courage, generosity, and healing. It brings the possibility of a renewed and stronger relationship, and it can also bring peace.

Equally important for maintaining and restoring relationships is to forgive others. Give people the benefit of the doubt and make sure you treat them as "innocent unless proven guilty."

Do not assume the worst about people. Many caregivers discover that people in their lives whom they expected to be helpful are not. These people do not call or offer help. A common caregiver response is to be angry and to write these people off as not caring. In fact, a person might not call because they don't know what to do or say. They are afraid to approach you because they know that the relationship has changed or that you might ask them to do something they cannot do or are not willing to do. As hard as it might be, if the relationship is important to you, reach out. Call the person, suggest you get together for coffee or that the person come over for coffee while your care partner is sleeping. People do not just know what to do. Sometimes they need to be guided.

When someone offers you an apology, accept it as graciously as possible and be ready to tell them how they can make amends. Sometimes, if you are wronged and the other person does not apologize, whatever happened grows larger and larger in your mind. Maybe the relationship is over but the feeling of being wronged still upsets you. In this case, work on forgiveness for your own peace of mind. This does not mean you have to rekindle that relationship (unless, of course, you want to). Rather it means that the past wrong no longer weighs you down.

Advocating Thoughtfully to Get Help

We use the word advocating because this is often what caregivers do: They advocate on behalf of their care partner. Usually the caregiver needs and is asking for something specific. When this type of communication is difficult, consider the following. First, review the situation. Exactly what is bothering you? What are you feeling? Most important of all, what specifically do you want?

Getting and giving help are part of life and especially critical for caregivers. Even though everyone needs help sometimes, few people like to ask for it. You may not want to admit that we are unable to do things for yourself. You may not want to be a burden on others. When you finally do ask for help, you may hedge or make a very vague request: "I'm sorry to have to ask this . . . ," "I know this is asking a lot . . . , or "I hate to ask this, but . . ." Hedging tends to put the other person on the defensive: "Gosh, what's he going to ask that's so much, anyway?" To avoid this response, be specific. A general request can lead to misunderstanding. The person being asked to help may react negatively because not enough information is given. This leads to a further breakdown in communication and no help. A specific request is more likely to have a positive result. Consider the following examples:

General request: "I know this is the last thing you want to do, but I need help shopping. Will you help me?"

Reaction: "Uh . . . well . . . I don't know. Um . . . can I get back to you after I check my schedule?" (probably next year!)

Specific request: "I need help shopping. Would you call me when you are going to the grocery store, and I can give you a short list? Then either I or my daughter will pick them up at your house and pay you for my groceries."

Reaction: "Of course, I am happy to do this, and I can just drop your things off as you are right on my way home. Would once a week be often enough?"

If you are the kind of person who hesitates to ask for help, try imagining yourself as the person being asked by a friend for help. How do you feel? Probably pretty good. Most people like to be helpful. It makes them feel useful. Providing help is also a way to show friendship. Now, think again about asking for help. Instead of feeling you are a bother or burden, think of it as giving that person a gift. Family and friends want to help, they want to feel good, but they may not know what to do and may not want to offend.

Here is an example. Neema is a caregiver and needed someone to help her by cutting the lawn. She called her brother-in-law, Malcolm, for help. The following conversation took place:

Neema: "Malcolm, our yard is really a mess. Could you help?"

Malcolm: "Uh, maybe. When would be a good time?"

Neema: "Terrific. How about Sunday morning?"

Malcolm: "You know we go to church on Sundays."

Neema: "Oh, never mind. Everything else is always more important."

Malcolm: "Well, if you cannot be reasonable, I cannot help."

In this conversation, neither Neema nor Malcolm stopped to think about what was really happening. The conversation ended with both feeling annoyed and the yard work did not get done.

The following is the same conversation but with both people using more thoughtful communications:

Neema: "Malcolm, our yard is really a mess. It would help a lot if you could come over and cut the grass."

Malcolm: "I can probably do that. When would be a good time?"

Neema: "Terrific! How about Sunday morning?"

Malcolm: "Gosh, I'm sorry, but we go to church on Sunday mornings. Would Sunday afternoon be OK, or maybe I could come over some evening after work?"

Neema: "I'm sorry, I totally forgot about church. Anytime in the afternoon would be fine. Thanks!"

Malcolm: "See you at about two. Maybe I will bring Paul to help. He would love to see his aunt."

In this second example, Neema was more specific about what she wanted done. This made it clear to Malcolm that she wanted an hour or so of grass cutting, not a whole day of weeding. Notice that after Neema mentioned coming on Sunday, Malcolm did not say "you know." He said, "we go." Malcolm did not consider this a thoughtless request and he made some alternative suggestions.

Neema admitted she was not thinking when she asked about Sunday morning, and they reached a happy conclusion. Neither blamed the other nor took offense. This is thoughtful communication.

Unfortunately, we are often in situations where the other person uses blaming communication. Maybe we are not clear, or not listening, and then we use blaming communication. This is what happened to Malcolm and Neema in the first example. In the second conversation, neither blamed the other.

You should know that even if the other person uses blaming communication, you can still use thoughtful communication and save the day. Look at the following example:

Jan: "Why do you always spoil my plans? At least you could have called. I am really tired of trying to do anything with you."

Neema (the caregiver): "I understand. When Raj [her care partner] gets into one of his moods, I just can't leave him. When my anxiety acts up at the last minute, I am confused. I keep hoping I can go and so I don't call you because I don't want to disappoint you. I really want to go. I keep hoping things will get better."

Jan: "Well, I hope that in the future you will call. I don't like being caught by surprise."

Neema: "I understand. If it is OK with you, let's go shopping now. I think I can leave Raj for a couple of hours today. I will call him while we are out. I do want us to keep making plans. In the future, if things are getting off track, I will let you know sooner."

In this example, only Neema uses thoughtful communication. Jan continues to blame. The outcome, however, is still positive. Both people got what they wanted.

The following are some suggestions for using thoughtful communication when seeking help and at other times too. Note that they are like the communication basics example at the beginning of this chapter.

- **Be clear.** Describe a specific situation or your observations using the facts. Avoid words like "always" or "never." For example, Neema said, "When my anxiety acts up at the last minute, I am confused. I keep hoping things will get better, so I don't call." This is specific and clear communication about her feelings and the reason behind her actions.
- **Show respect.** Always show respect and regard for the other person. Try not to preach or be excessively demanding. Avoid demeaning or blaming comments, such as "Why do you always spoil my plans?" The use of the word "you" is a clue that your communication might be blaming. Tact and courtesy can go a long way in defusing sensitive situations.
- **Listen and listen some more.**
- **Check assumptions.** Ask for more details. Jan did not do this. She assumed that Neema was rude because she did not call. It would have been better if she asked Neema why she hadn't called earlier. Assumptions are the enemy of good communication. Many arguments arise from people expecting other people to read their minds. One sign that you are making assumptions is

when you think, "They should know what I need. . . ." Direct, specific expression of needs and feelings is key. It is also important that you ask questions if you don't understand. Gathering more information is more effective than mindreading.

- **Open up.** Try to express your feelings openly and honestly. Don't make the other person guess what you are feeling. Chances are they will be off-base. Neema did this. She talked about wanting to go, not wanting to disappoint Jan, and hoping that Raj's mood would get better.
- **Accept and recognize others' feelings.** Try to understand what other people are feeling. This is not always easy. Sometimes you need to think about what was said instead of answering right away. You can always stall a bit by saying, "I think I understand," or, "I don't fully understand; could you explain some more?"
- **Use humor.** Sometimes gently introducing a bit of humor works wonders. But don't use sarcasm or demeaning humor and know when to be serious.
- **Do not be a victim.** You deserve respect, and you have a right to express your wants and needs. You become a victim when you expect that someone else *should* act in a certain way. Unless you have done something to hurt another, you should not apologize. Apologizing all the time is a sign you might be feeling and acting like a victim.

As a caregiver, you may often hear "How can I help?" And the answer is often, "I don't know," or "Thank you but I do not need any help." But all the time, you might be thinking, "They should know. . . ." or, "If they cared, they would know. . . ." Next time be prepared to accept these offers of help by being specific about the type of help you need or want. For example, "It would be great if we could go for a walk together once a week," or "Could you please take the garbage can to the curb tonight? I can't lift it." You could even ask if they could come over for a couple of hours twice a month to watch your care partner while you do other things in the house.

Remember that people cannot read your mind, so you'll need to tell them what help you want and thank them for it. Think about how each person can help. If possible, give them a task that they can easily accomplish. You are giving them a gift when you accept their help. People like being helpful and feel rejected when they cannot help you, especially if they care about you. Also, when someone helps you, do not forget to say thank you. It is important and healthy to express your gratitude (see "Practice Gratitude" in Chapter 5, Using Your Mind to Manage Stress, pages xx and xx).

Often, and as caregivers, you will get offers for help that you do not want or need. In most cases, these offers come from important people in your life. These people care for you and genuinely want to help. A well-worded "I" message allows you to decline the help without embarrassing the other person. "Thank you for being so thoughtful, but today I think I can handle it myself. I hope I can take you up on your offer another time."

Advocating for Yourself When You Are Not Being Treated Well

There is another type of advocacy which is a little more difficult than advocating to get help. *Self-advocacy*, which means speaking up for yourself when you feel that someone is not treating you well, can be even more of a challenge. Let us say some long-time friends let it be known that they no longer wish to see you because they say you are not fun anymore. Or maybe you are concerned because your provider seems to make unwarranted assumptions about older people or those with dementia. Maybe a friend supports a political candidate you do not like or tries to convert you to their religion. These examples may call for you to use self-advocacy.

Self-advocacy means being assertive without losing your cool. Here are some things to consider. When you feel you are being seen as less competent, morally bad, stereotyped, disrespected, or physically attacked, the brain interprets this as a threat, and you may respond with anger and want to fight back. The brain cannot instantly distinguish between physical threats and verbal threats. Thus, people often say or do things they would later like to take back. When confronted with direct or even more subtle verbal attacks, try the following:

- Remind yourself that you are not in immediate danger.
- Pause by taking several deep breaths or count to ten. This gives your brain the 30 seconds or so it needs to catch up. It also prevents you from cutting the other person off and from hearing the rest of what they are saying. It is important to use this time to think about what to say as well as the cost or benefit of what you say. Sometimes you may not care if a relationship ends. This is the cost. Other times, the benefits of the relationship may outweigh the hurt and anger you may feel. This is something only you can decide. If you need more time to think about how you might respond or choose not to respond, you might just leave the room.
- Sometimes you can let something go the first time and then have more time to think things over. If this is the case, think about what you want and make a list of possible actions. For example, someone has been with a dentist a long time but found them to be disrespectful and constantly upselling. When this happened again, they decided to complete the dental appointment and find a new dentist. When called several months later for a follow-up appointment, the person let the dentist know that they had moved on and why.
- Respond with an "I"" message. Here are some examples. "When you will not talk to me about my caregiving or aging concerns, I feel unheard, unimportant, and disrespected." "When you talk only to me and do not include my care partner, I feel hurt and disrespected. Please include both of us in your conversations." "I value our friendship and hope we can find some way for it to continue."

Saying No

How should you respond when you are asked to help? It is probably best not to answer right away. You may need more information. If a request leaves you feeling negative, trust your feelings.

Communicating with an In-Home Caregiver

Having someone new in the home may be difficult for you and your care partner. Here are some tips.

- Have a job description. That way both you and the caregiver are clear on what is expected.
- If possible, the caregiver should be of a gender and ethnicity/race acceptable to your care partner. This is not always possible. Remember that excellent caregivers can be of any gender and ethnicity. What might be most important is that you, the caregiver, and your care partner have a common language.
- Keep a notebook where both you and the caregiver can write observations. It may be that both of you see the same thing and interpret it differently.
- Have regularly scheduled check-in times with your caregiver away from your care partner where you can discuss what is going well and share concerns.
- Schedule time when you are in the house at the same time as the caregiver(s) so you can observe and listen from a distance.
- If there are problems, describe what you observed and what you would like to happen.
- Be open to listening, discussion, and joint decision-making. It may be that your paid caregiver has good ideas that come from experiences that are just different than yours.

The example we discussed earlier about help with shopping is a good one. "Help me shop" can mean anything from picking up a few groceries to being responsible for picking up their dry cleaning, medications at the pharmacy, and groceries all the time. Using your communication skills to get more specific information will help you avoid problems. It is important to fully understand any request before responding. Asking for more information or restating the request in your own words will help you understand. Start by saying, "Before I answer . . ." and then ask key questions. This will not only clarify the request, but also prevent the person from assuming you are going to say yes.

If you decide to say no, it is important to acknowledge the importance of the request. In this way, the person can see that you are rejecting the request rather than them. Your turndown should not be a putdown. For example, here is a polite way to say no: "I would like to help you with your shopping, but Raj has several appointments this week and I won't have the time." Again, specifics are the key. Try to be clear about the conditions of your turndown. Give them information. Let them know if you will always turn down this request, or is it just today, this week, or right now that is inconvenient? If you are feeling overwhelmed and imposed upon, saying no can be a useful tool. You may wish to make a counteroffer such as, "I won't be able to drive today, but I will next week." But remember, you have a legitimate right to decline a request, even if it is a reasonable one.

Communicating with Members of Your Health Care Team

One of the keys to getting good health care for yourself and your care partner is to communicate well with health care providers. This can be a challenge. You may be afraid to talk freely, or you think there is not enough time during the visit. Health care providers might use words you do not understand. You may not want to share personal and possibly embarrassing information. These fears and feelings can block communications with providers and harm your care partner's health as well as your own health.

Providers share the responsibility for poor communication. They sometimes feel too busy to take the time to talk with and get to know their patients and their caregivers. They may ignore or tune out our questions. Their actions or inactions might hurt or offend.

Although you do not have to become best friends with your providers, you should expect that they are attentive, caring, and able to explain things clearly. This is especially important if you or your care partner has an ongoing health condition. You might think that you can only get the best care by going to specialists. This may sometimes be true, but it can also greatly complicate care. You may be seeing several specialists. They may not get to really know you and might not be aware of what the other care providers are doing, thinking, or prescribing. These are good reasons to have a primary provider or a medical "home." Establishing and maintaining a long-term relationship with a provider may take some effort, but it can make a large difference to your health and that of your care partner.

Your provider probably knows more personal details about you and your care partner than anyone else. You should feel comfortable expressing your fears, asking questions that you think are stupid, and negotiating a treatment plan that satisfies you both.

To successfully communicate with your health care providers, you must be clear about what you want. Many people would like their providers to be warm-hearted computers—gigantic brains, stuffed with knowledge about the human body and mind. You may want your providers to analyze the situation, read your mind, make a perfect diagnosis, come up with a treatment plan, and tell you what to expect. At the same time, you may want them to be warm and caring and make you feel as though you and your care partner are their most important patients.

Most providers wish they were just that sort of person. Unfortunately, no one provider can be all things to all patients. Providers are human. They have bad days, they get headaches, they get tired, and they get sore feet. Many have families who demand their time and attention. They might be caregivers themselves, and they may also get frustrated by paperwork, insurance companies, electronic record keeping, and large bureaucracies.

Most doctors and other health care providers entered the health care system because they wanted to help sick people. Despite their years of training, they often must be satisfied with improvements rather than cures for their patients. Sometimes all they can do is slow the decline of someone's condition. Undoubtedly you have been frustrated, angry, or depressed from time to time about your care partner, but bear in mind that your health care providers have probably felt similar emotions because they cannot make your care partner well. In this, you are truly partners.

Taking PART

Another source of unclear communication with health care providers can be the lack of time. This is an obstacle to a good patient-provider relationship. If you or your provider had a wish for your relationship, it would probably be for you to have more face-to-face time. When time is short, the resulting anxiety can bring about rushed communication. "You" messages and misunderstandings are common.

Take P.A.R.T.

P = Prepare
A = Ask
R = Repeat
T = Take action

Most doctors and other providers are on very tight schedules. They try to stay on schedule, but things happen. This is painfully clear when you have a long wait in the doctor's office because of an emergency or late patient. Delays like this can cause both patients and doctors to feel rushed. A good strategy to get the most from your visit is to take PART (Prepare, Ask, Repeat, Take action).

Prepare

Before visiting or calling your health care provider or that of your care partner, prepare. What are the reasons for your visit? What do you expect from your doctor?

Make a written list of your concerns or questions. These can be concerns about your care partner's health and your concerns about being a caregiver. After you've walked out of the doctor's office, have you ever thought to yourself, "Why didn't I ask about . . . ?" or, "I forgot to mention. . . ." Making a list before your appointment helps ensure that your main concerns get addressed. Be realistic. If you have 13 different problems, your provider probably cannot deal with all of them in one visit. Star or highlight your two or three most important questions or concerns.

Give the list to your doctor at the beginning of the visit and explain that you have starred your most important concerns. Be silent and allow your doctor a few minutes to review the list. By giving the doctor your list, the doctor knows which items are the most important to you. The doctor also sees everything in case there is something medically important that is not starred. If you wait until the end of your appointment to bring up concerns, there will not be time to discuss them.

Here is an example: The provider asks, "What brings you in today?" You might say something like, "I have a lot of things I want to discuss this visit (the doctor looks at the clock, thinks of the appointment schedule, and immediately begins to feel anxious), but I know we have a limited time. The things that most concern me are that Emiko [your care partner] is not sleeping and can no longer find the toilet." The doctor feels relieved because the concerns are focused and potentially manageable within the appointment time available.

In addition to the starred list, there are two other things to prepare before your visit. Bring a list of all your or your care partner's medications and the dosages. If writing a list is difficult, put all the medications in a bag and bring them with you to the appointment. You might be able to download the list from your electronic medical record (EMR) on your providers' website where you or your partner have a patient portal. If all the providers you and your partner see use the same medical record, this may not be necessary. If you or your care partner take vitamins and over-the-counter medications and supplements, make sure the doctor knows about these as well.

The final thing to prepare is your story. Visit time is short. When the provider asks how you and your care partner are feeling, some people go on for several minutes about this and that symptom. It is better to say, "I think that overall Emiko's anxiety is less, but now she has more trouble sleeping." You should be prepared to describe your or your care partner's symptoms:

- When the symptoms started
- How long they last
- Where they are located
- What makes them better or worse
- Whether you or your care partner have had similar problems before
- Whether you or your care partner have changed diet, exercise, or medications in a way that might contribute to the symptoms
- What worries you most about the symptoms
- What you think might be causing the symptoms

If you or your care partner started a new medication or treatment since your last visit, be ready to report how it went. If you are seeing several providers and they are not all using the same electronic medical record, bring with you any test results from the past six months. (If all your providers use the same electronic medical record system, this may not be necessary.)

When telling your story, talk about trends. Are things getting better or worse, or are they the same? Also mention if your or your care partner's symptoms are more or less frequent or intense. For example, "In general, Emiko is slowly getting better, but today she does not feel good."

Be open and share your thoughts, feelings, and fears. Remember, your provider is not a mind reader. If you are worried, explain why: "I am worried that my care partner will get worse and I may not be able to work," or "My father had similar symptoms before he died." The more open you are, the more likely it is that your provider can help. If you have a problem, don't wait for the provider to discover it. State your concern immediately. For example, "I am worried about this mole on Emiko's back." Share your hunches or guesses about what might be causing the symptoms because they often provide vital clues to an accurate diagnosis. Even if it turns out that your guesses are not correct, it gives your doctor the opportunity to reassure you or address your hidden concerns.

The more specific you are (without adding unnecessary details), the clearer the picture you give the doctor of your problem. If you share specific information, you waste less of both your and the doctor's time.

Ask

Your most powerful tool in the doctor-patient partnership, and especially as a caregiver, is the question. Asking questions can fill in important missing pieces and close gaps in communication. Also, asking questions shows that you are an active manager of your own care and that of your care partner. This is critical to restoring and maintaining health. Getting answers and information is key to self-management and good caregiving.

Be prepared to ask questions about diagnosis, tests, treatments, and follow-up. The following are some guidelines for asking questions:

- **Diagnosis.** Ask what's wrong, what caused it, if it is contagious, and what the outlook (or prognosis) is. What can be done to prevent or manage it?
- **Tests.** If the doctor wants to do tests, ask how the results are likely to affect treatment and what will happen if the test is not done. For example, say your care partner is due for a colonoscopy. If this test finds cancer, is this something you or your care partner would want treated? If yes, a colonoscopy is a good idea. If no, then there is no reason to have a colonoscopy. If you decide to have a test, find out how to prepare for the test and what it will be like. Also ask how and when you will get the results.
- **Treatments.** Ask if there are any choices in treatments and the advantages and disadvantages of each. In considering treatment for someone with dementia, the question to ask is if treatment will give a better quality of life. Ask what will happen if no treatment is chosen instead. (See Chapter 12, Managing Your Treatment Decisions and Medications.)
- **Follow-up.** Find out if and when you should call or return for a follow-up visit. What symptoms should you watch for in between visits, and what should you do if they occur?

Repeat

One way to check that you have understood everything that comes up in an appointment is to briefly report back the key points. For example, "You want my care partner to take this pill three times a day with meals." Repeating back gives the provider a chance to quickly correct any misunderstandings.

If you don't understand or remember something the provider said, say that you need to go over it again. For example, "I'm pretty sure you told me some of this before, but I'm still confused about it." Don't be afraid to ask what you think might be a stupid question. Such questions are important and may prevent misunderstanding.

Sometimes it is hard to remember everything. Take notes or bring another person to important visits. You can even record the visit with a smartphone if your provider grants permission. Many providers give you a written summary of the visit. Your provider may give you a copy of this at the end of the appointment, or you may be able to get it online in your electronic medical record or through your patient portal.

Take Action

At the end of a visit, you need to understand what to do next. What action do you need to take? This includes scheduling treatments, tests, and return visits. You should also know any danger signs to look out for and what you should do if they occur. If necessary, ask your provider to write down instructions. You can also ask your providers to recommend reading material or online resources.

If, for some reason, you can't or won't follow providers' advice, say so. For example, you might say, "I didn't take the aspirin. It gives me stomach problems," or "My care partner's insurance doesn't cover that much therapy, so we can't afford it," or "I've tried to exercise, but I can't seem to keep it up." If providers know why you can't or won't follow advice, they may be able to make other suggestions. If you don't share the reasons why you are unable to take actions, it's difficult for your providers to help. Also, if you or your care partner doesn't take the medication or follow providers' recommendations, it is difficult for the providers to know which treatments work or don't work and what to recommend in the future.

Asking for a Second Opinion

Sometimes you might want to see another provider or take your care partner to get a second opinion. Asking for this can be hard. This is especially true if you or your care partner have had a long relationship with your provider. You may worry that asking for another opinion will anger your provider. Maybe your provider will take your request the wrong way. Requests for second opinions seldom bother providers. If a condition is complicated or difficult, the doctor may have already consulted with another doctor (or more than one). This is often done informally. Asking for a second opinion is perfectly acceptable, and providers are taught to expect such requests. However, asking for third, fourth, and fifth opinions may be unproductive.

Ask for a second opinion by using a non-threatening "I" message such as the following: "I'm still feeling confused and uncomfortable about this treatment. I feel another opinion might reassure me. Can you suggest someone I could see?" Express your own feelings without suggesting that the provider is at fault. Also, confirm your confidence in your provider by asking for their recommendation. You are not bound by your doctor's suggestion though.

Give Positive Feedback to Providers

When you are pleased with your care, let your providers know. Everyone appreciates compliments and positive feedback, especially members of a health care team. They are human, and your praise can help nourish and console these busy, hardworking professionals. Letting them know that you appreciate their efforts is one of the best ways to improve your relationship with them. Plus, gratitude and praise make them feel good! Likewise, if you do not like the way you or your care partner have been treated by any of the members of your health care team, let them know.

Share in Medical Decisions

Many medical decisions are not clear-cut. Often there is more than one option. The best decisions, except in life-threatening emergencies, depend on your values and preferences. The decision should not be left solely to your doctor. For example, if you have high blood pressure, you might say, "I'm very conservative about taking medications. What's a reasonable period for me to try exercise, diet, and relaxation first, before I start taking the medication?" Or, "I know that my care partner is not going to get better. Will this medication really help his quality of life? If not, will *not* taking it harm his quality of life?"

No one can tell you which choice is right for you and your care partner. But to make an informed choice, you need information about the treatment options. Informed choice, not merely informed consent, is essential to quality medical care. The best medical care for you and your care partner combines a doctor's medical expertise with your own knowledge, skills, and values.

To make an informed choice about any treatment, you need to know the cost and risks of the treatment. This includes the likelihood of possible complications, such as drug reactions, bleeding, infection, injury, or death. It also includes the personal costs, such as absences from work, and financial considerations, such as how much of the treatments your insurance will cover. You should also know the risks of doing nothing.

You also need to understand how likely it is that the proposed treatments will benefit you or your care partner in terms of relieving symptoms, improving function, or prolonging life. Sometimes the best choice may be not to treat or to delay a decision about a treatment in favor of watchful waiting.

Making decisions about treatments can be difficult. For some suggestions on how make decisions see "Making Decisions: Weighing the Pros and Cons" on page ••• in Chapter 2, Becoming a Better Caregiver: The Basics, and see "Asking Questions about New Treatments" on page ••• in Chapter 12, Managing Your Treatment Decisions and Medications, for help on how to evaluate new treatments.

Working with the Health Care System

Most providers work in larger systems such as clinics. Someone other than your provider usually decides on policies relating to appointment times, billing, and telephone and email use.

If you are unhappy with your health care system, don't suffer in silence. Do something about it. Find out who is running the organization and who makes decisions. Then share your feelings in a constructive way by letter, phone, email, or message through your organization's online portal. Most health care systems want to keep you as a patient, and therefore, they usually respond to feedback. The problem is that the people who make the decisions tend to isolate themselves. It is easier to express our feelings to the receptionist, nurse, or doctor. Unfortunately, these people have little or no power to change the system. But they can tell you whom to contact. If something is a problem for you, it might also be a problem for your provider and other patients. If you work closely in partnership, you and your provider may be able to improve the system.

In Canada, the province or territory sets health care policies. Patient care quality offices can address complaints about care and health care providers. Other terms for patient quality care offices are patient relations or patient ombudsman. You can also contact your provincial or territorial health ministry.

If you do decide to write or email, here are some suggestions. Keep your letter short and factual. Share what actions you would find helpful. For example:

Dear Ms. Brown:

Yesterday, my mother and I had a 10:00 a.m. appointment with Dr. Zim. She did not see us until 12:15, and our total time with the doctor was eight minutes. I was told to make another appointment so we could get our questions answered.

I know that sometimes there are emergencies. I would appreciate being called if my doctor is running late so I don't make the trip to the clinic. If we are already at the clinic, I would like to be told I can leave and when to return. We would also like 15 or more minutes with my mother's doctor.

I would appreciate a reply within two weeks.

Thank you.

The following are some common issues that come up with health care systems. We offer a few tips for addressing these issues and working with the health care system. Not all these problems and suggestions will apply to all systems, but most do.

- **"I hate the phone system."** Often, when you call for an appointment or information, you reach an automated system. This can be frustrating. Unfortunately, you cannot change this. However, phone systems do not change often. If you memorize or write down the numbers or keys to press, you can move more quickly through the menu of options. In some systems, pressing the pound key (#) or 0 will get you to a real person. Once you do get through, ask if there is a way to do this faster next time. Many systems now let you make appointments online. This often saves time and prevents frustration.
- **"It takes too long to get an appointment."** Ask for the first available appointment. Take it. Then ask about how you can be on a wait list to be called if other people cancel their appointment. Some organizations will call you when they have an empty spot or put you on their electronic wait list that notifies you by text or email if there is a cancellation. In others, you may have to call them once or twice a week or look online to check for cancellations. Ask the scheduler what you can do to get an earlier appointment. Ask for a telephone number so you can reach the person making appointments directly. Some systems set time aside each day for same-day appointments. If these appointments do become available, know when to call to get one. It is usually early in the morning. If you are in distress or believe you must see a doctor right away, tell the scheduler. No matter how frustrated you are, be nice. The scheduler has the power to either give you an appointment or not. If you feel you can't wait, some health care systems in the United States and Canada have drop-in or urgent care clinics. These clinics can provide care that doesn't require you to go to the emergency department at the hospital.
- **"I don't want to travel to the clinic."** A trip to the clinic can be difficult for you and your care partner. It requires planning and time. One good thing that the COVID pandemic

gave us is the availability of video visits. These visits are conducted on a computer screen or tablet via Zoom or other secure application. Video visits for some provider visits can be a good alternative to travelling to the clinic. They may not be appropriate, however, if the provider needs hands-on evaluation, but it never hurts to ask.

- **"Between myself and my care partner we have so many providers. I do not know whom to ask for what."** One of those providers is in charge. Your job is to find out which one. Ask each provider who is coordinating your care or that of your care partner. It is most likely that your primary care doctor or general practitioner (GP) is the coordinator. Check with that doctor to confirm that they are coordinating your care. Ask how you can help make communication and coordination of care smoother among the different providers. One way might be to let this doctor know when someone else orders a test or new medication. Keeping the coordinating doctor informed is especially important when not all providers are in the same system and using the same electronic medical record.
- **"I can never reach my doctor."** It is hard to get a provider on the phone, but you might be able to email. Many systems now have ways that doctors and patients can communicate by secure text or email. The next time you see your provider, ask about this. Or visit your care provider's internet portal to review your options. One good thing about electronic systems is that routine things such as prescription refills can be done quickly.

In a medical emergency, do not waste time trying to contact your doctor directly. Call 911 (in the United States and Canada) or go to a hospital emergency department.

In Canada, because of COVID-19, there are companies that provide virtual health care, and you can have an appointment with a doctor that may be covered by provincial or territorial health insurance or your workplace health plan. You can Google "virtual health care in Canada" to find available companies.

Walk-in clinics to see a doctor may be available in your area of Canada if you are unable to make an appointment with your family doctor in a timely manner or you don't have a family doctor.

In all provinces, pharmacists can do much more than just deliver medications. They can often advise on minor conditions, renew prescriptions, and give injections and vaccinations.

- **"I have to wait too long in the waiting room or the examination room."** Delays caused by emergencies happen. Or when every patient before you takes an extra five minutes, this can also cause a wait. If your schedule is tight and it may cause a problem if your appointment is delayed, call your doctor's office before you leave home and ask how long you will have to wait. If you learn that your doctor is running late, you can decide whether to take a book to read or ask to reschedule. You can also show up with your book and ask about the wait. Rather than getting upset, let the receptionist know that you are going to step out for a little while to run a quick errand nearby or for a cup of coffee. Tell the receptionist that you will return at a specific time.

There are two ways you can help prevent this problem. First, use your time with the provider wisely. Be prepared for your visit. Try hard not to take extra time. If every patient takes five extra minutes, it means two or three extra hours of extra work for the provider and extra waiting time for the patients whose appointments are later in the day. Second, if you do not need all your time, do not chitchat. When you have what you need, thank the doctor. Say you have gotten what you needed and that you are going to give your extra five minutes to the next patient. This is a big gift and will be appreciated and remembered.

- **"My care partner and I don't have enough time with the provider."** This may be a system problem since someone other than your provider often decides how many patients to schedule and for how long. The decision is sometimes based on what you tell the scheduler. If you say your partner needs a blood pressure check, you will be given a short visit. If you say your care partner seems very depressed and cannot function, you might be given a longer appointment. When making the appointment, ask for the time you want, especially if you want more than 10 or 15 minutes. Be prepared with the reasons why you need more time. You can also ask for the last appointment of the day. You may have to wait a while, but at least the provider will not rush your visit to get to other waiting patients.

In Canada, depending on your province or territory, your family doctor may provide you with a longer appointment if you have chronic health conditions. Check with your family doctor's office for more information.

- **"What is an electronic medical record (EMR) anyway?"** Most of your medical information is stored on a secure computer. Any provider who is in the same system can see your information. Very few doctors today keep paper charts. You should know what information is in your EMR. In some systems, the EMR includes just test results. In other systems, the EMR has test results and medication information. In most systems, it has everything your provider knows about you. Like a paper record, an EMR does no good if your providers don't read it. For example, when you have a test, the doctor ordering the test knows when the test results are ready. However, your other doctors will not know anything about the test unless you tell them to read the results. Learn about the medical records system your provider uses so you can help all your providers use it more effectively.

In the United States and many other countries, you have the right to a copy of almost everything in your record. Many times, you can get this information online through such apps as MyHealth or MyChart. Before you visit a provider outside your regular health care system, ask for copies or download your tests and medications to give to the new provider.

In Canada, there is a difference between an EMR and an EHR. An EMR (electronic medical record) has information from a single care provider and stays in the office system, while EHRs (electronic health records) are designed to be used by multiple care providers and health-care organizations, providing a full picture of person's health and their medical history. With an EHR, your family doctor can share medical records with your specialist, the lab, the drug store, and your computer at home.

The use of health information technologies has been slowly increasing in Canada. Provinces and territories are responsible for developing their own electronic information systems and are working at improving the sharing of information. Ask your family doctor about accessing your health information online as this varies depending on where you live. More than half of residents of British Columbia, Alberta, Saskatchewan, and Ontario have accessed electronic health information. In June 2024, the federal government introduced the *Connected Care for Canadians Act*, a plan to enable a modern, connected care system with health information that can be securely accessed by patients and shared between providers, when needed.

What to Do If You or Your Care Partner Live in Canada and Do Not Have a Family Doctor

- Many Canadians do not have a family doctor. There are several ways to find a family doctor, but the process can vary depending on where you live in Canada.
- See if your province or territory has a patient registry where you can go on a wait-list that will match you when a family doctor becomes available or aid in finding a family doctor open to new patients.
- Ask family members or friends to see if their family doctor is open to new patients.
- Ask your specialist if they can recommend a family doctor open to new patients.
- Ask clinics in your community if they have a waitlist.

If you need care and you don't have a family doctor, consider the following options:

- Depending on where you live, you may have walk-in clinics where you can see a doctor without an appointment. The Medimap website lists most of the walk-in clinics in Canada.
- Depending on where you live, you may have access to an urgent or primary care centre. These centres provide care for non-life-threatening conditions when you need to see a healthcare provider within 12 to 24 hours but don't need to go to a hospital emergency department.
- Pharmacists in all provinces and the Yukon can treat and prescribe medications for some common medical ailments and may also be able to adjust medications, provide vaccinations, and order lab tests.
- All provinces and territories except Nunavut have an 811 provincial health access line. You will often speak with a nurse who will try to triage the issue or suggest you visit the hospital emergency department for further assessment.
- There are companies that provide virtual health care, and the appointment may be covered by provincial health insurance or your workplace health plan. Many virtual care options are available, such as a doctor's

appointment by phone or video. Depending on whether you are covered by your provincial health or your workplace health plan, the appointment may or may not be free. You can search online for "virtual health care in Canada" for companies providing this service.

- See other healthcare providers, such as physiotherapists or dietitians, to help you with your health issues. Some healthcare providers can be seen for no charge through hospital programs, or you may have coverage from your employee benefits.

The following are some parting words of advice for dealing with the health care system:

- In Canada, the Canadian Dental Care Plan (CDCP) is a federally delivered public plan to help ease financial barriers to accessing oral health care for eligible Canadian residents. It is intended to provide dental coverage for low- and middle-income Canadian residents who do not have access to dental benefits. Eligibility includes having an adjusted family net income of less than $90,000, being a Canadian resident for income tax purposes, and having filed a tax return for the previous year. You must see a dentist who is participating in the CDCP. You can visit the website to confirm your eligibility and to apply online. if you are unable to apply online, you can apply by phone by calling 1-833-537-4342. Ask your dentist for more information.
- **If something in the health care system is not working, ask how you can help to make it work better.** Very often, if you learn how to navigate the system, you can solve, or at least partially solve, your problems.
- **Be nice—or at least as nice as possible.** If the system or your provider sees you as a difficult patient, life will become more difficult.

Many people think that things should not be this way. It is not fair to place this burden on the patient. Health systems should be responsive and patient friendly. Many health care systems are already striving to be better. In the meantime, use the suggestions in this chapter to help you deal more effectively with difficult situations.

For a complete list of suggested further readings, useful websites, and other helpful resources, please see:www.bullpub.com/resources.

Chapter 7

Getting Help

A MAJOR PART OF CAREGIVING is knowing when you need help, what help you need, and how to find help. Seeking help is a sign of strength, not weakness, and getting help is one of the best things you can do to reduce your stress. Unfortunately, getting help can be challenging for many caregivers. The following example shows what too often happens to many caregivers.

Minh is overwhelmed. She hasn't been sleeping much because her care partner, Tran, has been getting out of bed in the middle of the night. Minh hasn't had time to do anything except watch her care partner. She is stressed, angry, and even has cross words with Tran. Minh knows that she needs help, but she thinks that there is no one available to help. Because she does not know how to get help, she decides that no one can do a better job at caregiving than her anyway. At this point, she just continues doing what she is doing and becomes more and more overwhelmed until some crisis occurs.

This story could have a happier ending, and in this chapter, we will give you some tools to make a better ending possible.

The first step is to figure out what you need help with. As we mentioned in Chapter 6, Communicating Effectively, it is important to be as specific as possible when you ask for help. Start by writing a list of what help you would like. Do not worry whether that help is available or possible: Just write the list. At the end of this section on page 103, you will find a tool for thinking about the help you need and who might give it.

Thinking about resources for getting that help is the second step. Who can help? As caregivers begin to look for help, most people start by asking family or friends. Sometimes this can be difficult to do. You may be afraid that others will see you as weak. Sometimes your pride gets in the way. The truth is that most people want to be helpful but do not know how. Your job is to tell them what you need. Finding the right words to ask for help is discussed in Chapter 6, Communicating Effectively. You might argue that no one has offered help and assume that this means that no one wants to help. But sometimes the offers don't come because you have not asked for help or you were not specific about what help you needed. A good way to start recruiting help is to hold a family meeting.

Holding a Family Meeting

Sometimes the best way to get help is to hold a family meeting. This may seem like a big step or like something that shows neediness or weakness on your part. While it might be a big step, it is not a sign of weakness. Calling a family meeting shows strength. The objective is to get the care your care partner needs while maintaining the mental and physical health of the caregiver(s). When you have this meeting, not everyone must be in the same place at the same time. You can hold the meeting by conference call or via a video calling program such as Zoom, Google Meet, Skype, or FaceTime. On pages 102 and 103 you will find some tools to help you set up family meetings. The following are some additional tips:

- **Invite everyone who might be interested or helpful.** This meeting is not just for immediate family. It may include extended family, such as in-laws, and close friends. As you make the list of the people you want to invite, don't forget relatives who are far away. They might not be able to come to your house to help, but they could have good ideas or be able to help pay for support. Even if that is not possible, they may be interested as they are part of the family. Do not exclude them. Invite them to sit in on the phone or computer video conference if they cannot attend the meeting in person. Most family meetings do not include the care partner. Find a friend, volunteer, or care companion (see page 110) to take your care partner out while you attend the meeting.

- **Find a professional or another neutral party to run the meeting.** This may be a professional, such as a social worker or religious leader, or could even be a friend who has experience in running complex meetings. The person does not need to know much about you, your care partner, your family, or the situation. Their job is to facilitate. By having an uninvolved party run the meeting, there is more chance that everyone will participate and be heard. It will also be easier to limit the input of any not-so-helpful family members.
- **Avoid serving alcohol during the meeting.** Alcohol tends to change the thinking and emotions of even social drinkers, and there always seems to be someone who has a little too much. Stick with nonalcoholic drinks. One way to make this easier is to hold the meeting in the morning or early afternoon.
- **Write an agenda and share it with everyone before the meeting.** Everyone then has a chance to prepare and can avoid surprises. It can also help focus the discussion and keep the meeting from going off topic.
- **Set ground rules.** Listening is hard and even harder when the topic is emotionally charged. Listening to everyone else may be the hardest part of the meeting for attendees. One way you can make this easier is with ground rules such as the following:
    1. Begin the meeting by allowing each person to talk in turn for as long as they want for an agreed-upon time without interruption. At the end of this time, the person speaking says, "I have spoken," and the others say, "I have heard" (or some other pre-arranged phrases).
    2. There is no discussion until everyone has spoken. After everyone has said how they feel, then you can have a discussion but never an interruption.
    3. Use the words "our" and "we," not "me" and "I."
- **Start the meeting with a status report.** Tell the group about your care partner's present condition. Be specific and clear and factual. Unless the group sees your care partner every day, they may not know what is really going on. Short visits, as you know, can be deceiving.
- **Let all members of the group express how they feel about the situation.** Remember the ground rules. No interrupting.
- **Avoid expressing anger and pushing emotional buttons.** All families have emotional issues, and many family members are experts on how to "get to" another family member. Family members may be likely to overreact because of stress.
- **Clearly express the problem and the specific help that you want.** If there are distractions or excuses, use your broken record tool (see page xx in Chapter 4, Dealing with Difficult Emotions). Repeat your phrase, whether it is, "Thank you for your input," "Let me think about this," or "I would rather talk about something else." No matter what they say, repeat your phrase. You might have to do this several times. Remember, do not express anger.

Family Meeting Checklist

- ☐ Invite everyone who might be interested or helpful. This may include in-laws and close friends.
- ☐ Find a professional or other neutral party to run the meeting.
- ☐ Don't serve alcohol.
- ☐ Write and share an agenda before the meeting.
- ☐ Establish ground rules and make sure everyone agrees to them.
- ☐ Start the meeting with a current report on your care partner's status.
- ☐ Let everyone express how they feel about the situation.
- ☐ Use the words "our" and "we," not "me" and "I."
- ☐ Avoid expressing anger.
- ☐ State the problem and the help that you want.
- ☐ Do not tell people what they should do.
- ☐ Ask for solutions.
- ☐ Record offers of help.
- ☐ Following the meeting, send everyone a summary of agreements resulting from the meeting.
- ☐ Regularly schedule family meetings, if possible.

- **Ask what each person can contribute.** Do not tell people what they should do.
- **As help is offered, write it down and repeat it back to the group.** Be flexible and open to offers. Say, for example, "Mary, I understand that you cannot come here to help, but your offer to pay for a housekeeper one day a week would be a great help."
- **After the meeting, send everyone a copy of the written plans agreed to in the meeting.**
- **Family meetings work best when they are scheduled to happen regularly.**

Finding Resources in the Community

Some caregivers do not have family or close friends or cannot bring themselves to ask family for help. Often even when they are willing to help, family or friends cannot provide all the help that is needed. Thankfully, you have another wonderful resource: your community.

Finding community resources can be a little like a treasure hunt. As in a treasure hunt, creative thinking wins the game. Finding what you need may be as simple as making a couple

Family Meeting Planning Tool

This tool will help you plan a family meeting. On the form, give a name to each category, and under each category, write what you need. Do not leave the meeting until the right-hand column is filled out!

The following are sample categories of the help you may need:

- Household chores, such as repairs, grocery shopping, meal preparation, gardening, pet care, or housecleaning.
- Financial support, such as paying the mortgage, the rent, or other bills, or buying or renting equipment such as shower stools, walkers, or wheelchairs.
- Financial organization, such as keeping track of financial records, taxes, and insurance forms and claims, or setting up accounts and making sure bills are paid.
- Health care, such as making medical appointments, providing transportation to appointments, submitting insurance forms and other forms related to medical care, or drafting and executing durable power of attorney for health care.
- Family communications, such as keeping family members informed or arranging family meetings.

Family Meeting Planning Tool		
Category:		
Name of task	Who will do it	When they will do it
Category:		
Name of task	Who will do it	When they will do it
Category:		
Name of task	Who will do it	When they will do it
Category:		
Name of task	Who will do it	When they will do it

of phone calls or searching the internet. Other times it might require some digging. A community resource detective must find clues and follow them. Sometimes this also means starting over when a clue leads to a dead end.

The first step in tapping into your community is defining the problem and the cause of the problem. Evaluate the situation. Then ask yourself what you can and want to do to improve the situation. If you cannot do something you want to do, then figure out why so you can find the solution. For example, suppose the problem you need help with is meal preparation. You would really like to have an evening meal prepared three times a week but do not always have the time. You might start by asking friends and neighbors for help. You could also call your local information and referral agency, such as United Way or the local Area Agency on Aging (these are located in most communities across the United States). In Canada, call 211, or visit https://211.ca/about-211/index.html (Please note that most Canadian-specific content is shaded throughout the book.) These services can help you find information and/or a referral for most issues you might have.

After a few days, you might have a whole list. For example, you learn that the local church has a program that supplies one meal a week to local community members. You also learn that you can order delivery services from many local restaurants and grocery stores on the internet. The Area Agency on Aging shared information about Meal on Wheels, which serves lunch at your local community center every Monday, Wednesday, and Friday. Another friend told you about a business that allows you to order pre-prepared meal kits that you can cook at home. Finally, one of your neighbors shared your need with a friend who is a teacher. The friend said that providing some meals for you might be a good project for her middle-school cooking class. You decide to go with the group at the local church and one meal a week from Meals on Wheels. And one night you will order food from some of your favorite restaurants.

There are people in every community who are natural at finding resources. These "naturals" or "connectors" seem to know everyone and everything about their community and connect people to the help they need. These folks usually have lived a long time in the community and have been involved in local organizations. They are also natural problem-solvers. These people are the ones that others turn to for advice. They always seem to be helpful. Your connector might be a friend, a work colleague, the mail carrier, your physician, your pet's veterinarian, the checker at the corner grocery, the pharmacist, a bus or taxi driver, a real estate agent, the Chamber of Commerce receptionist, or the librarian. Think of this person as an information resource and don't be shy about asking them about your specific need. Sometimes they will take on the thrill of the hunt and, like a modern-day Sherlock Holmes, announce that "the game is afoot!" and promptly join you in your search.

You may be a member of a neighborhood, school, church, or internet group. These groups are also helpful for finding resources.

As this example illustrates, the most important steps in finding community resources are:

1. Identify the problem.
2. Identify what you want or need.

3. Search for resources.
4. Ask friends, family, and neighbors for ideas.
5. Contact organizations that might have experience with your issue.
6. Identify and ask the "naturals" and "connectors" in your community.

One last note: The best sleuth follows several clues at the same time. This will save you time and shorten the hunt. Watch out, though—once you get good at thinking about community resources creatively, you may become a connector in your own right!

Resources for Resources

When you need to find goods or services, there are certain resources you can call on. One resource often leads to another. The connector is one of those resources, but our community resource detective's kit needs a variety of other useful tools.

Internet search engines (such as Google, Bing, Yahoo, etc.) are the most frequently used tools. These are particularly helpful if you are looking for someone to hire. For most searches, this is where to start.

Organizations and Referral Services

Almost every community has one or more information and referral services. Sometimes these are related to a geographic area such as a city or county. Other times they are specific to an age group, such as the Area Agency on Aging or the Government of Canada Programs and Services for Seniors. Sometimes the organizations are specific to a disability or health condition, such as Alzheimer's or Parkinson's disease.

Several types of agencies operate these services. Try using search terms such as "United Way information and referral," "senior information and referral" (or "Area Agency on Aging" or "Council on Aging" in Canada), or "information and referral" or "211" in Canada. If you are using a telephone directory, be sure to check your county or city government or municipality or province listings.

Once you have the telephone number or email address of a reliable information and referral service, your searches become easier. These services maintain huge files of referral addresses and telephone numbers for just about any help you might need. Even if they don't have the answer you seek, they are usually able to refer you to another agency that can help.

Voluntary agencies such as the American Heart Association or Alzheimer's Association are great resources. There are similar organizations in most other countries. For example, Canada has the Heart and Stroke Foundation and the Alzheimer Society. These agencies are funded by contributions from individuals and from corporate sponsors. They provide up-to-date information about health issues, as well as support and direct services. They also fund research intended to help people live better with their illness and to someday lead to a cure. For a small fee, you can become a member of one of these organizations. Often, this puts you on the list to receive regular bulletins by mail or email.

But you do not have to be a member to qualify for their services. They are here to serve the public. Many of these organizations have wonderful websites. Websites can be accessed anywhere at any time if you have internet access. In our modern, globally connected world, you can live in rural North Dakota or the Canadian Artic and get help online from the Parkinson's Foundation in Victoria, Australia.

There are other organizations in your community offering information and referral services along with direct services. These include the local chapter of AARP (formerly known as the American Association of Retired Persons), CARP (formerly the Canadian Association for Retired Persons), senior centers, community centers, and religious and social service agencies. These organizations offer information, classes, recreational opportunities, nutrition programs, legal and tax help, and social programs.

Don't overlook your local senior center. Most senior centers have a social worker who is very knowledgeable about available resources. You do not need to be a senior to use this resource. There is probably a senior or community center close to you. Your city government office or local librarian can tell you where such resources are and how you can contact them. Also, the calendar section of the local newspaper may list current information about programs these organizations offer.

Most religious groups offer information and social services to persons who need it. They provide services directly through the place of worship or through groups such as the Council of Churches, Catholic Diocese, Jewish Family Services, or the Muslim Social Services Agency. To get help from religious organizations, start with the local place of worship. People there will either help you or refer you to someone who can. You usually need not be a member of the congregation or even of the religion to receive help.

Another option is to call your local hospital, clinic, or health insurance plan and ask for the social service department. Doctors and their staff are also good resources. They know about the physical and mental health services available through their health care organizations. The Veterans Administration offers services to those whose care partner is a US military veteran. Every Veterans Administration hospital has a caregiving coordinator.

Libraries

Your public library is a particularly good resource if you are looking for information. Libraries are not just collections of books. The resources your library can connect you to are vast and varied. Even if you think you are an excellent library detective, it's a good idea to ask the reference librarian to make sure you haven't overlooked something. Librarians see volumes of material cross their desks daily and are knowledgeable about the community. If you cannot get to the library, you can call or contact them online.

In addition to city or county libraries, some communities may have other, more specialized health libraries. Ask your information and referral service if there is a health library in your area. These libraries, such as the Government of Canada Health Library, specialize in health-related resources. They usually have a computerized database of information available along with the usual print and digital materials. Health libraries are usually maintained by nonprofit organizations and hospitals and sometimes charge a small fee for use. Even if there is no health library in your community, you can contact most health libraries online. They are used to getting questions from around the world.

Universities and colleges also have libraries open to the public. By law, the regional government documents sections of these US libraries must be open to the public at no charge. US government publications exist for just about any subject, and health-related publications are particularly extensive. You can find everything from information on organic gardening to detailed nutritional recipes. Public university and college librarians are usually very helpful, and these publications represent your tax dollars at work.

If you are fortunate enough to have a medical school in your community, you might be able to use its medical library. This is a place to go to for information rather than to look for help with tasks. Naturally, you can expect to find a great deal of information about disease and treatment at a medical library. Unless you have special knowledge about medicine, however, the detailed information you find in a medical library can be confusing and even frightening. Use medical libraries with care.

Most everyone knows about search engines like Google. But many don't know about Google Scholar, which lists peer-reviewed science articles. Peer-reviewed articles are checked for accuracy and trustworthiness by panels of professionals in the field. You can use Google Scholar just like Google to find scientific literature on almost any topic. In your search results, you can always see the short abstracts for the articles, and sometimes the entire article as well. Once you find an article title or abstract that interests you, you can go to your library's reference librarian to ask how to get a copy.

Books

Books can be useful (indeed, you are reading a book now!). Many caregiving-related books contain reading and resource lists, either at the ends of chapters or at the backs of books. These lists can be very helpful. We have a resource list that is updated regularly at www.bullpub.com/resources.

Newspapers and Magazines

Your local newspaper, especially if you live in a smaller community, can be an excellent resource. Most newspapers publish both paper and online versions. Be sure to look for a local calendar of events page. On this page you can get an idea of the organizations that are active in your community. Even if you are not interested in a featured event, calling the contact telephone number may help you find what you are looking for. News stories might also be of interest, especially local stories in the pages around the calendar section. Also, look in other logical places for topics that might also be of interest. For example, if you are looking for an exercise program, check out the sports and fitness section.

Sometimes you can find clues in the classified section. Look under "announcements," "health," or any other heading that seems promising. Review the index of classified headings to see which headings your newspaper uses.

At the local bookstore or newsstand, there are a variety of general magazines that might be useful. For example, some publications focus on specific health conditions, such as Alzheimer's, diabetes, or arthritis. Often you can find many of these on the internet as well.

The Internet

Most people have access to the internet. If you are not an internet user, you probably know an internet user. Even if you do not have a computer, smartphone, or tablet, you can use one in your local library. The internet is the fastest-growing source of information. New information is being added every second of every day. The internet offers information about caregiving and anything else you can imagine. It also provides several ways in which you can interact with people all over the world. For example, someone who has Gaucher disease, a rare health condition, might find it difficult to locate others nearby who have the same disease. The internet can put a person in touch with a group of such people. It doesn't matter whether these people are across the street or on the other side of the world.

The good thing about the internet is that anyone can maintain a website, a Facebook or other social network page, a blog, or a group. That is also the bad thing about the internet. There are virtually no controls over who is posting information. There is also no agency ensuring information is accurate or even safe. This can mean that even though there is a lot of information out there that might be very useful, you may also see incorrect or even dangerous information. You should never assume that information found on the internet is entirely trustworthy. Approach information obtained online with skepticism and caution. Ask yourself, is the author or sponsor of the website clearly identified? Is the author or source reputable? Does the information contradict what everyone else seems to be saying about the subject? Does the information make common sense? What is the purpose of the website? Is someone trying to sell you something or win you over to a particular point of view?

One way to determine the purpose of the website is to look at the URL (the address located at the top of the screen, starting with http://). The URL will usually look something like this:

https://act.alz.org/ OR https://alzheimer.ca/

At the end of the main part of a US–based website's URL, you will most commonly see .edu, .org, .gov, or .com. For non-US websites, the very last letters can represent the country of origin. Many Canadian-based websites end in .ca, so you will have to investigate if that site is affiliated with a school, nonprofit organization, government agency, or a commercial enterprise. You may also see other endings, such as .biz or .info. This will give you a clue about the nature of the organization that owns the website. College or university website addresses end in .edu. Nonprofit organization website addresses end in .org. US governmental agency website addresses end in .gov. In Canada, the ending .gc.ca is used by federal government sites. Commercial organization website addresses end in .com.

As a general rule of thumb, .edu, .org, and .gov are usually trustworthy sites. Although, be aware that a nonprofit organization can be formed to promote just about anything. A website address with a URL that ends with .com is usually a commercial organization trying to sell a product or service or is selling advertising space on its site. This doesn't mean that a commercial website can't be a good one. On the contrary, there are many outstanding commercial sites dedicated to providing high-quality, trustworthy information. They are often able to cover the costs of providing this service only by selling advertisements or by accepting grants from commercial firms. The URLs for some of our favorite reliable websites are listed at www.bullpub.com/resources. Please note that this is a commercial site owned and curated by the publisher of this book.

Never give your financial information, such as a credit card number, bank account number, or social security number to a person who contacts you online or on the phone. Only give your credit card information to reliable merchants that you know are legitimate. You should also avoid entering personal information into forms online, such as your birthdate, unless you are familiar with the site and know it is secure. Likewise, if you receive an unsolicited email from what looks like an organization you know, do not click a link in the email but go directly to their website instead. One way to confirm whether an organization that is trying to reach you is legitimate is by checking for spelling errors or strange characters in their message. If things don't seem correct, terminate the conversation and contact them using phone numbers or email addresses listed on official websites only. If you're unsure about the person you're talking to or what you're being told, ask a friend or family member before you give out any information. Do not allow anyone to have remote access to your computer.

The Internet and Social Networking Sites

Social networking sites and blogs are everywhere on the internet. Sites such as Facebook, X (formerly Twitter), Instagram, and Nextdoor are currently very popular, but everything may change by the time this book is published. These sites enable the average person to communicate easily with others who want to listen (or read). Some sites, such as Facebook, require that users determine who will be allowed to read the thoughts they post on their page. Others, such as Blogger, are more like personal journals that are open to anyone who finds them on the internet.

You can find other caregivers who are eager to share their experiences on these sites. Some have discussion forums where groups of people get together to share information, suggestions, and opinions. The information and support on these sites can be valuable, but again be cautious because some sites may propose unproven or even dangerous ideas.

Online Discussion Groups

Facebook, Yahoo!, Google, and other websites offer discussion groups for just about anything you can imagine. Anyone can start a discussion group about any topic. The people or organizations that start the groups run these groups. For any health condition, you will probably find dozens of discussion groups. You can join them and the discussion if you wish or just lurk (read without interacting). Online support groups operate differently than online discussion groups. Support groups involve interaction with others in real time or not, on camera or through chat rooms, or 24/7 text or telephone calls, or message boards. Online support groups are also facilitated by trained group leaders.

For caregivers, there are various online discussion and support groups. These allow caregivers to connect and share their experiences with others, encourage and support one another, and exchange practical advice and information. For some, this could be the only opportunity to talk with someone else. Smart Patients, for example, has an excellent online group at: https://www.smartpatients.com/communities/caregivers.

To find other online groups, search for a link to "groups" or "online caregiver support groups" or "online caregiver discussion groups." Check to see that the group has a moderator who enforces the rules of the group.

Keep in mind that the internet is changing all the time. Our guidelines reflect conditions at the time this book was written. Things may have changed by the time you read this.

Getting Caregiving Help

One thing many caregivers need help with is figuring out how to get the help they need or want. Earlier in this chapter, we outlined how to organize a family meeting to ask for help from family and friends. Sometimes, however, family and friends may not be able to provide help or more help is needed. In this section, we provide some information to help you decide what help you need and how to find it.

In-Home Care: What Is It?*

Many different types of people and organizations offer in-home help. The following list can help you think about what you and your care partner want and need.

- **Housekeeper/yard worker**: This is someone who can help with the household and/or outdoors chores. Some of these chores might include housecleaning, doing the laundry, ironing, cleaning, or they could be seasonal chores such as lawn care and snow shoveling. These workers do not usually interact much with a care partner. They help free up caregiver time and make caregiver life less complicated.
- **Care companion**: A care companion provides an extra pair of eyes, ears, and hands. They can help your care partner do as much as possible for themselves and help out with the following tasks:
  - Driving your care partner on errands or to social outings
  - Grocery shopping
  - Taking your care partner to the doctor
  - Cooking and/or filling the freezer with healthful, prepared meals
  - Light housekeeping such as vacuuming and bathroom and kitchen cleaning
  - Organizational projects such as cleaning your garage, closets, or junk drawer
  - Keeping your care partner company by playing cards, looking at photo albums, or even just sitting and chatting

*The material in this section was adapted from Caring.com's website.

- **Home aide or personal care assistant:** Personal care assistants provide care that involves physical assistance. They usually have some training and can help your care partner with everyday tasks such as:
    - Bathing
    - Toileting
    - Getting dressed
    - Shaving
    - Dental hygiene
    - Nail care
    - Walking
    - Incontinence

  If needed, some personal care assistants will also help with driving, shopping, cooking, light housekeeping, and keeping your care partner company.
- **Respite care in your home:** Sometimes you just need a break and a little time for yourself. Having someone come in just once or twice or on a regular basis can provide this help. This can be a relative or friend. You can also check with your place of worship, senior center, Area Agency on Aging, or some other community agency to see if they have suggestions for people who can fill this role for you. Neighborhood email lists may be another resource. In-home care agencies can also help. You can call them to arrange care for just one time or to schedule someone to come on a weekly or monthly basis. If your care partner is a veteran (even if they do not use veteran's services), you can call the caregiver support person at your local branch of the US Department of Veterans Affairs or Veterans Affairs Canada. In Canada, depending on your province or territory, respite may be available on a short-term basis in a long-term care home, hospice or other community care setting. You can get more information on how to get a referral from your family doctor or your Home and Community Care Office.
- **Live-in care:** Many in-home care agencies can help you arrange round-the-clock care. A caregiver like this can provide care for and protect your care partner and allows you, the main caregiver, to take care of other responsibilities and get rest or sleep. You might arrange for one caregiver to live with you or a set of caregivers to work in shifts throughout the day or on different days of the week. You can find live-in care in the same way you can find respite care.

  In Canada, programs are offered through provincial and territorial health ministries and private companies. Check with such resources as the Canadian Seniors Directory or the Canadian government's "Programs and Services for Seniors" page to learn about respite services. The federal government supports the Veterans Independence Program (VIP) through Veterans Affairs Canada. Also, all the provinces and territories offer a limited amount of publicly funded home care services from both public and private agencies. The types of services offered vary across the country. Support may be based on a sliding scale based on income.

In-Home Help Options

Two types of organizations offer in-home services; these are in-home care agencies and in-home care registries. A third option is to hire someone directly. These three options are explained here:

1. **In-home care agencies** assume all the employer responsibilities. An agency hires and pays the caregiver, pays the Social Security and payroll taxes, carries the insurance, and so forth. The agency also provides some training and supervision; it may also send a substitute when your usual assistant is unavailable. Be sure to get all the details about each agency's policies as these can differ from one agency to the next.
2. **In-home care registries** are referral services that can help you find different types of in-home care. Most of these agencies supply home aides as well as licensed staff such as certified nursing assistants (CNAs), licensed vocational nurses (LVNs), or registered nurses (RNs). Unless your care partner is bedbound or requires some procedure that must be done by someone with a certain category of license, a home aide will most likely be the appropriate choice.

   The people referred by these registries usually have experience and may have required training. You pay a fee to the registry for this service, but, unlike an in-home care agency, they do not employ these care providers. If you hire someone from a registry, that person is *your* employee (that is, an independent contractor). This means you might be responsible for paying taxes and Social Security for this person, and you must buy your own liability insurance. In Canada, you may be responsible for paying taxes, Canada Pension Plan, and Employment Insurance. When you contact a registry, ask about the training and experience of the people they refer to you as well as what you will be expected to do as the employer of an independent contractor.
3. Another way to find help that is less expensive is to **hire someone recommended by a friend or found through a help wanted ad or posting on a website**. If you choose this option, know that it involves more time. Also, you will be responsible for checking all references and doing all the screening. This person can work for you as an employee or independent contractor. You will want to talk to your lawyer or get some legal advice about the implications of both choices when considering such things as employment taxes and insurance.

In Canada, all the provinces and territories offer a limited amount of publicly funded home care services from both public and private agencies. The type of services offered vary across the country.

If you want to explore hiring in-home help, check the Caring.com website (www.caring.com) or CaregiverJobs.ca (www.caregiverjobs.ca) in Canada. These sites provide lists of agencies, reviews from families, and checklists to guide you through the process. Other resources include local senior centers and centers serving the disabled, community bulletin boards, and neighborhood newspapers. They often have listings of people looking for work as home care assistants. The best source of help is usually word of mouth. It is great to get a recommendation from someone who has worked for a friend or relative. Putting the word out through your family and social network may lead you to that jewel of a person.

Home sharing can also be a solution. If you have space, you can offer a home to someone in exchange for help. This works best if the help needed consists mainly of household and garden chores. Some people, however, may be willing to provide care such as running errands, helping with dressing, bathing, and meal preparation. Some communities have agencies or local government bureaus that help match up home sharers and home seekers.

Again, remember every county in the United States has an Area Agency on Aging that can help. In Canada, every province and territory has an agency that offers resources for seniors. You can find caregiver resources by province and territory online by visiting The Canadian Centre for Caregiving Excellence.

Adult Day Care

Not all help needs to be provided in your home. There are many adult day care centers throughout the country. These often provide transportation and are sometimes partially financed by government programs. For example, your care partner could attend an adult day care center for a half or full day one or more days a week. These centers provide activities, including exercise and socialization. They can typically address the needs of adults who require continuing supervision, such as those with dementia. In addition to providing the caregiver with some much-needed respite, these centers offer your care partner an opportunity to socialize and learn new skills.

One word of caution, though. Your care partner may not want to go to such a center. It is a new and unknown experience that does not include you. Therefore, before bringing this option up with your care partner, talk with the center director or social worker about how to handle this discussion with them. Remember that your care partner's mental functioning may have changed due to their condition. They might not be able to be an equal partner in decision-making or they might not be able to make rational decisions. For you, this could be a very difficult decision to make. It may be another reminder to you that things are not as they used to be, and you may feel guilt, grief, and loss. These are normal feelings but can be challenging for you to deal with at the same time.

Caring.com has information about this option as well.

Moving to a New Residence

The time may come when your care partner needs to move to a new residence. This may be due to your care partner's declining health or because of your own health needs. It might be because you find it too difficult to care for your care partner as you think you should. Perhaps you've reached the end of your physical or emotional energy. Whatever the reason, caregivers often feel guilty about this. Sometimes your care partner is upset about leaving familiar surroundings and will let you know, potentially adding to the guilt. Again, these feelings are normal. To manage these emotions and thoughts, remember to adapt how you think about the situation as discussed in Chapter 4, Dealing with Difficult Emotions (see page xxx). Rather than dwelling on the negatives, recognize that your care partner will receive better care and that you will be able to take better care of yourself as well.

This is a difficult decision to make regardless of the reason, and the decision-making tool discussed in Chapter 2, Becoming a Better Caregiver: The Basics, can help you with this process. Once you make the decision, you can then begin to look for the type of community that provides the care your care partner needs. The following are the different types of residences.

- **Independent living senior communities.** If either you or your care partner is a senior (usually over 50), this option is open to you. These may be owned or rental units that provide a more protected setting with security and emergency response services. These communities usually offer meals in a dining room and weekly housekeeping. They sometimes also offer laundry service and transportation. They often host a variety of activities and field trips. This kind of community is an option if you no longer want to cook and clean but do want to be around others every day. These communities usually do not offer personal assistance to you or your care partner.

  There are almost always waiting lists for this type of community, often even before they are built and ready for occupancy. If you think such a place would be right for you, get on a waiting list right away, or at least a couple of years before you think you plan to move. You can always change your mind or decline if you are not ready when a space is offered. To find these communities in your area, call your senior center or search the internet for senior independent living or retirement communities near you. If you have friends living in any of these nearby communities, ask to be invited for a visit and meal. This will help you get a better idea of what they are like before you decide. Some communities may even have guest accommodations where you can arrange to stay for a night or two before you commit to a lease or contract.
- **Assisted living residences.** An assisted living residence usually offers all the services that independent living residences do plus some personal care assistance and/or help with taking medication. Personal care assistance typically includes help with daily living tasks such as showering and dressing. However, your care partner must be able to get to the bathroom, in and out of bed, and to the common dining room on their own. You can choose to live with your care partner in assisted living, but you may have to eventually move out if your care partner must move to a skilled nursing facility or dies.
- **Skilled nursing facilities (SNF).** Sometimes called "nursing homes," "convalescent hospitals," or "long-term care facilities," a skilled nursing facility provides the most complete care for severely ill or disabled people. These facilities provide medically related care for people who can no longer function without such care. This means that there may be medications to be administered by injection or intravenously or monitored by professional nursing staff. The patient is

In Canada, senior housing costs and programs vary by province and territory. There are different laws governing the operation of some types of housing and differences in access to subsidized units for low-income seniors.

Here are the three major types of seniors' housing in Canada:

1. Independent living means that a person is looking after themselves in their own place. They might hire someone for household tasks or pay for a meal delivery service. Some provinces and territories have programs, benefits, or tax credits for seniors who are making changes to their homes to make them more accessible so they can remain in their homes.
2. Supportive housing/assisted living/retirement home is a large housing category that goes by different names. The common feature is that residents have support services as part of their housing, ranging from meals, assistance with bathing, to an on-call nurse. Facilities are owned and operated by for-profit companies; not-for-profit organizations, such as service clubs or churches; and by the government. Some provinces and territories provide government support to make this more affordable for low-income seniors. For-profit retirement homes are not subsidized in many provinces and residents fully cover the cost of housing and any additional services at rates set by providers.
3. Long-term care/nursing home is a type of housing usually for people who need high levels of ongoing personal or medical care because of a chronic health condition or disability. They may need to be assessed by their doctor or other health care provider to get access.

How Much Does Housing Cost?

There is a wide range in costs. Differences in cost come from the different types and levels of services offered. Prices vary depending on where you are in Canada, from a subsidized spot for under CAN$1000 a month to a private retirement home with services costing more than CAN$10,000 per month.

usually very physically limited, needing help getting in and out of bed, eating, bathing, or dealing with bladder and bowel control. Skilled nursing facilities can also manage the care of feeding tubes, respirators, or other higher-tech equipment. A person who has had a stroke or a hip replacement may be transferred from the acute care hospital to a skilled nursing facility for rehabilitation before going home.

Many people have negative feelings about skilled nursing facilities. You might have read or heard negative stories. Unfortunately, these reports and stories help to create anxiety and fear. There are organizations that monitor local skilled nursing facilities. Also, each facility is required by law to post in a noticeable place the name and phone number of the ombudsman, a person assigned by the state licensing agency to assist patients and their families with problems related to their care. In Canada, provincial ministries of health monitor all care facilities. You may want to visit several facilities to see all the options. Although some of these stories may be true, all the excellent care received in skilled nursing facilities never makes the news.

Skilled nursing facilities provide a type of care and facilities that you may not be able to provide or afford in your current living situations. However, not all nursing homes provide all types of care. Some specialize in rehabilitation, others in long-term custodial care, and others provide memory and dementia care. Some provide high-tech nursing and others do not. Skilled nursing facilities have doctors, nurses, physical therapists, social workers, psychologists, occupational therapists, and nutritionists available on site. If your care partner must have 24-hour care from a professional staff, skilled nursing is usually the best option.

When you are searching for a facility, ask friends, senior center social workers, and hospital discharge planners about good facilities in your area. Do your research. Tour the facility, ask questions, visit again, and look around more closely. Visit during a busy time such as mealtime or a shift change. Is everything clean? How does it smell? How many beds are in each room? Is there space to do more than just sleep in the bedrooms? Is everyone in bed, or do you see residents in common areas or outside on the patio? Does the staff seem happy? What is the facility's rating on the Five-Star Medicare Quality Rating System? To learn more out your options, try contacting a local nursing-home ombudsman. Every state has ombudsmen to investigate residents' concerns and some help families evaluate facilities. Websites that offer directories and ratings of nursing homes can be found in the resources listed at the URL address at the end of this chapter.

Skilled nursing care can be expensive. Explore options for financial assistance and find out the facility's policy on taking Medicaid if your care partner's money runs out. If you or your care partner is a veteran, you may qualify for care and assistance funds from the Veterans Administration.

- **Continuing care retirement communities (CCRC).** These facilities offer all three types of services mentioned already (independent living, assisted living, and skilled nursing) at one site. The advantage of these communities is that if you and your care partner need different levels of care, the facility can accommodate both of you. Another advantage is that should the care needs of you or your care partner change, you can remain in the same facility.
- **Residential or board-and-care homes.** Board and care homes are licensed by the state or the county social services agency. Residential care homes are also known as assisted living in Canada. These are usually small homes in residential areas that provide non-medical care and supervision for individuals that cannot live alone. Homes have about six residents who live in a family-like setting. Each person usually has a private room, but residents eat together. The larger homes may have more residents who live in a boarding-house or hotel-like setting.

These residential homes offer personal care, meals, housekeeping, and sometimes transportation. They differ from assisted living in that they do not offer the wider range of other activities. The larger board and care homes have more staff and may offer some other types of planned activities. Residents in larger facilities usually need to be more independent because they will not receive as much personal attention as in the smaller homes.

In most states, these homes are licensed for either "elderly" (over 62) or "adult" (under 62). The adult category is further divided into facilities for those with mental illness, developmental disabilities, and physical disabilities. When considering a residential or board-and-care home, be sure to evaluate the type of residents already living there to make sure they have conditions and needs similar to your care partner. Checking on the license status of a residential home is advisable. Some might not be licensed and therefore not regulated.

Although all homes are required to provide healthy meals, make sure that the food is to your care partner's liking and can meet their nutrition and health needs.

The monthly fees for residential care homes vary, depending on whether they are simple or more luxurious. The simpler facilities cost about the same as the government Supplemental Security Income (SSI) benefit and will accept SSI beneficiaries, billing the government directly. The more luxurious the home is, with respect to furnishings, neighborhood, and services, the greater the cost. However, even the nicest of these typically cost less than full-time, 24-hour, 7-days per week at-home care. In Canada, costs vary from province to province. Government subsidies may be available depending on your income.

Whatever options you consider for your care partner, this requires a lot of thought and research. It's a big decision. Use the decision-making tools on pages xxx–xxx and consider holding a family meeting to discuss this with and get ideas and help from close family members and friends.

For a complete list of suggested further readings, useful websites, and other helpful resources, please see: www.bullpub.com/resources.

Chapter 8

Preventing Injuries

No one wants to have an accident or an injury. Studies have shown that the risk of injury is higher for caregivers and care partners. As a caregiver, you might be able to imagine reasons for this:

- You may be exhausted and worried about your care partner and trip on a throw rug because you were distracted.
- You may be rushing to leave for a medical appointment and twist your knee or back when helping your care partner get up from a chair.
- You may have let your routines for self-care and relaxation go by the wayside because of limited time and notice you feel down and distracted during caregiving and miss a chance to prevent a care partner fall.
- You may have experienced other challenges that make taking care of yourself and preventing injuries difficult to attend to in your busy caregiver life.

In this chapter, we teach you about your injury risks and offer specific ideas to reduce them. By paying attention to risks and making small changes, you can reduce the chance of injuries. The focus in this chapter is on the caregiver, but we do not ignore potential care partner injuries. If you have previously experienced injury as a caregiver, this chapter may help reduce future risk.

Understanding the Injury Cycle

The injury cycle (Figure 8.1) illustrates factors that can increase the risk of injuries for caregivers. These include physical and emotional care burden/fatigue, poor body mechanics, being out of condition (decrease in physical abilities), and unsafe surroundings. The following are some examples of each factor.

- Physical and emotional care burden/fatigue. When you are tired or feeling overwhelmed, your reaction time might be slower. When you reach out to guide your care partner into the car, both of you end up injured.
- Poor body mechanics. When you repeatedly bend at the waist and twist your body to help your care partner get out of bed, it is common to develop pain in your back or legs.
- Being out of condition (decrease in physical abilities). Being less active because of caregiving demands can result in decreased strength and balance. Similarly, changes in your hearing or vision can increase injury and fall risk.
- Unsafe surroundings. Clutter or cords stretched across the floor can create unsafe surroundings making it easy to trip or fall.

Each factor of the cycle can be related to or influence other parts of the cycle. If your body is out of condition and weak, your posture is likely poor, and it will take more effort to do the daily caregiving tasks. If you are tired, you are less likely to notice hazards in your surroundings. All these factors may lead to strains,

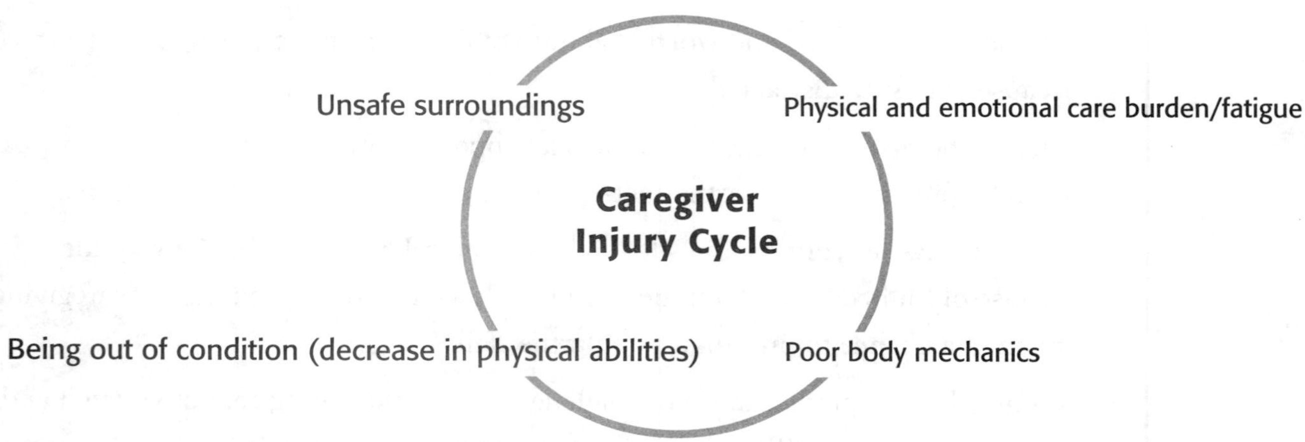

Figure 8.1 **Caregiver Injury Cycle**

sprains, and pain. As you can see, this cycle feeds on itself.

In the next section, we discuss injury prevention tools in detail so you can use them as a daily part of your caregiving activities. Not all injuries can be prevented. However, the rate and severity of injury can be dramatically reduced. There are tools you can use to break the injury cycle. In the Injury Risk Assessment Exercise on page 122, you can ask yourself the list of questions to determine your risks of injury. You will notice that the prevention tools listed in the last column overlap and often address more than one type of injury risk.

Reducing Injury Risk

To reduce your risk of injury, start by taking the following risk assessment on page 122. it will highlight your risks, what might happen, and what you can do to lower your injury risk. Knowing your risks, you can start using the following toolkit below. We discuss each of the tools in detail in the material that follows.

Exercising and Being Physically Active to Address Physical Changes

You might have physical limitations due to illness, chronic health conditions, and/or aging. These limitations can affect your safety and increase your injury risks. We all know that exercising is good for you. However, finding the time and energy to exercise can be a challenge. Caregiving can be demanding. When faced with caregiver responsibilities, even regular exercisers may stop their programs and non-exercisers might find it hard to start a program. It is important to know, however, that just thirty minutes of exercise two or three times a week can make

Toolkit for Reducing Injury Risk

- Exercise.
- Use proper body mechanics during caregiving activities.
- Emphasize your own self care needs.
- Build calm and positive connection with care partner.
- Use mindful movement approaches.
- Modify home and surroundings.
- Use special equipment.
- Seek health professional guidance.

Injury Risk Assessment Exercise

If you answered yes to the questions here . . .	Your injury risk is . . .	And these are prevention tools to reduce your injury risk:
◆ Are you edgy and short-tempered with your care partner due to fatigue and exhaustion? ◆ Do you have difficulty making enough time to care for yourself? ◆ Are you feeling down or depressed?	Physical and emotional care burden and fatigue	◆ Meet own physical and emotional needs. ◆ Promote calm and positive connections. ◆ Stay attentive and focused. ◆ Use proper body mechanics. ◆ Modify your home and surroundings. ◆ Use special equipment. ◆ Seek health professional guidance. ◆ Exercise. ◆ Ask for specific help from friends and family.
◆ Do you frequently get into awkward positions and experience body pain during caregiving activities? ◆ Do you do over 50% of the lifting during transfers with your care partner?	Poor body mechanics	◆ Exercise. ◆ Use proper body mechanics. ◆ Use special equipment. ◆ Modify home and surroundings. ◆ Seek health professional guidance. ◆ Promote calm and positive connections. ◆ Stay attentive and focused.
◆ Are you afraid of falling? ◆ Have you noticed changes in your vision or hearing? ◆ Do you use your hands to push up from a chair? ◆ Do you take medications that increase your risk of a fall?	Being out of condition (decrease in physical abilities)	◆ Exercise. ◆ Modify your home and surroundings. ◆ Consider an evaluation by a physical therapist to get a "body tune up" even if you have not had an injury. ◆ Seek health professional guidance. ◆ Use proper body mechanics.
◆ Are there hazards and clutter in your home that increase risk of fall or injury? ◆ Do you have furniture that is too low, too soft, or without arms? ◆ Do you frequently wear slippers and shoes with no backs? ◆ Do you think your care partner uses a cane or walker improperly?	Unsafe surroundings	◆ Use special equipment. ◆ Modify your home and surroundings. ◆ Seek health professional guidance. ◆ Consider a home safety evaluation by an occupational therapist. ◆ Promote calm and positive connections.

a big difference in your physical abilities and health as a caregiver. In Chapter 9, Exercising for Health and Wellness, we explain the importance of physical activity in increasing energy, managing stress, improving fitness, and controlling chronic health conditions. Some people are afraid that exercise will cause injury. The truth is that the risks associated with inactivity are greater than the risks of injury during exercise.

Exercising to Reduce Body Pain and the Risk of Injury

Building flexibility, strength, and endurance reduces back injury and body pain. Back pain is more common among people who are not physically fit. When you bend and reach, it puts you at further risk for increased back pain. And if your care partner is overweight, there is an even greater risk for pain and musculoskeletal discomfort for both the care partner and their caregiver.

If your care partner gets stuck coming to stand, you might be required to grip hard with both hands and hold on tight, keeping your forearm muscles contracted, to keep your care partner from falling. Over time, gripping tight and holding muscles in a contraction can result in shortening of the muscles of your wrist at your forearm (near your elbow), and you may get into this position or similar ones repeatedly. Short muscles put tension on ligaments and tendons and result in immediate or eventual pain. The pain can feel like a severe muscle cramp. Flexibility, strength, and endurance exercises are described in detail in Chapter 9, Exercising for Health and Wellness. Specific exercises to reduce injury risk are listed in Table 8.1 and shown in Chapter 9.

Exercising to Reduce the Risk of Falls

Researchers have found that exercise to improve strength and balance is the most effective strategy to reduce risk of falls for you and your care partner. As people age, they have less coordination, flexibility, strength, and balance, and reaction time diminishes. This is often due to inactivity. At any age, exercise can improve all of these.

One of the biggest risks for falls is muscle weakness. Stiff, weak muscles limit motion and increase the risk of strain or pain. You can increase your stability by building strength in your muscles around the hips, knees, and ankles. See Table 8.1, Exercises to Reduce Injury Risk, on page 124 for specific exercises to build strength. Walking is often included as part of a fall-risk reduction program to improve endurance but walking alone won't reduce fall risk. See Table 8.1 for balance exercises to add to your plan such as heel and toe walking. If you have poor balance, you can easily fall while exercising. As you practice these exercises, be sure you have support, such as a chair, kitchen counter, or table.

In Table 8.1, there are twenty-nine exercises to improve flexibility, strength, and balance to reduce injury risk. If you are looking for general injury prevention, select exercises from all three areas. Tailor your program to your own needs. Try two or three and assess how you feel. You can also use this list to determine if group exercise programs you participate in include exercises that have the potential to reduce your injury risk. You will know the exercises or physical activities are making a difference if you can do more repetitions, use less support, and continue for longer with fewer rest breaks.

You can also work on your strength and balance, by repeating a difficult daily task, such as getting up from a chair or climbing stairs. Repeatedly doing chair squats or chair rises by coming from sitting to standing without using your arms can improve your fitness. Walking and stair climbing can also improve with practice. Leisure activities such as tai chi, yoga, dancing, and gardening can improve physical fitness too. Make sure to tune in to your posture, your balance, and how you feel during daily tasks for safety and success.

If you have a history of body pain or falls, it is best to speak with your health care provider before you start any exercise program. You may want to consult with a physical or occupational therapist. Physical therapists can create and supervise an exercise program and help you carry it out correctly. If you have injuries or pain related to smaller muscles, such as arm and hand, occupational therapists similarly can create and supervise your exercise program.

Exercise Programs

We know it may be hard to get out of the house, but you might prefer a group exercise program to exercising on your own. The good news is that many of these can now be taken virtually using Zoom or a similar video meeting program. A Matter of Balance; Stepping On; Stay Active and Independent for Life (SAIL); Tai Chi for Arthritis; Tai Ji Quan: Moving for Better Balance; and The Otago Exercise Program are group programs researched and found effective in reducing risk of falls. Community-based organizations in most US states, as well as in Canada, Australia, and other countries offer these programs. To find a program, contact your

Table 8.1 **Exercises to Reduce Injury Risk**
(The page numbers in this table refer to detailed descriptions of these exercises that you can find in Chapter 9, Exercising for Health and Wellness.)

Flexibility	
Back and Neck	
Heads up	p. 143
Neck stretch	p. 144
Cat and cow pose in seated position	p. 144–145
Knee-to-chest stretch	p. 145
Pelvic tilt	p. 145
Back lift	p. 145
Low-back rock and roll	p. 146
Arms and Legs	
Pat and reach	p. 146
Shoulder shape-up	p. 146
Good morning (with wrist stretch down and wrist stretch up)	p. 147
Hamstring stretch	p. 147–149
Achilles stretch	p. 148
Better posture	
Shoulder-blade pinch	p. 148–149
Curl-up	p. 149
Roll-out	p. 149
Leg strength	
Straight-leg raises	p. 150
Back kick	p. 150
Hip hooray	p. 150
Knee strengthener	p. 151
Power knees	p. 151
Ready-go	p. 151
Tiptoes	p. 151–152
Sit-to-stand	p. 152
Balance	
Beginning balance	p. 153
Swing and sway	p. 153
Toe walk	p. 154
Heel walk	p. 154
One-legged stand	p. 154
Walk-the-line	p. 154–155

local senior center or Area Agency on Aging. In Canada, you can call 211. (Please note that most Canadian-specific content is shaded throughout the book.)

Using Proper Body Mechanics During Caregiving Activities

Your care partner may have difficulty moving. This can come on slowly. For example, it could begin with your care partner just needing more help to get dressed. Or it can come on suddenly, and all at once your care partner needs help with everything. The amount of help your care partner needs might be the same every day or it might vary day-to-day. One of the most familiar challenges for care partners is changing positions, such as getting on and off the toilet or getting in and out of bed. These position changes are called *transfers*.

If you help your care partner transfer out of bed, without attention to your body position, your back is likely to twist in an unnatural direction. You might not be in this twisted position for much time, but you might be doing it multiple times a day or week. Often caregivers sacrifice their own bodies to keep their care partners safe. The way you move while you are helping your care partner transfer or get up can not only hurt you (resulting in back pain, falls, or muscle pain), but it can also hurt your care partners. If you are not stable, your care partner might fall. Helping your care partner manage daily activities requires teamwork. In this way, it is much like dancing. To prevent injury to both you and your care partner, establish ways to help your care partner that are consistent, safe, and efficient. The following sections on posture and body mechanics and care partner transfers can lead you in the right direction.

Practicing Good Posture and Body Mechanics

Good posture and body mechanics will reduce the risk of pain and injury. Good posture strengthens your body, but only if you make it a habit. Paying attention to how you use your body is especially important during transfers. This is the time when you or your care partner are likely to twist, get into awkward positions, and lose your balance.

Proper posture involves maintaining the three natural curves in the spine at the neck, upper back, and lower back. When these curves are maintained, the spine is the strongest. The natural curves help the body absorb the "shock of movement" and the strain of holding positions with the least strain. Proper posture also requires that all body parts are in alignment. Proper alignment prevents strain on muscles, ligaments, tendons, and joints. Figures 8.2–8.4 illustrate good sitting and standing posture.

Good standing posture is characterized by the following:

- Ears over shoulders
- Shoulders over hips (shoulders even and relaxed)
- Hips over knees
- Knees over feet (knees straight but not locked)
- Feet shoulder-width apart (even weight on both feet)

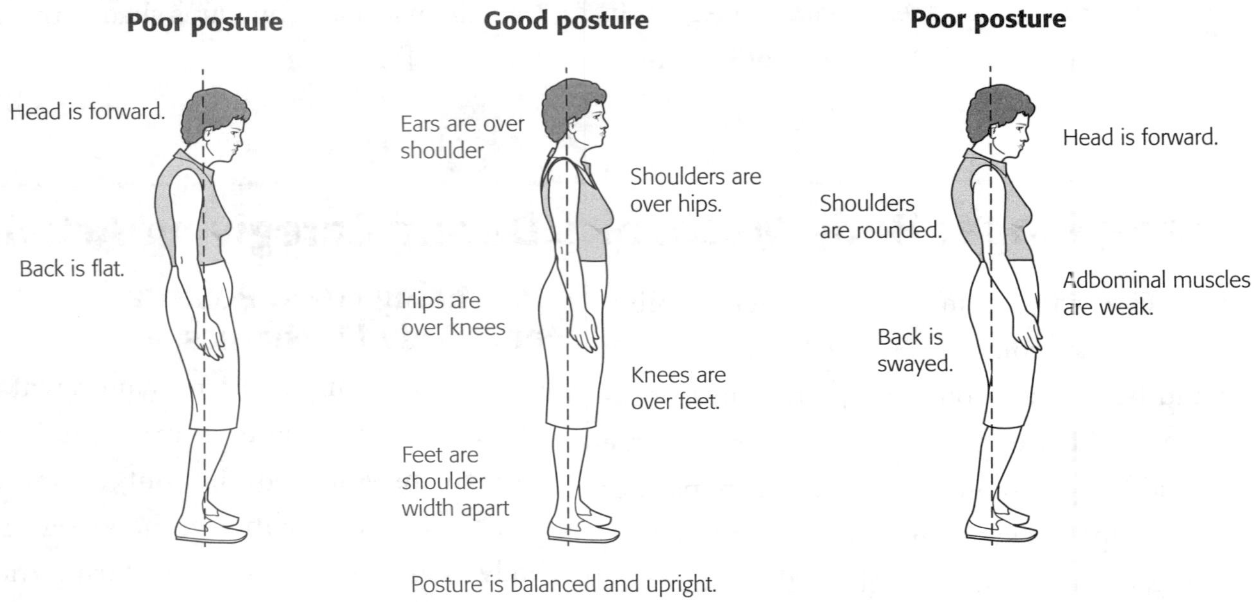

Figure 8.2 **Standing Posture**

If you have upper back or shoulder pain, even when you are not moving or assisting your care partner, think about what else might be causing it. For example, many people experience pain that stems from poor posture while using a computer. Compare your posture to the suggestions in Figure 8.4 and consider making a change to improve your posture.

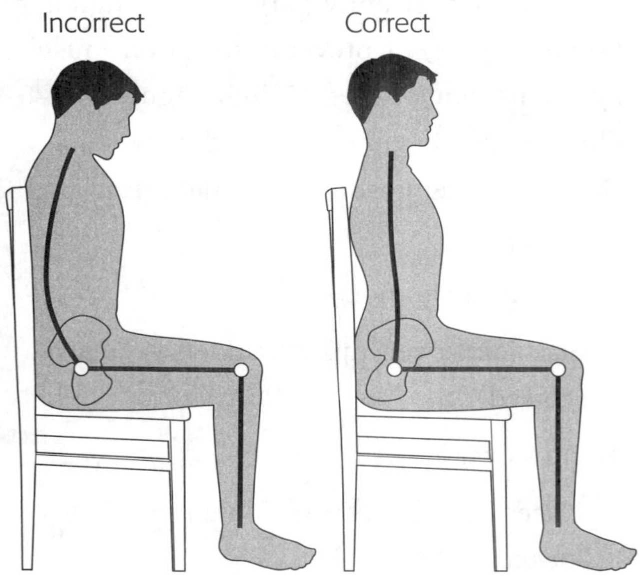

Good sitting posture is characterized by the following:

- Ears over shoulders
- Shoulders relaxed but not elevated
- Upper back relaxed and over hips
- Hips bent 90 degrees
- Knees bent 90 degrees
- Buttocks flat on seat with even weight on both hips
- Feet flat on floor or foot rest

Figure 8.3 **Sitting Posture**

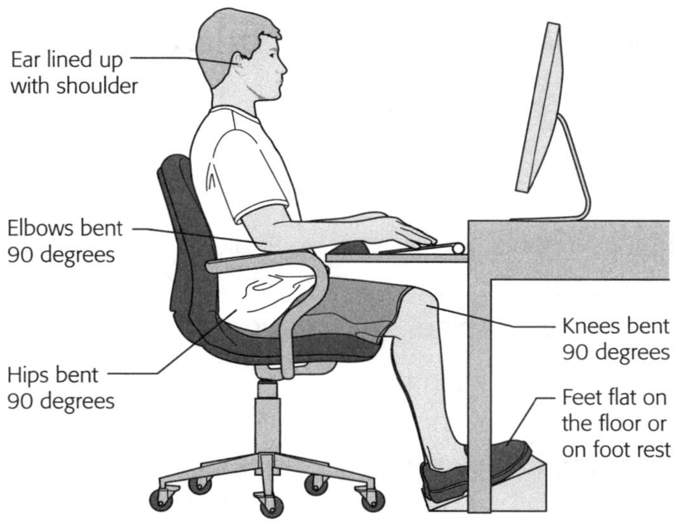

Figure 8.4 **Good Sitting Posture for Computer Use**

Using Recommended Transfer Posture

Encourage your care partner to actively participate, even if this takes more time. Use the tips discussed in the previous section to protect your back and limbs. If your care partner cannot help and needs a total assist, get help or use equipment. Do not try to lift your care partner by yourself.

In this section, we illustrate transfers for getting in and out of a chair or bed and getting up from the floor. Carefully review the complete instructions before practicing with your care partner.

First, we list general tips and then we explain specific transfers.

Adjust the instructions so that you and your care partner feel safe, steady, and balanced. If these instructions do not work for you, consult an occupational or physical therapist.

Moving from Sitting in an Arm Chair to Standing

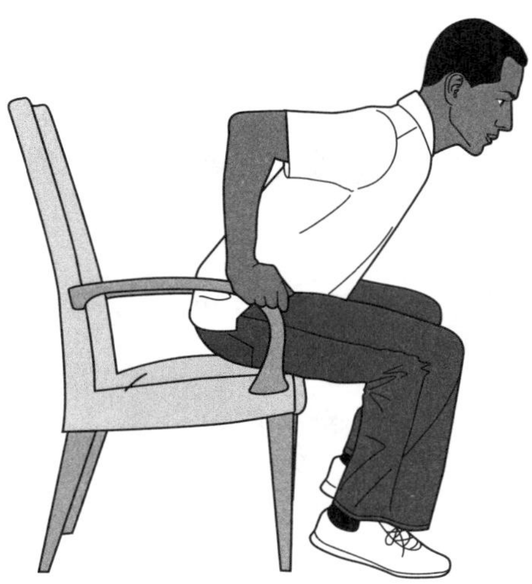

1. Ask your care partner to slide their hips forward to sit near the front half of the chair. If your care partner has trouble scooting forward, ask them to lean to one side to slide the opposite hip forward and repeat with the other side and hip.
2. Make sure care partner's feet are on floor (making a 90-degree angle with knees).
3. Ask your care partner to lean forward (nose over toes).
4. Ask your care partner to push from chair arms to come to a standing position. (If assistance is needed, consider using a gait belt; see Table 8.2 on pages 138–140.)

Body Mechanics for Daily Caregiving Activities

Good body mechanics involve using good posture when helping your care partner with activities such as getting dressed, taking a shower, or changing position. The following tips can protect your back and limbs:

- Bend your knees and hinge (bend) at the hips if you need to lean forward. Do not bend at the waist as it strains your spine.
- Use equipment or change your position to avoid awkward body posture. For example, consider sitting on a low stool to help your care partner put on shoes or socks. Use a long-handled sponge to reduce bending and twisting while helping your care partner shower.
- Reduce twisting, especially bending forward and twisting. One helpful trick is to think of your belt buckle or imagine one. Keep your belt buckle and your feet pointing in the same direction.
- Avoid assisting your care partner with your arms outstretched. Make sure you are close to the bed when you assist your care partner with transfers.
- Make sure both you and your care partner feel steady. Place your legs about hip distance apart with one foot a few inches further forward than the other.
- Gently tighten and lift your stomach muscles to support your spine.
- Use a gait belt (see Table 8.2 on page 138) to increase safety as needed.

Incorrect

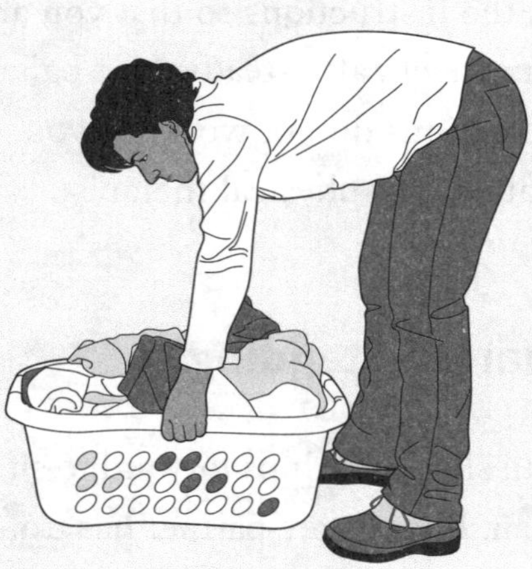

Do not bend at the waist.

Correct

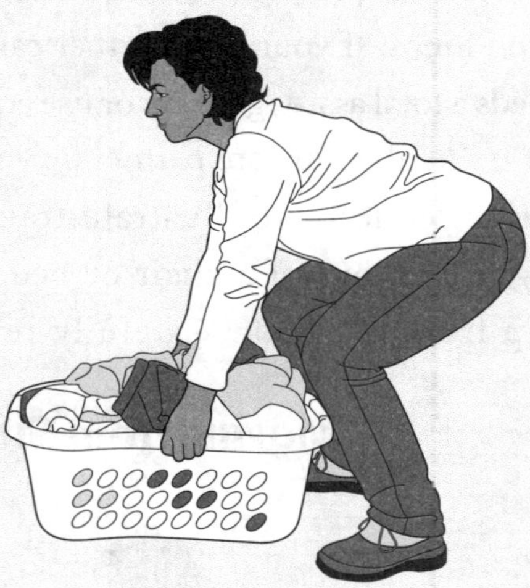

Protect your back by bending your knees and bending at your hips.

Getting into Bed

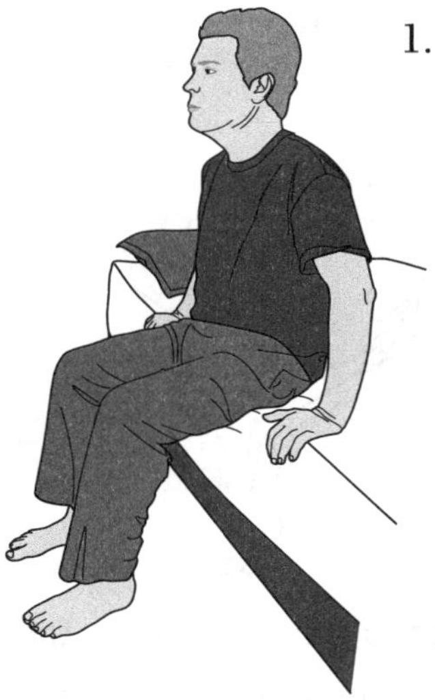

1. Ask your care partner to sit on the bed about a foot below the pillow.

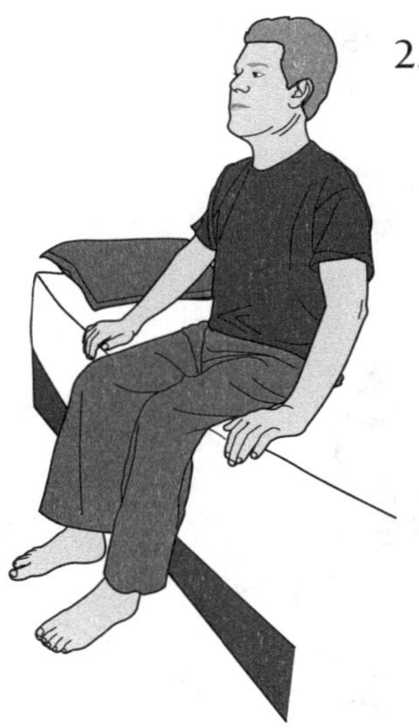

2. If needed, ask care partner to not sit on the very edge of bed (or assist care partner to move away from edge). The backs of your care partner's knees should be touching the mattress..

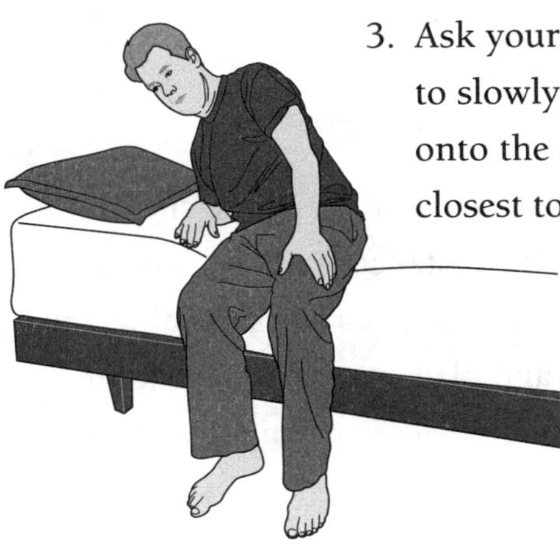

3. Ask your care partner to slowly lower body onto the arm that is closest to the pillow.

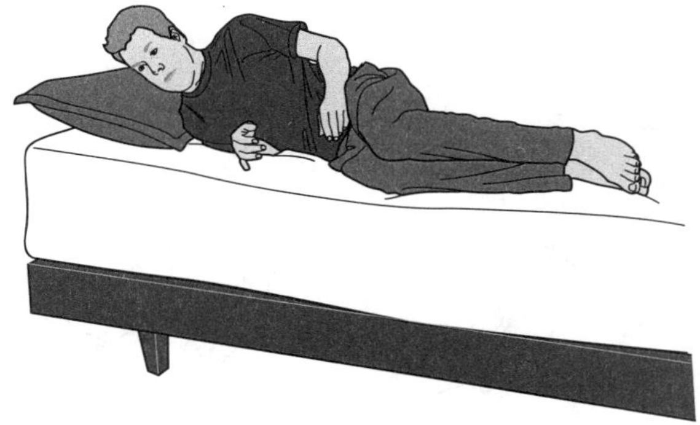

4. Ideally, at the same time, ask your care partner to bend knees and pull them onto the bed. (If assistance is needed, guide your care partner's legs into the bed, keeping knees bent.)

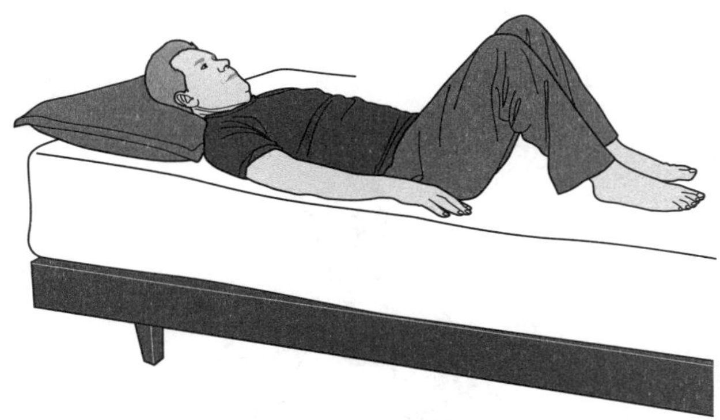

5. Ask care partner to roll onto back.

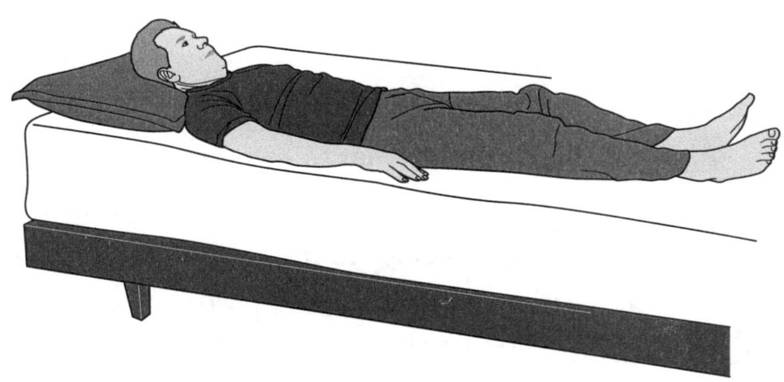

6. Encourage care partner to relax legs and get comfortable.

Getting out of Bed

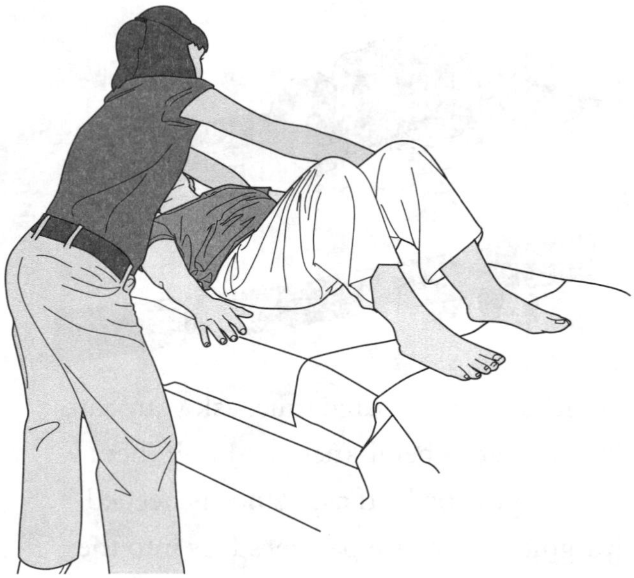

1. Ask care partner to bend knees while lying on back (or bend knees for them).

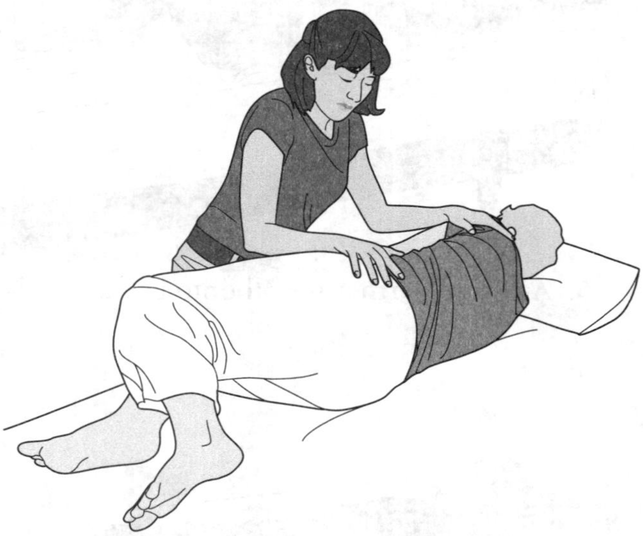

2. Ask your care partner to roll toward you as you stand at the side of bed. (If assistance is needed, get as close to the bed as possible and gently guide your care partner with one hand on their shoulder and the other on their hip. Make sure care partner does not roll onto their hands.)

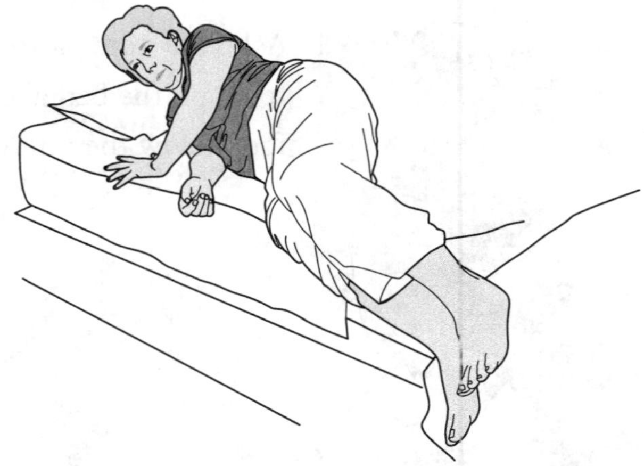

3. Ask your care partner to move feet over the edge of the bed while pushing up onto one elbow. (If assistance needed, guide care partner's feet over the edge.)

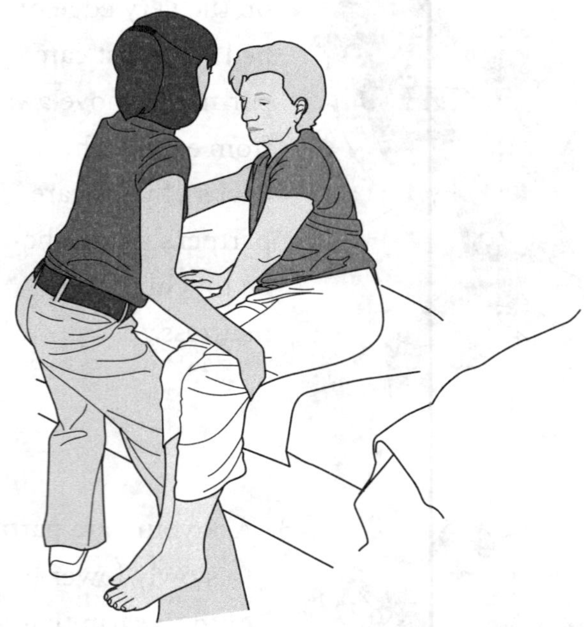

4. Ask care partner to move to the sitting position. (If assistance is needed and you are able, cradle care partner's shoulders in one hand and place your other hand on their hip to guide care partner up to sitting position.)

Trouble Shooting Tip for Transfers

- Sometimes one side of the bed is easier than the other.
- Consider installing a safety rail on the side of the bed to help with pushing up.
- If using an assistive device (for example, a walker or a cane), push up from a steady, permanent surface rather than the device, as it is safer.
- **DO NOT LIFT** care partners even if they are small enough to make this possible.
- If you find yourself bending at the waist during transfers, consider changing your partner to a bed that is height adjustable or a hospital bed.
- To view videos of transfers, search online sources such as YouTube. Look for videos from physical therapy practices, medical institutions, and patient education websites. Use search terms such as "safe patient transfer techniques," "wheelchair transfer demonstration," or "transferring a person with limited mobility."

Getting up from the Floor

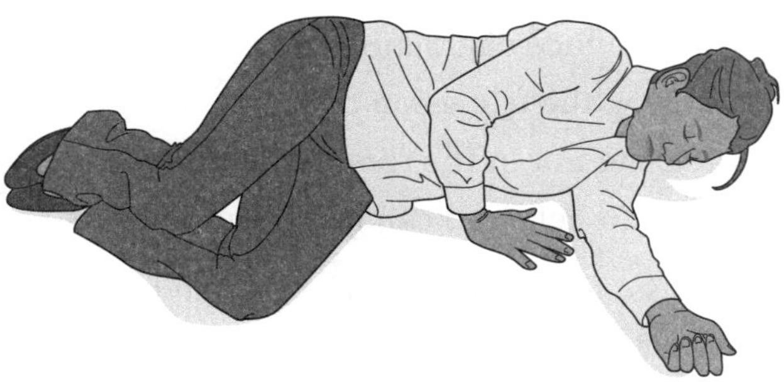

1. Roll onto one side.

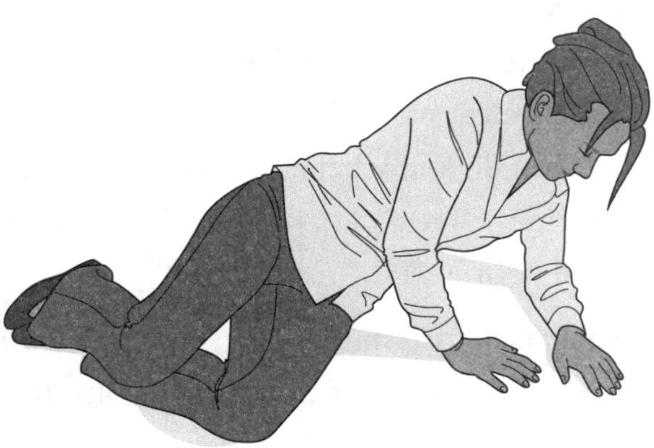

2. Push up with upper hand enough to get lower elbow under the body.

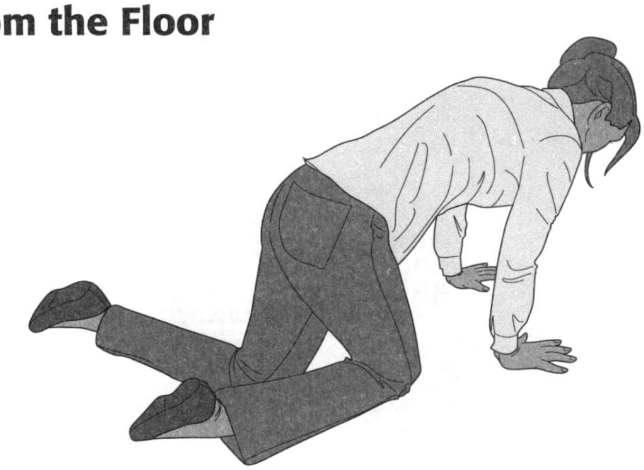

3. Tuck knees under the body and roll to all fours.

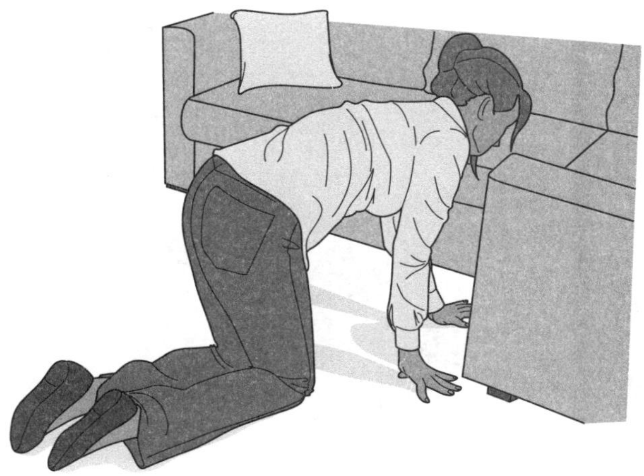

4. Crawl toward the bed or a sturdy chair.

Continues ▶

Getting up from the Floor

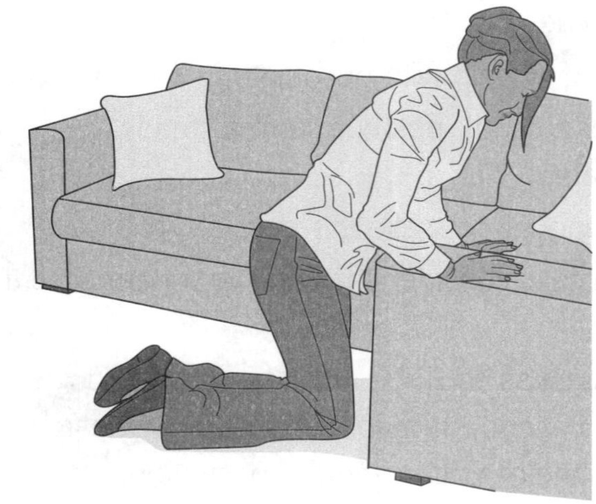

5. Place hands on sturdy surface (chair or bed).

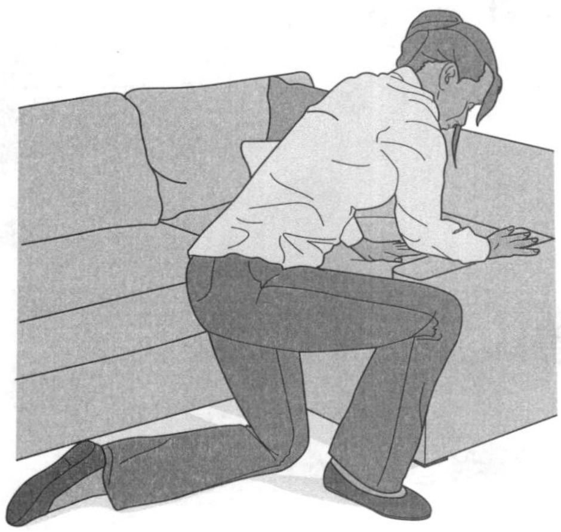

6. Bend stronger leg and put the foot of that leg flat on the floor.

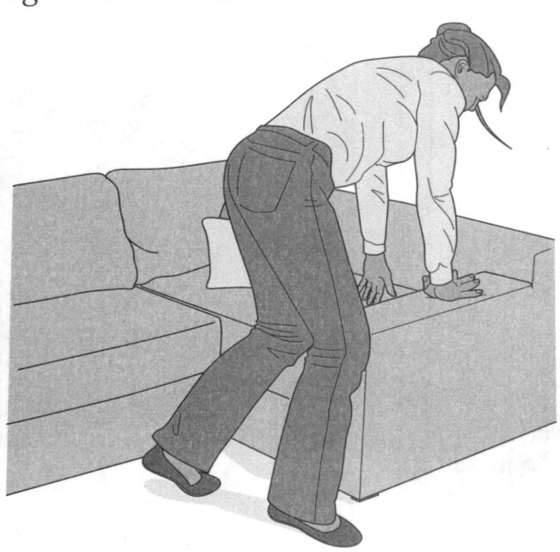

7. Push up to standing position.

Staying Safe During Transfers and Daily Activities

Preparation, communication, and moving with teamwork is a three-step strategy for assisting your care partner. This strategy can be applied to transfers and other difficult daily tasks, such as dressing or bathing.

Step 1. Prepare

- *Stress assessment.* How calm are you? What is your and your care partner's state of mind? Consider using mindful breathing (see Chapter 5, Using Your Mind to Manage Stress) and take a few breaths prior to each transfer. Or use another mindfulness tool to check in and manage your stress level. Ask your care partner to take a few deep breaths too. Reduce distractions by turning off or muting the television or music. It is best if pets are not in the room. They sometimes want to help and can get in the way.
- *Assistance assessment.* How much help do you and your care partner need? If it has been a bad day due to illness or mood, you or your care partner may need more assistance. If two people are required for the transfer, have a plan so that neither person is injured. Think ahead about the task and have a clear picture of what your care partner can do and what assistance you need to provide. Have a plan in place for when you need help.
- *Equipment assessment.* What equipment will you need today? We discuss gait belts, transfer boards, and mobility aids later in this chapter (see Table 8.3 on pages 141–144). One or all of these could help improve safety and prevent injury.

- *Safety assessment.* What can you do to make your surroundings safer? If your care partner uses a wheelchair, make sure to lock it and swing away or remove the legs before you start. Safe transfers start and end with a stable surface.

Step 2. Communicate and Create Calm

There are many right ways to communicate with your care partner. The important thing is that the two of you work together. It is a dance. Communicating clearly and calmly is always helpful.

- *Be partners.* If possible, be sure your care partner helps. Talk about your ideas and your care partner's ideas. Decide who will give the cues and what each of you will do. You might need to have this discussion only once, or you might have to go over this several times a day. Remember, in most cases, your care partner is trying to do it right.
- *Agree on cues.* Decide on commands. Give quick, clear, simple commands that the two of you have agreed on. Keep them the same every time and make sure all caregivers use them. Too many words and repetition tend to result in confusion and frustration. Consider cues such as "take a breath," "push," "up," or "turn." If you like the recommended transfer postures, consider using shortened versions of those cues.
- *Keep talk to a minimum.* Avoid the urge to repeat the commands too much or too often. During transfers, keep conversation to a minimum. Limit distractions such as television, phone, or music to improve focus.

Step 3. Move with Teamwork

This step is like a complicated dance and requires putting all the steps together.

- *Give direction.* Either you or your care partner needs to state aloud what is being done and what each of you are expected to do. Encourage your care partner to do as

Safely Swinging Away Wheelchair Leg Rests

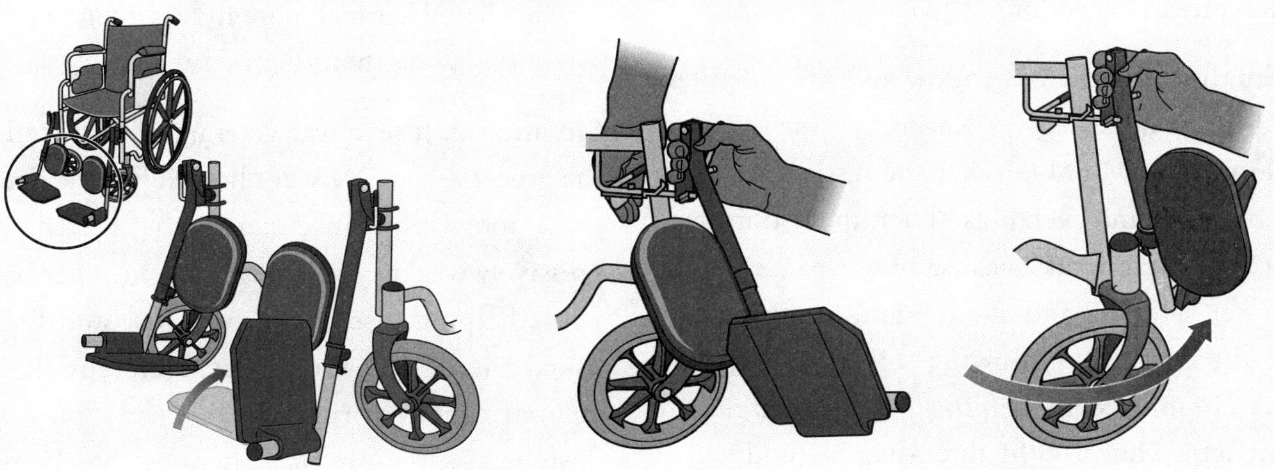

1. Lift foot rest and calf support in the middle so they fold toward the metal leg rest.
2. Lift/release lever at top of leg rest.
3. Swing away or remove leg rest.

much as possible. You will have less to do and your care partner will use their muscles which helps them to maintain muscle strength. Even if you are strong enough to get the job done, repeatedly lifting your care partner increases your risk of injury and your care partner's dependence. Try to work out consistent ways of moving so you both know what to expect. This will decrease frustration and increase efficiency. Do not expect your care partner to remember their "dance steps." Reminders may need to be repeated each time you make a transfer.

- *Tune into your body.* Do a quick body scan to tune into pain or soreness. Small twinges of pain in your back and arms are easily overlooked, but pain can add up. If you have aches or pain, try some stretches or some ice (not more than 20 minutes at a time). You may also find a few deep breaths help prevent the hurry and carelessness that can lead to injury.

The following two examples show the three-step process in action:

Situation 1: Leila is a widow and her daughter, Karina, is her caregiver. Karina became so afraid her mother would fall that she restricted Leila's movement and even picked her up for transfers. Leila became weak because of not participating in her self-care and she fell and was admitted to the hospital. Following this accident, Karina committed to helping her mother regain strength. They use the three-step method.

1. *Preparation:* Before a transfer, Karina takes a few deep breaths to relax and reminds herself that her mother needs to do more. Both agreed to use a gait belt (see Table 8.2 on pages 138–140) so that Karina can help if needed. Leila agreed to use the two-wheeled walker and feels safe after having physical therapy and occupational therapy both at the hospital and for a few times at home.
2. *Communication:* After the fall, Karina expressed her worry and her mother expressed her desire to regain her independence. Together they decided that Karina will stay nearby during transfers, and Leila will use her walker all the time. Both agreed to use the gait belt. Karina agreed to remain quiet unless a command is needed. They turn off the television or put it on mute during transfers. They make sure the dog and the cat are not in the room.
3. *Moving together:* Leila needs assistance with shower transfers and dressing. Karina stands by and remains calm and quiet as Leila transfers herself to a shower chair. Karina pays attention to maintaining her posture and Leila does too. Leila requests assistance while dressing but does most of it herself. This helps her feel more independent as well as strengthens her body.

Situation 2: Jose, a war veteran, recently fell at the grocery store. He went home after the emergency room visit. Since then, he has gotten progressively weaker. His wife, Elena, hurt her back while helping Jose out of bed. Jose and Elena asked the doctor for physical therapy. Jose's commitment to a brief regular exercise program designed by the physical therapist has helped him increase his strength. The physical therapist also taught Jose and Elena to work together for transfers.

1. *Preparation:* Before a transfer, Elena asks Jose how he is doing today. When he says he is feeling tired, she puts on the gait belt (see Table 8.2 on pages 138–140) so she can help him. Jose always keeps his walker near his chair or bed. Elena takes a couple of deep breaths as a cue to remind herself to use good body mechanics and to stay focused.
2. *Communication:* The physical therapist taught Elena to break the transfer into steps because Jose is forgetful. Jose is very agreeable to Elena using cues for each step of the transfer. He reminds her to pay attention to her posture because he doesn't want her to injure her back again.
3. *Moving together:* Elena puts a gait belt on Jose when he feels he needs it. She says: "Slide hips forward," "Feet under knees," "Nose over toes," and "Push up." She is careful to use the body posture position shown in Figure 8.2 on page 126 as it takes strain off her back. After the transfer, she does a quick body scan, and if her back is at all sore, she does a few stretches that the physical therapist gave her.

Meeting Your Self-Care Needs

Caregiving is time consuming and stressful. You might not be meeting your own needs or making time for yourself. You might be edgy or short tempered. Think about your own needs and set priorities. What are the current activities that cause you the most frustration and fatigue? Which activities bring you satisfaction or calm you down? Explore the advice and suggestions offered in this book. Select ideas that appeal to you. Review setting priorities on pages 46–47. Consider trying one or two suggestions in Chapter 5, Using Your Mind to Manage Stress.

Some of the activities to build positive connections and calming experiences described in the following sections may help you meet your own needs while helping your care partner. One caregiver we know has included a daily 15-minute mindful meditation in her schedule. She finds that setting aside this time is possible on most days. The meditation leaves her more refreshed and energized to deal with the many requirements of caregiving. She reports that she is less likely to lose her temper with her care partner and more optimistic about the future.

Asking for Specific Help from Friends and Family

Another way to reduce stress is to ask for help from others. See more about this in Chapter 6, Communicating Effectively, and Chapter 7, Getting Help.

Building Calm and Positive Connections and Experiences

Caregiving comes with many frustrations. Frustration makes daily tasks more challenging. This causes tension and adds to frustration. This, in turn, can increase the risk of an injury.

Remaining calm and connected while still managing the changes in life is not always easy.

Listed below are some options that allow you to relate to your care partner and provide pleasure for both of you:

- **Music creates a mood.** Choose music you both enjoy. Play music that is calming to reduce agitation, or upbeat to promote participation. If your care partner has memory issues, music can be organizing and might enhance positive mood and increase participation in daily activities. Not everyone likes calming music. If your care partner likes Gilbert and Sullivan, marches, pop, or jazz, play those. Select music that will create a positive mood for both of you.
- **Enjoy nature.** Observing nature does not require memory or physical ability. Taking your care partner for a wheelchair walk in the park is an opportunity to be outside. Observing nature can be both stimulating and calming. There are botanic gardens, greenhouses, and garden centers you can visit. Even a care partner with limited memory can participate and enjoy the experience in the moment. If you are confined indoors, ask a friend or family member to put up a bird feeder or birdbath and stock it regularly. The action around a bird feeder viewed through a window can entertain and calm the viewer.
- **Shared activities.** Games offer an opportunity to relate. If your care partner was a game player in the past, choose the games they played then. If games of the past are too hard, try simple games such as Go Fish or Parcheesi. Adult coloring books are another idea for an activity you might be able to do together.
- **Laugh together.** It is easy to get wrapped up in required activity or the frustrations of the day. Make some time to laugh. Maybe you have funny memories you share. Maybe you can read jokes from an online source. Sometimes you can just find the humor in life and laugh about everyday things. Humor is a wonderful outlet for frustration.

Staying Attentive and Focused

Do you find yourself rushing through tasks? Rushing might mean speeding to a doctor's appointment because getting ready took longer than expected, running to answer the phone, or hurrying through your care partner's shower. Rushing can lead to accidents and problems. When you rush, you focus on a future task and it is easy to lose sight of the current task. When you are rushing, you might not notice your care partner's faltering balance or their bumping into furniture until it's too late. You may overlook fall hazards on the floor and trip over something. Rushing can also create a silent tension between you and your care partner.

It is easy to get caught up in thinking about the next thing on your to-do list. Being mindful is the opposite of being rushed or preoccupied. Recall from Chapter 5, Using Your Mind to Manage Stress, that mindfulness is a way of calmly and consciously observing and accepting whatever is happening in that moment of your life. When you are mindful, you can be more present and pay closer attention while doing your daily tasks. To practice being more mindful, consider the following suggestions.

- **Reduce rushing.** One way to reduce rushing is to gain control of predictable tasks and allow extra time to complete them. Start breakfast early if you have an appointment that morning. Try to schedule planned appointments at your care partner's best time of day or a time of day that doesn't require a mad dash for you to make it. Even if rushing is still a problem sometimes, it is a win if you can disrupt the rushing cycle some of the time.

Making Activities Easier and Safer with Special Equipment

Assistive equipment and mobility aids make your job easier while giving more support and safety to your care partner. The important questions to ask and answer are: "What devices are available?" "How do I choose the right one?" and "How do I use the device properly?"

Using Mobility Aids

Mobility aids such as walkers, canes, and wheelchairs are common. If you or your care partner are experiencing any of the following, think about using a mobility aid:

- You or your care partner are touching furniture or steady surfaces as you move around the house.
- One leg is weaker than the other for you or your care partner.
- You or your care partner are unsteady outside of the house or when walking on uneven surfaces.
- You or your care partner have fallen due to poor balance, weakness, or slow reaction times.

Falls of almost any type could signal the need for mobility aids. Not using a mobility aid correctly, or using a wrong or improperly fitted aid, can also lead to falls and injury. If mobility changes, you may need to change aids. If you have any questions about which aid is right for you or how to use it, ask a health care professional, such as a physical therapist, and get proper training. Take a short video with your cell phone during the training so that you remember how to use the mobility aid correctly when you get home.

If you or your partner have not been told to use a walking aid but you feel you or they may need one, review Table 8.3 which lists commonly used mobility aids and tips to prevent injuries. This is general information to get you started and show you a range of options. It does not replace individualized guidance and training from a health professional.

Reducing Caregiver Strain and Effort with Assistive Devices

Assistive devices can decrease caregiver effort. For example, if your care partner can stand up by holding onto a grab bar, it takes less effort from you to keep them upright.

Table 8.2 lists and describes devices that reduce the effort needed to physically support your care partner. You will not need all these devices, and it is not a goal to own all these devices. Select only the devices that allow you to complete tasks with greater ease or that solve a problem that other strategies or tools do not. In addition to the devices listed in Table 8.2, there are many other types of equipment that have the potential to improve your care partner's independence in daily living tasks.

Table 8.2 **Special Equipment**

Device	Purpose	Tips
Gait belt 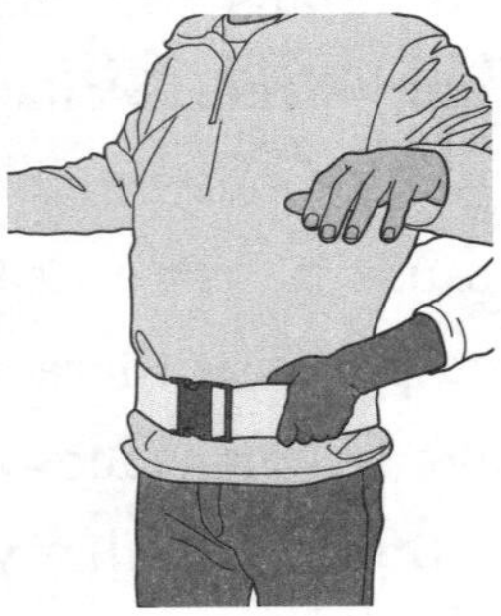	• Assists with transfers and unstable walking • Allows you to grasp the belt in order to assist in transferring or moving a person	• Place the gait belt low around your care partner's waist. • Fasten the belt tight enough so it does not slide but loose enough so you can slip a finger under the belt. • When you put the belt on your partner who is sitting, fasten tighter than you might think is necessary as it will loosen up when you partner becomes more upright.
Mobility bed rail 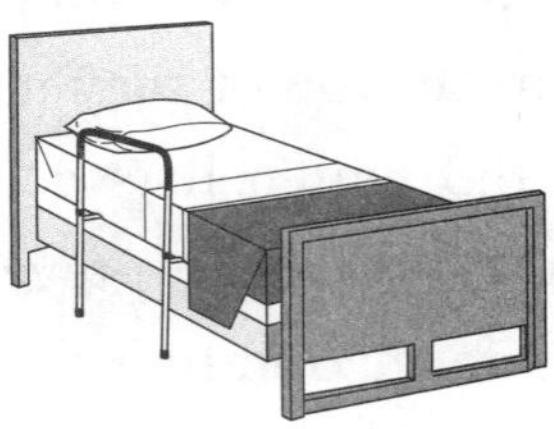	• Helps with sitting up or getting out of bed • Prevents falls from bed • Allows you to exert less effort to sit your care partner up in bed if the care partner has strength in upper extremity	• Place on your care partner's stronger side. • Test that the rail is secure before your care partner grasps it. • May need more than rail if care partner puts excessive weight on the rail. • The rail is not designed to keep people in bed, rather to help them sit up and to prevent them from falling out of bed accidentally.
Hoyer lift 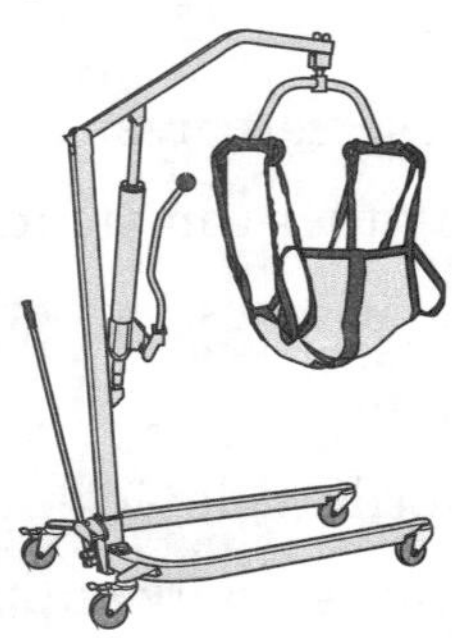	• Assists with getting out of bed or chair • Useful in reducing injury if your care partner needs full assistance and/or is too heavy for you to lift	• Seek professional guidance from your health care team before purchasing. • Proper use is critical and requires special training.
Chair lift up 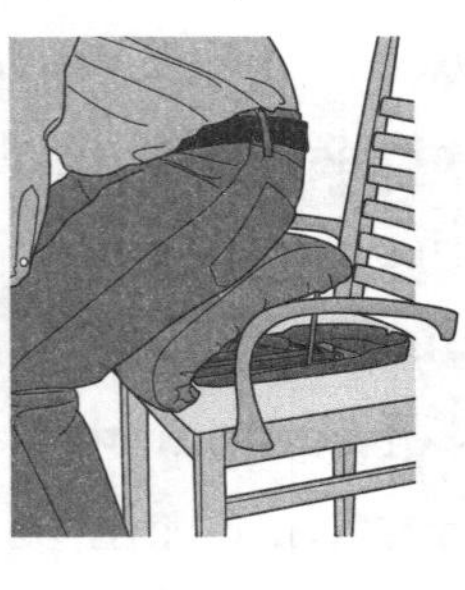	• Assists with safely standing from a seated position • Best if used in a rigid chair, not for use on a soft chair or couch.	• Test the seat yourself before your care partner uses to make sure that the seat is stable and not sliding.

Device	Purpose	Tips
Raised toilet seat/ uplift commode assist 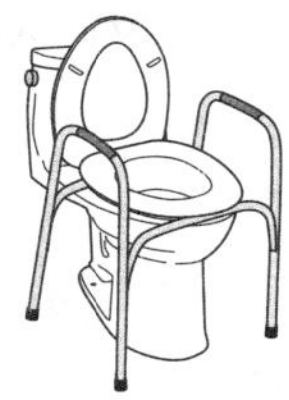 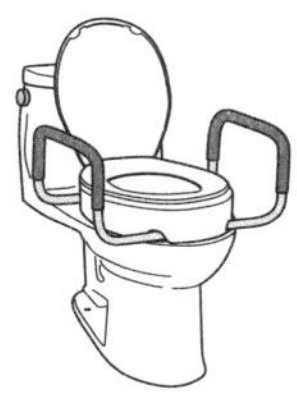	◆ Higher seat assists with safely standing from a seated position ◆ Allows one to follow precautions, if needed after hip replacement	◆ Make sure the seat fits securely. ◆ Assess for stability before care partner uses. ◆ If only one bathroom, consider a toilet seat that is easy to remove so guests and family do not need to use it.
Toilet safety rails 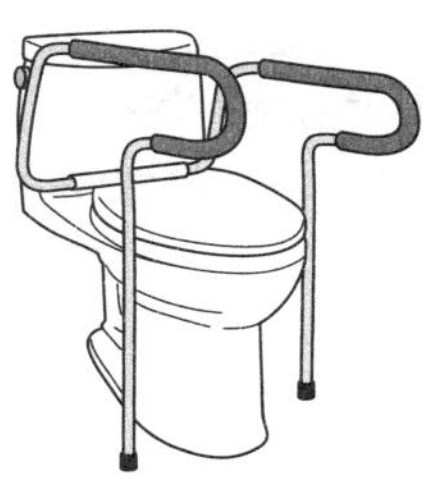	◆ Assist with safely standing from a seated position ◆ Assist with safely sitting from standing position ◆ This is a suitable alternative to the raised toilet seat/uplift commode assist described above if care partner only needs the armrest but not the raised toilet seat	◆ Assess to make sure this is sturdy enough to hold care partner's weight when pushing up. ◆ Measure current toilet (width and height) to make sure the rails will fit before purchasing.
Grab bars 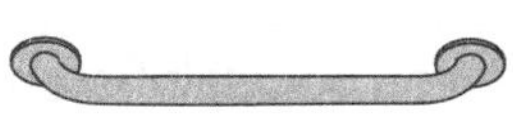 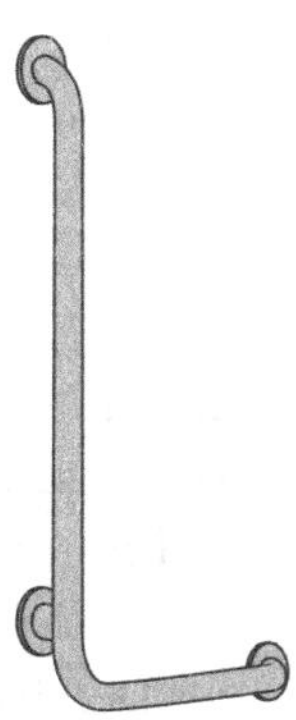	◆ Assist with getting out of tub/shower ◆ Assist with slowly and safely assuming a seating position from a standing position ◆ Provides stability and supports longer standing time (for example, so caregiver can wash entire body)	◆ Use to enter the shower, to get up from the toilet seat, or get over a step or two in a hall, not just in a bathroom. ◆ See the "Tips for Installing Grab Bars in the Bathroom" box on page 146. ◆ Have grab bars professionally installed so they will not pull out of the wall. ◆ Request assistance and a home visit with an occupational therapist for guidance on where to place and install bars. ◆ Avoid suction grab bar options as they may pull away from the wall unexpectedly. ◆ Use professionally installed grab bars, NOT towel bars; a towel bar is not a grab bar and with repeated pressure, it will unexpectedly pull out of the wall.

Table 8.2 **Special Equipment** (*continued*)

Device	Purpose	Tips
Shower chairs/bench 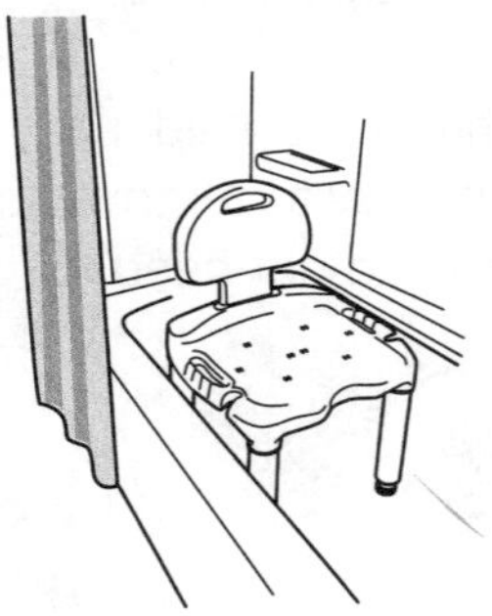	• Provides stability and prevents falls in shower/tub • A shower stool or folding shower seat is adequate if care partner only needs a place to rest • Choose a shower chair with armrest/back if care partner needs more support • Choose a shower chair without armrest if you are using a transfer board (described below) • Choose a tub transfer bench if care partner cannot safely step over the tub edge • Portable chairs are available for travel	• Install a handheld shower head to increase care partner's independence and control over water flow.
Handy bar 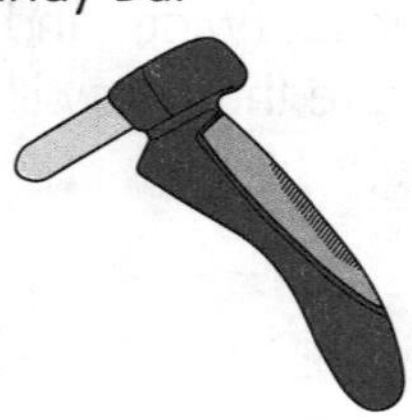	• Assists with getting in and out of car 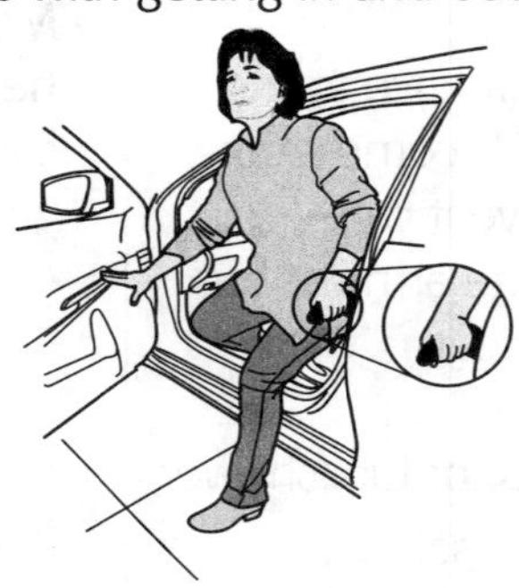	• Before care partner uses the handy bar, make sure to assess its sturdiness.
Swivel cushion 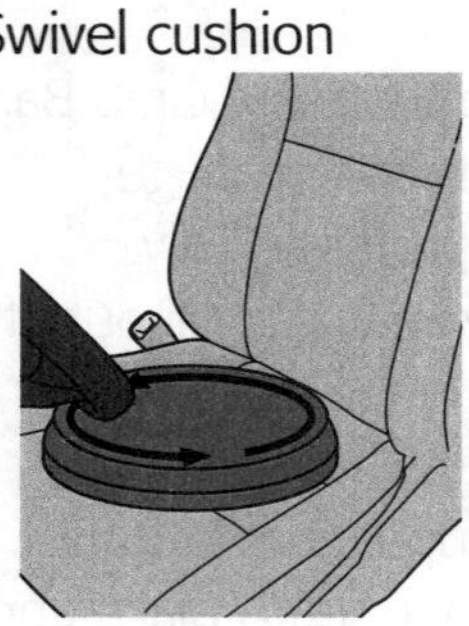	• Assists with getting in and out of cars • Helps with swiveling around when one is in a chair or car seat	• Evaluate the cushion yourself before care partner uses.
Transfer board 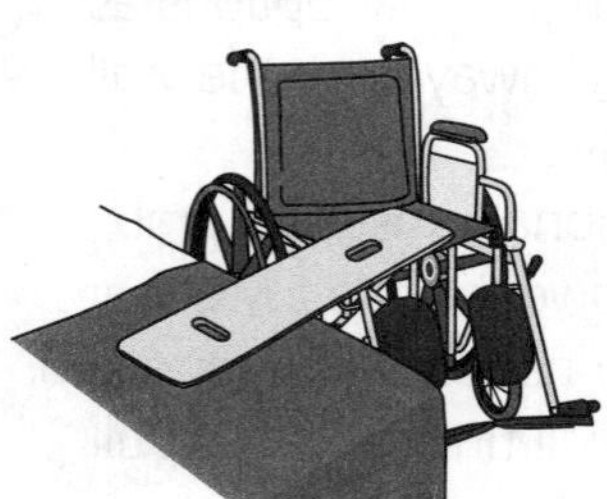	• Assist chair-to-chair transfer (wheelchair-to-car, -tub bench, -bed, -chair) • Allow your care partner to slide over the board instead of lifting him/her	• Make sure care partner has good arm and trunk strength before using transfer board. • Before using with care partner, try the transfer board yourself and seek instruction from a health care professional to make sure you understand how it works.

Table 8.3 **Mobility Aids and Injury Prevention Tips**

Mobility Aids	Qualities	Injury Prevention Tips
Walking sticks 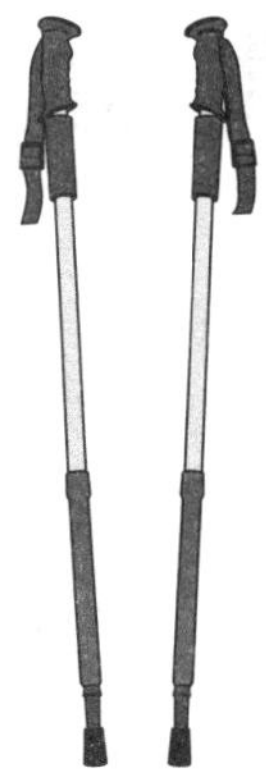	◆ Often longer than a conventional cane ◆ Can use one or two ◆ Use two walking sticks on uneven or rough terrain ◆ Two sticks provide a standing rest break ◆ Designed for people who have adequate balance on flat ground ◆ Tends to hold less stigma than a cane	◆ Use of two sticks is helpful when hiking or on uneven terrain. ◆ Choose cork or molded rubber hand grips; plastic grips tend to get sweaty.
Single-point cane or straight cane 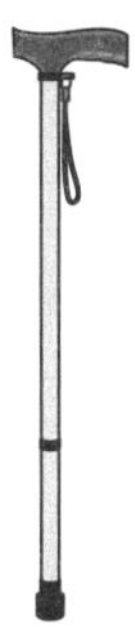	◆ Good for people who need more stability while walking ◆ Increases safety and balance compared with no assistive device ◆ Helps maintain mobility when pain or weakness is on one side of the body	◆ Hold vertical with upright posture. ◆ Keep the cane close to your body. ◆ Do not drag the cane. ◆ A cane is not useful if held in air and not touching ground. ◆ Hold the cane in hand opposite weak or injured leg; step out with injured or weak leg and cane at same time. 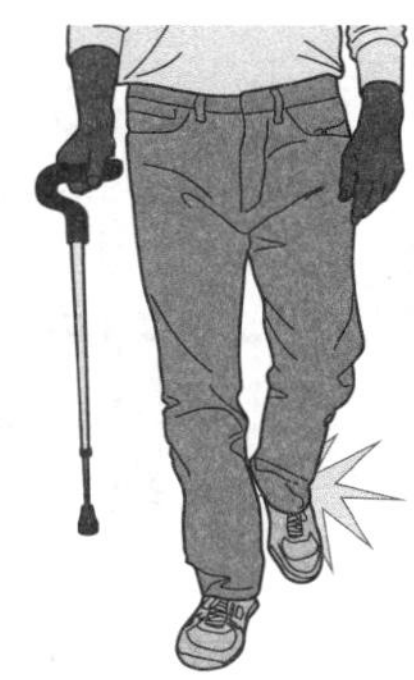 ◆ Use the cane at the right height for optimal function. Look for an adjustable height cane so you can get the proper fit. ◆ The top of the cane should come to your wrist crease with arm straight at your side. During use, your elbow should be bent at a comfortable angle, about 15 degrees. ◆ Pick a handle that feels comfortable. If you have hand pain, a larger grip is better. ◆ Canes vary in weight; aluminum is lightest. If you fatigue easily choose a lightweight cane.

Table 8.3 **Mobility Aids and Injury Prevention Tips** (*continued*)

Mobility Aids	Qualities	Injury Prevention Tips
Quad cane 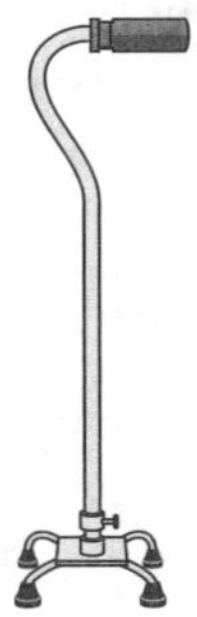	• Good for people who need more stability than a straight cane • Can stand upright so it does not have to be picked up from the floor • Provides a broader base of support and has a larger base • Commonly used for people with function in only one hand (for example, post stroke) • Tends to be heavier than other canes	• User tips are the same for the quad cane as the straight cane. • Be aware of the larger base and make sure you do not trip on it. • Pick up and place the cane for each step to make sure that all four feet touch the ground at the same time.
Tripod cane 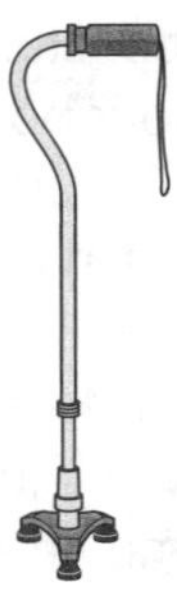	• Good for people who need more stability than a straight cane • Can stand upright so it does not have to be picked up from the floor • More stable than a straight can • Not as stable as a quad cane because it has a smaller base • Easier to use than a quad cane • Has rubber tips	• User tips are the same for the tripod cane as the straight cane. • Be aware of the larger base and make sure you do not trip on it.
Hemi walker 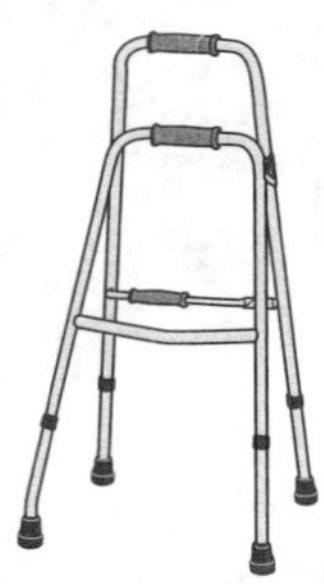	• Good for people who have had a stroke and/or need more support than a cane • Most stable device for people with use of one arm • Large base of support • Folds for storage • Bulky/heavy	• Advance the walker as you advance the affected side, then take a small step to bring it in line with other foot. • Have someone close by for balance if concerned about falling.
Rollator with 4 wheels 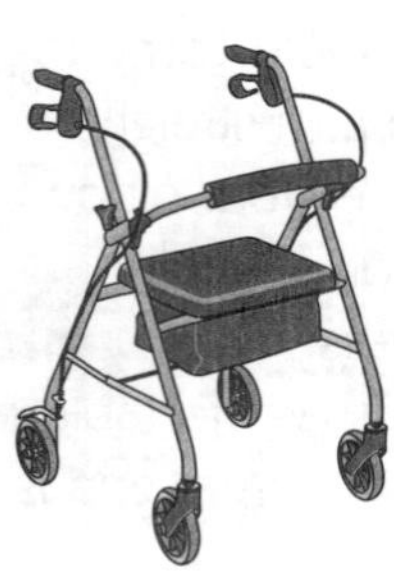	• Good for people who have more balance but reduced endurance • Fastest walking speed • Offers seat for rest break and basket to carry items	• Stand tall. • Stay close to walker. • Handles of walker should be at user's wrist height (arms hanging straight at side). • Lock the brakes before you sit down or go from chair to standing. • Can tip if you put full weight on the hand rests.

Mobility Aids	Qualities	Injury Prevention Tips
Rolling walker with 2 wheels 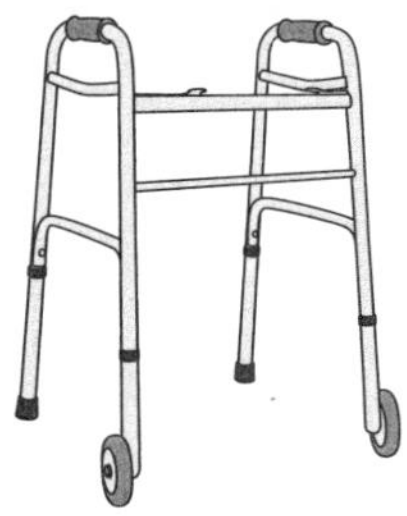	◆ Good for people with some balance issues who need some support to walk ◆ Moves faster than standard walker ◆ Glides forward only	◆ Stand tall. ◆ Stay close to walker. ◆ Handles of walker should be at user's wrist height (when arms are hanging straight at side). ◆ Consider attached tennis balls or glides to back legs to allow back legs to slide. 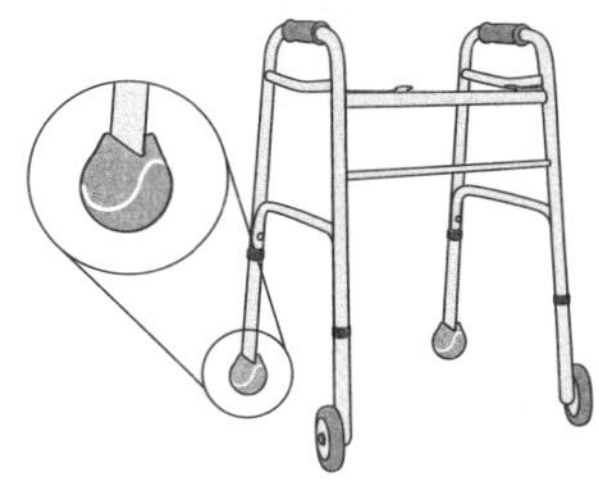
Standard walker 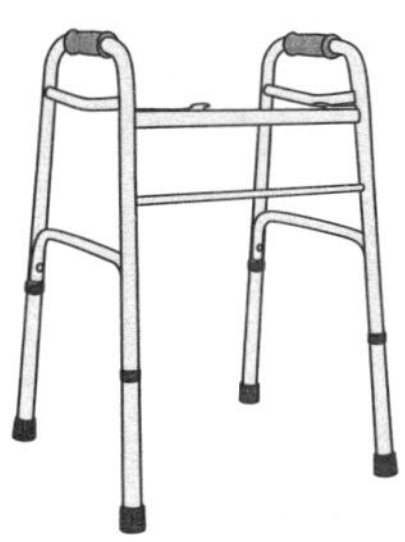	◆ Good for people with limited balance who need a lot of support to walk ◆ Slow to move ◆ No wheels ◆ Need to pick up	◆ Stay close to walker. ◆ Handles of walker should be at user's wrist height (when arms are hanging straight at side). ◆ Keep all four legs in contact with the ground when walking. ◆ Stand tall.
Manual wheelchair 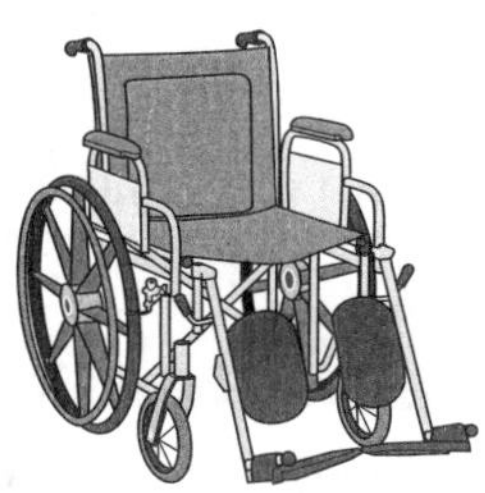	◆ Good for people with enough upper body strength to propel the wheelchair ◆ Good for people who lack the endurance to use a walker or cane for outings (museums and outdoor gardens often have wheelchairs available if you call ahead) ◆ Good for people who have someone to push them	◆ Always lock the brakes before getting in and out of the wheelchair. ◆ Swing away the wheelchair legs for a safer transfer (see box content on page 133). ◆ Avoid putting heavy loads on the back of a wheelchair. ◆ Avoid going up or down steep inclines. ◆ If there are no curb cuts, consider backing up wheelchair to go up/down to/from a curb.

Table 8.3 **Mobility Aids and Injury Prevention Tips** (*continued*)

Mobility Aids	Qualities	Injury Prevention Tips
Scooter 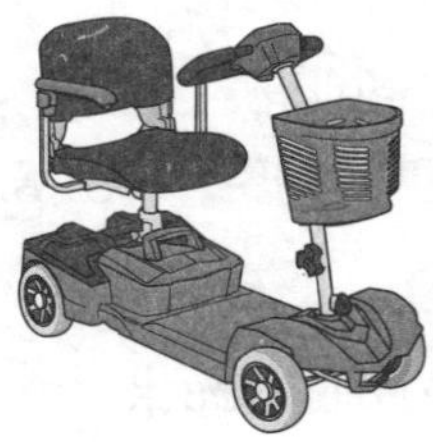	◆ Good for people who don't require a power wheelchair full time.	◆ Always ride solo. ◆ Wear seat belt. ◆ Keep track of battery charge indicator so battery is fully charged.
Power wheelchair 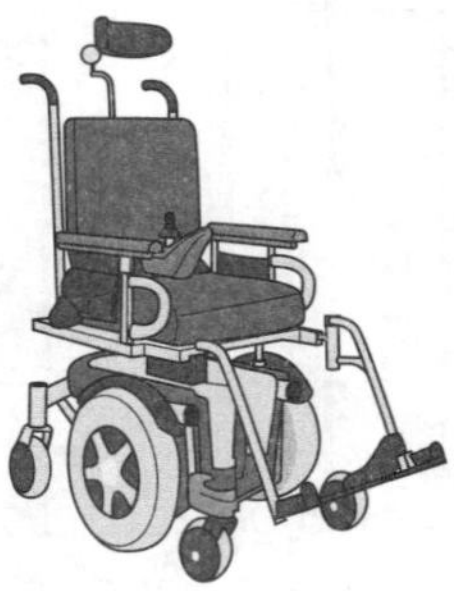	◆ Good for people who cannot push a wheelchair with their own arm strength ◆ Power wheelchairs with standing options are available that allow people with paraplegia to stand independently	◆ Turn the power off before transferring. ◆ Avoid riding in the rain. ◆ Avoid going up or down steep inclines. ◆ Keep track of battery charge indicator so battery is fully charged

Assistive devices that can make tasks easier include equipment specifically made for people with physical limitations. These are often commercially available. A small change in how you do something or the use of a piece of equipment can make a task less frustrating and safer. Consider the following examples, some of which are shown in Figure 8.5.

- If your care partner struggles to get clothes or shoes on, consider buying new items a size bigger and look for clothes with larger neck openings. You can also add Velcro closures to clothing or shoes or use elastic shoelaces.
- If your care partner has reduced balance or mobility, they can use a long-handled shoehorn while sitting.
- When bathing, your care partner can use a long-handled sponge. This can help address reduced balance, motion limitations, and motion restrictions. Installing a handheld shower head and using a pump dispenser for shampoo or body wash can also make bathing easier.
- *Dycem* is a nonslip substance you can purchase to keep plates from moving. This can help at mealtimes. Utensils with built-up handles or other special utensils, such as a rocker knife, can also increase your care partner's independence during eating. A scooped plate can prevent food spills. To find these devices, check a local medical supply store, drug store, or online retailers. Often the easiest way to purchase them is

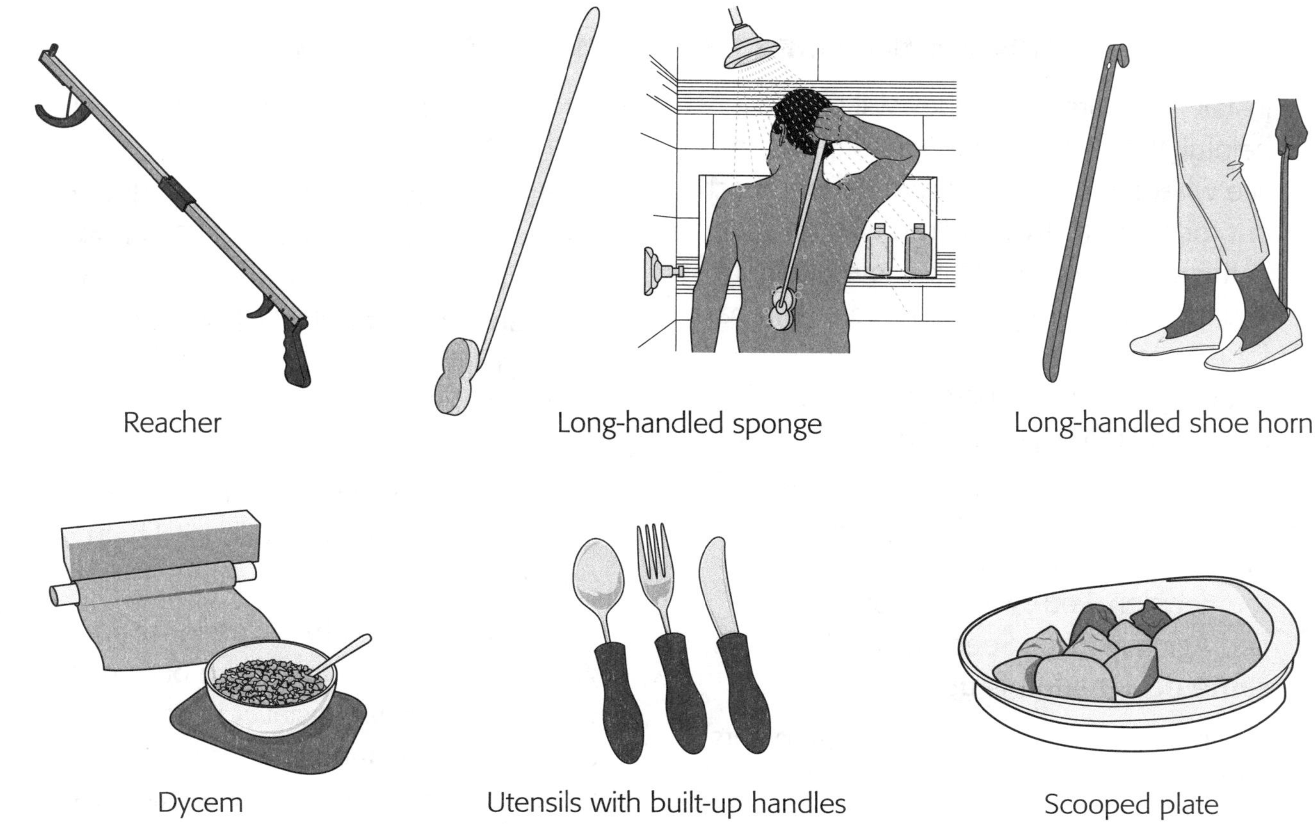

Figure 8.5 **Tools to Make Tasks Easier**

online. Search for them on the internet by the specific names listed in Table 8.2 and Figure 8.5. You can also use search terms such as "assistive devices," "assistive equipment," "adaptive equipment," "adaptive devices," or "mobility aids." If you are not sure if the device is the right choice or if you know that you will only need a device temporarily, you might be able to borrow it. Look for a lending closet, senior center, or community organization in your area that rents or loans out equipment.

Adapting Your Home and Surroundings

You may not have noticed injury hazards in your home and surroundings. But there are often many small changes that can make your home safer and help you worry less. Increased awareness can help you manage risks outside your home, such as uneven surfaces, damaged sidewalks, or streets without curb cuts. In this section, we introduce some ways you can make your surroundings safer. Most of them are general tips that can help both you and your care partner. Walk around your house and see how these tips apply.

Tips for Installing Grab Bars in the Bathroom

- Install grab bars where they will be most helpful. When you use the bathroom, notice where you and your care partner reach out for support. Try a dry run without water in the shower or tub. Make note of where you and your care partner need a grab bar for maintaining balance. If either of you put weight on towel bars, replace towel bars with grab bars. Test the best location around the toilet as well. If you are unsure, consult with an occupational therapist or physical therapist to receive help with the decision. Look for one that is a Certified Aging in Place Specialist (CAPS). **This same designation is used in Canada.**
- The most common locations for grab bars are:
  - Bath or shower along the back wall and between shower and valve
  - Toilet along the side wall and behind the toilet tank
- Pairing a vertical and horizontal grab bar can make bars more versatile. This makes it easy for you and your care partner to use the grab bars comfortably if you are of different heights. Some people also prefer an angled grab bar.
- Mount horizontal grab bars 33″–36″ (840–915 mm) from the floor for better leverage around the toilet and bath or shower.
- Hire someone who has experience with grab bar installation to put the bars in for you. Make sure the installer uses anchors or attaches the grab bars to studs so they are secure. Following the installation, ask someone to pull the grab bar with all their strength to evaluate its holding power.

Rearranging the Layout and Setup of Your Home

Reducing hazards and clutter and rearranging furniture and daily items can make your home safer. Your goal is to establish a clear pathway without obstacles to areas where you and/or your care partner frequently walk, such as the bathroom, bedroom, and kitchen. A wide pathway allows you and your care partner to move straight through a narrow space. Twisting to avoid obstacles or clutter can increase fall risks. Take the following steps to clear the high-traffic areas in your home:

- **Remove or organize cables or cords.** Cables on the floor are major tripping hazards. Use cable covers or cord covers to hide cords.
- **Remove (or secure) throw rugs.** Throw rugs tend to slip, slide, and bunch up and are easy to trip over. The best option is to not use them, but if you want to keep them, secure with nonslip padding or rug anchors. Bathmats are dangerous in the same way.
- **Rearrange the layout of furniture.** Strategically place furniture so it can be used as support. For example, place a sturdy cabinet at waist height on the path to the bathroom so there is something to grab if you or your care partner lose your balance. Make sure tripping hazards, such as low coffee tables, are not near or in pathways. Place sturdy chairs throughout the house. A chair in the bedroom can support balance during

Explore Modern Technology to Make Caregiving Easier

- Motion-activated lights inside and outside the home
- Lights set to come on or turn off in the house synchronized with your routine
- Smart speakers that use AI assistants, such as Google Nest and Amazon Echo, to call for help, set times, and read daily schedule
- Smart watches, such as the Apple Watch, that offer fall detection and emergency calls
- Other wearable devices that detect falls or wandering

dressing and one in the kitchen allows rest while waiting for the water to boil.

- **Re-organize items in your cabinets** to prevent repetitive bending or reaching every time you need an item. Put the most frequently used items in the front of the cabinet and store them between shoulder and hip height.
- **Keep frequently used items in each room or on each floor** if you live in a multistory house. Keep canes, landline phones, reading glasses, or other important things in areas you often use them. Rushing to another room to answer the phone often results in a fall. Placing a phone in every room or keeping a cell phone with you will prevent you or your care partner from hurrying to answer it. At the same time, you will have a phone close at hand in emergencies. Check daily to make sure that cell phones are charged, and landline phones are on their chargers.

Changing the Lighting in Your Home

You need to see where you are walking. If your home is dimly lit, it is more likely that you or your care partner might trip over something.

- **Improve lighting.** Check the lighting in all areas in your home. Change the bulbs to brighter ones or add more lighting as needed. Do the same for entrances to your home.
- **Install nightlights.** Light is particularly important at night. People often fall when they go to the bathroom. Install nightlights or motion-sensitive lights throughout your home, particularly on the path to the bathroom. You may want to purchase lights that are motion or light sensitive and turn on when you walk by or when it is dark. These types of light don't require you to turn them off and on. They come on automatically when you need them so you do not even have to think about them.

Choosing Furniture to Help Reduce Strain

The type of furniture in your home can increase or reduce the amount of assistance your care partner needs.

- **Choose sturdy, firm chairs and sofas or couches with arms.** Unstable chairs are likely to cause falls. It is far more difficult to help your care partner stand from a soft recliner or sofa than from a kitchen chair with arm support.

- **Use beds and chairs at the right height.** Chairs or beds that are too low can be difficult to get into and out of without help. At the same time, chairs that are too high with limited support, such as stools, are not safe. Consider purchasing a bed that is height adjustable. If your care partner is suddenly having difficulty getting out of a bed or a chair, consider consulting a rehabilitation professional, such as an occupational therapist or physical therapist.

Providing Environmental Cues for Your Care Partner

You can create environmental cues and reminders that help keep both you and your care partner safe. These cues are particularly helpful if your care partner has visual or cognitive problems. However, a cue can help anyone in the household, especially in a busy environment where it is easy to lose track of things or become careless.

- **Apply brightly colored, nonslip tape on stairs** to prevent tripping or sliding. If you wear slippers at home, the risk of falling increases when walking on surfaces and stairs that are slippery (such as wooden floors and staircases). To prevent tripping, slipping, or missing steps, mark the edge of each step (or the last step only) with nonslip, brightly colored tape (for example, colored duct tape). There are also glow-in-the-dark tapes that are useful in darker areas such as stairs to the basement.

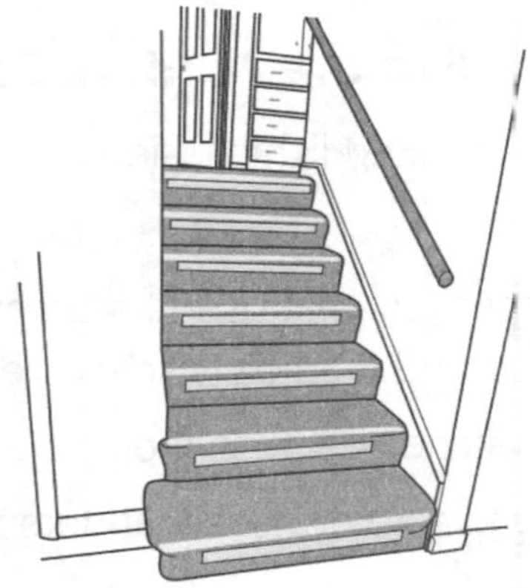

- **Use high contrasting colors** to make it easy to locate items or spaces. A care partner with dementia may wander at night and have difficulty finding the bathroom. You can paint the doors of the bathroom or bedroom a bright color; post signs on the doors; or use glow-in-the-dark tape to mark the path from the bed to the bathrooms. High-contrast colors also help when locating items. In a white bathroom, install or use special equipment or bathing items that do not blend in. For example, in the illustration below, the bathtub bench is dark, so it stands out in the all-white bathroom. Use of contrasting colors can improve your care partner's independence.

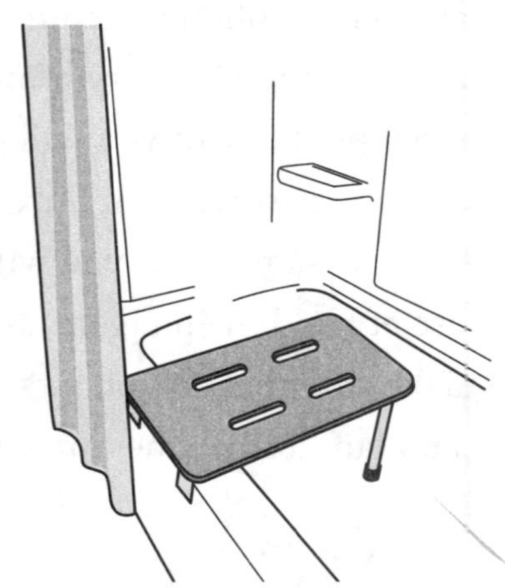

- **Post signs to prevent dangerous situations.** Care partners with cognitive or visual impairments are at risk of eating spoiled food or inedible materials. Lock and put up

What Can You Do to Prevent Falls?

There are specific ways you can reduce fall risk for yourself and your care partner. These strategies are supported by research.

- Both you and your care partner can exercise to improve leg strength and balance.
- Ask your doctor or pharmacist to review your and your care partner's medications.
- Ask to have your and your care partner's balance and hearing checked, especially if either of you are feeling dizzy.
- Check your and your care partner's vision and wear eyeglasses with a current prescription.
- Wear sturdy footwear with a back. Do not wear flip-flops or slippers.
- Make your home safer.
  - Install and maintain good lighting.
  - Remove trip hazards and clutter.
  - Install strong railings on all stairs.
  - Install and maintain safety equipment and grab bars in the bathroom.

"stop" or "no" signs on cabinets where you store cleaning materials to ease your mind about dangerous situations. Explore available safety aids designed to protect young children and see what might work for you. If there are guns in the house, store them in a locked gun safe. Always keep guns and ammunition in separate places.

Advocating for Accessibility in Your Neighborhood or Community

As we mentioned before, fall and injury hazards are not just problems at home. Being mindful about your surroundings can help you and your care partner avoid dangerous situations such as curbs and uneven pavement when you are out in the community. However, in the long run, it may be better if those hazards were removed, so they do not get in your and your care partner's way every time you get out in your neighborhood. Under the Americans with Disabilities Act (ADA), you and your care partner have the right to request evenly paved sidewalks and curb cuts at inaccessible locations. You can contact your city hall or alderman's office to request changes in your neighborhood. If you live in a large city, there might be a phone number to call to express complaints about inaccessible areas. Sometimes it takes a long time to get these fixed. Be assertive and regularly check on the progress so the job gets done to your advantage. In addition to working with your local government, you can work with your neighbors to help make the neighborhood more accessible for all. For example, if you have a neighbor with foliage that extends onto the walk, kindly ask them to cut it. They are probably unaware of the problem and will be happy to help.

The Accessible Canada Act (ACA) aims to remove barriers to accessibility for people with disabilities by 2040. The ACA applies to federal government organizations and federally regulated private organizations with at least ten employees. It requires businesses to create accessibility plans and regularly publish progress reports about seven priority areas including employment, communication, the built environment, goods, services, facilities, and transportation.

Seeking Guidance from Health Professionals

Self-management is always a good strategy, but you do not have to do everything alone. Both your primary health care provider and your care partner's provider should have access to a range of health professionals to support safety and well-being. It is best if you approach a health care provider with a specific problem and some possible solutions. For example, if your partner falls, you might say, "Omar keeps falling and I think he needs a walking aid. Can you refer us to someone who can give us advice on this?" Request a medication review to make sure none of the prescribed medications increase fall risk. This can be done by your physician or a clinical pharmacist. Many retail pharmacists can also review your or your care partner's medications for fall risk. If equipment is needed, find out if the equipment is covered by your insurance and if it can be ordered by your health care provider. Sometimes a nurse or care coordinator can assist you. Or call the number on the back of your insurance card.

In Canada, your province or territory may have home and community care where community nurses, occupational therapists, or physiotherapists can visit your home and assess your needs. Nonprofit organizations that lend equipment, such as the Canadian Red Cross, may be available in your area.

If you or your care partner needs rehabilitation services such as occupational therapy (OT), physical therapy (PT), or speech therapy, ask your health care provider or insurance company if a referral is needed. All therapy services begin with an evaluation. The following are some services you can expect from various therapists:

- *Speech therapy* focuses on enhancing communication and understanding, and on safe eating. Common services offered by speech and language pathologists include sustaining attention, enhancing problem solving and understanding, speech training, swallowing assessment, and safe eating practices (to reduce choking risk).
- *Physical therapy* focuses on teaching and restoring safe movement. Common services offered by physical therapists include instruction in exercise and proper gait; home exercise programming to increase flexibility, strength, balance, and endurance post-fall or post-injury; transfer training for you and your care partner; selection of mobility aids and training in their proper use; and manual therapy and other procedures for pain management.
- *Occupational therapy* aims to maximize independence and active participation in everyday activities. Common services offered

by occupational therapists include home safety assessment, transfer training, self-care training with an emphasis on proper body mechanics, problem solving to reduce safety risks, modifying home and surroundings, modifying tasks to make them safer, enhancing participation in activities, and guidance in selecting and using special equipment.

Putting It All Together: Utilizing Tools to Avoid Risks

In this chapter, we identified risks that contribute to accidents and injury and describe tools to reduce injury risks. These tools can make your caregiving experience easier and more positive. We discuss the tools individually, but you can combine tools and techniques to reduce your risk of injury.

For a complete list of suggested further readings, useful websites, and other helpful resources, please see: www.bullpub.com/resources.

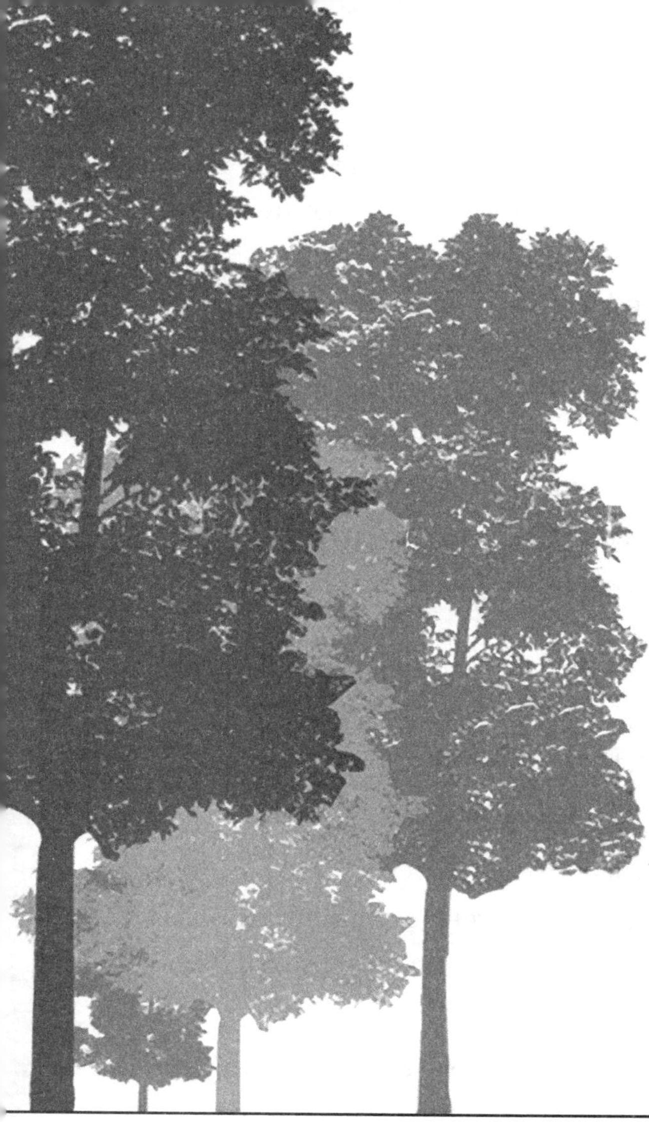

CHAPTER 9

Exercising for Health and Wellness

YOU PROBABLY ALREADY KNOW THAT REGULAR EXERCISE IS IMPORTANT for both you and your care partner, but when you care for another person or you have a chronic health problem, you might feel you are already too busy or too tired to add anything else to your day. You may want to exercise but don't want to do anything that could cause injury. You might wonder what you could possibly do to make a difference in your health and wellness. You might be worried about your current health and capacity, your limited skills, or natural ability. These are common concerns, but you (and often your care partner) can learn and do many activities that can make you feel better, increase your energy, and reduce your risk of injuries. The information in this chapter will help you get started and be successful.

When you are physically active and exercise, you improve your strength, flexibility, and endurance. You also reduce your risk of injuries from strained muscles, overstressed joints, fatigue, and poor balance. Regular exercise improves self-confidence and reduces feelings of stress, anxiety, and depression. In addition, regular exercise can help you sleep better and feel more relaxed and happier. Exercise can help you maintain a healthy weight, which takes stress off your back and legs. Exercise is also part of keeping bones strong. Published research, medical recommendations, and public health guidelines from many countries stress the effectiveness and importance of regular physical activity to improve health and fitness.

The good news is that it doesn't take painful, sweaty exercise to achieve health benefits. Even short periods of moderate physical activity can make a big difference in how you feel and what you are able to do. If you can exercise with your care partner, both of you can achieve physical, emotional, and relationship benefits!

What Exercise Can Do for You

In the same way that different types of food (such as vitamins, protein, fats, and fiber) provide different benefits for your body, different kinds of exercises have different positive effects. In this chapter, we outline four types of exercise: those that make you more flexible, those that boost strength, those that improve your endurance, and those that improve your balance.

- **Flexibility.** Being flexible helps you move comfortably and safely. Limited flexibility can cause pain, lead to injury, and make your muscles work harder and tire more quickly. You lose flexibility when you are inactive, or your daily movement is limited. Certain illnesses and diseases can also lead to less flexibility. However, you can improve flexibility by doing gentle stretching exercises such as the ones described in this chapter.
- **Strength.** Muscles need to be used regularly to be strong. Inactive muscles weaken and atrophy (shrink). When your muscles get weak, you feel weak and tire quickly. Much disability and lack of mobility is due to muscle weakness. Strengthening exercises (such as lifting a weight or pulling against a resistance band) require muscles to do more work.
- **Endurance.** Endurance depends on the fitness of your heart, lungs, and muscles. Your heart and lungs must work efficiently to send enough oxygen-rich blood to your muscles. Your muscles must be fit enough to use the oxygen. Endurance or aerobic ("with oxygen") exercise is exercise that uses the large muscles of your body in continuous activity, such as walking, swimming, dancing, mowing the lawn, or riding a bike. Numerous studies show that aerobic exercise improves endurance, promotes a sense of well-being, eases depression and anxiety, promotes restful sleep, and improves mood and energy levels.
- **Balance.** Strong and coordinated muscles in your trunk and legs are a key part of good balance. Flexibility, strength, and endurance

also contribute to balance. Of course, there are many causes of falls (poor vision, poor lighting, obstacles such as rugs on the floor, dizziness, or being tired or distracted), but being balanced, strong, and coordinated are very important and can help reduce fall risk. Certain exercises described in this chapter are especially good for improving balance.

The descriptions and illustrations in this chapter include all these kinds of exercise. You can select which activities you want to do depending on what you want to accomplish. The exercises illustrated in the following sections are arranged in groups of flexibility, strength, and balance. Suggestions and examples of endurance exercise are described later in this chapter. In Chapter 8, Preventing Injuries, there are more details of how exercise can help you protect yourself and your care partner from getting hurt. In that chapter, you will also find Table 8.1 on page 124 that lists exercises to reduce injury risk and references the exercises in this chapter.

Flexibility Exercises

Whole-Body Flexibility

1. The Whole-Body Stretcher

This exercise is a whole-body stretch to be done lying on your back. You can do it in bed first thing in the morning and last thing at night. Start the motion at your ankles as explained here (or you can reverse the process if you want to start with your arms first).

- Point your toes, and then pull your toes toward your nose. Relax.
- Bend your knees. Then, straighten your knees and let them relax.
- Arch your back. Do the pelvic tilt (Exercise 6 on page 157). Relax.
- Breathe in and stretch your arms above your head. Make gentle fists and then straighten your fingers and spread them apart. Breathe out and lower your arms. Relax.
- Stretch your right arm above your head and at the same time stretch your left leg by pushing down with your heel. Hold for a count of 10. Switch to the other side and repeat.

Neck and Back Flexibility

2. Heads Up

This exercise relieves jaw, neck, and upper back tension or pain. It also helps promote good posture. You can do it while driving, sitting at a desk, sewing, watching TV, reading, or exercising. Just sit or stand straight and gently slide your chin back. Keep looking forward as your chin moves backward. You'll feel the back of your neck lengthen and straighten. To help, put your finger on your nose and then draw your nose straight back from your finger. (Don't worry about a little double chin—you really look much better with your neck straight!)

The following are clues for finding the correct position when doing the Heads Up exercise:

Ears over shoulders, not out in front

Head balanced over neck and trunk, not out in front

Neck vertical, not leaning forward

Bit of double chin

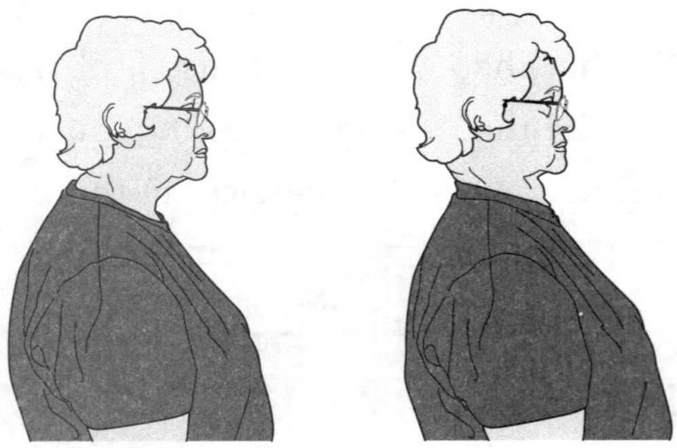

3. Neck Stretch

In heads-up position (Flexibility Exercise 2) with your shoulders relaxed, turn slowly to look over your right shoulder. Then turn slowly to look over your left shoulder. Next, tilt your head to the right and then to the left. Move your left ear toward your left shoulder and your right ear toward your right shoulder. Do not lift your shoulder up to your ear.

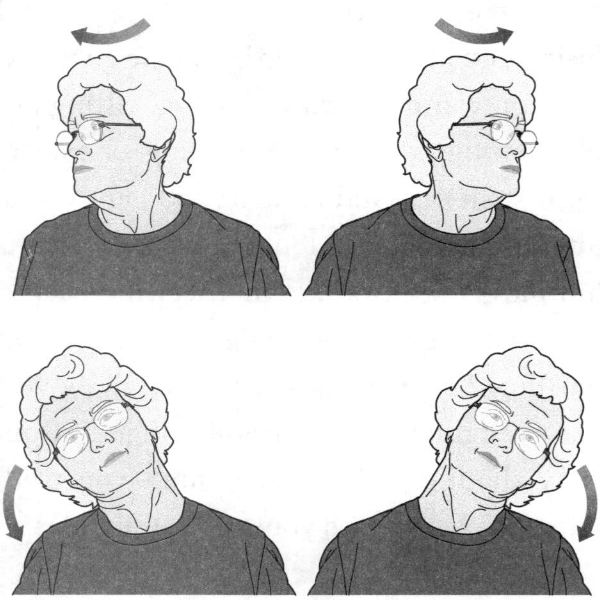

4. Cat and Cow Pose in Seated Position

This two-part exercise stretches and improves flexibility in the entire spine and opens the chest. It is a yoga exercise that can reduce tension and calm the mind. At first, keep your movements small so that you do not strain your lower back. If you have neck problems, make sure to keep your neck in line with your body, not letting your neck go too far back or too far forward.

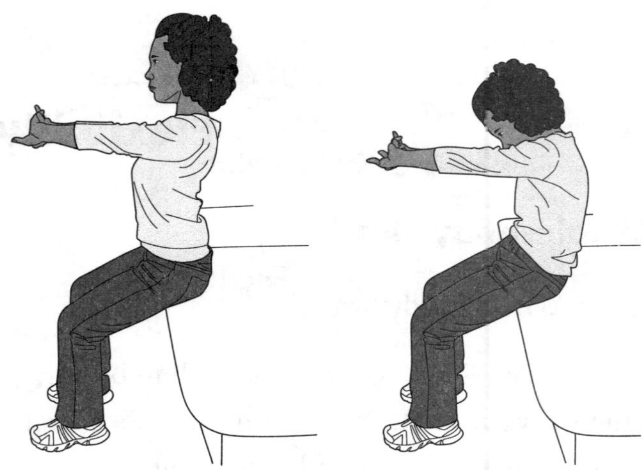

Sit in a straight-backed chair so that your back is not against the back of the chair. Sit with your head over your shoulders and shoulders over your hips. Place your feet flat on the floor with your knees over your heels and your hands rested gently on your thighs.

Imagine a string attached to the top of your head lifting your body to its full length. Start the "cat" by exhaling slowly as you bring your belly toward your spine and your back toward the back of the chair. Allow your back and shoulders to round and your head to come forward. Then move into the "cow" by inhaling and bringing the chest forward and up as you let the shoulders come up and back. As you do this, your head raises and gently looks up as far as is comfortable. This puts the back in a gentle back bend. Repeat the cat and cow several times at your own pace.

5. Knee-to-Chest Stretch

For a low-back stretch, lie on the floor with knees bent and feet flat. Bring one knee toward your chest, using your hands to help. Hold your knee near your chest for 10 seconds and then lower the leg slowly. Repeat with the other knee. You can also bring both legs to your chest at the same time if you wish. Relax and enjoy the stretch.

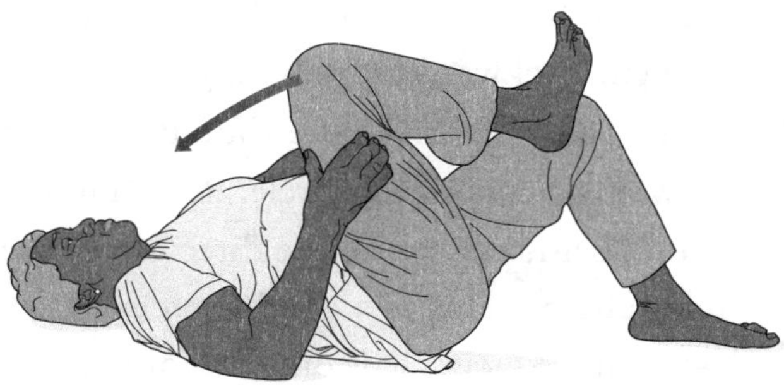

6. Pelvic Tilt

This is an excellent exercise for the low back and can help relieve low-back pain. Lie on your back with knees bent, feet flat on the floor. Place your hands on your abdomen. Flatten the small of your back against the floor by tightening your stomach muscles and your buttocks. When you do this exercise, you will be tilting your tailbone forward and pulling your stomach back. Think about trying to pull your stomach in enough to zip a tight pair of trousers. Hold the tilt for five to 10 seconds. Relax. Arch your back slightly.

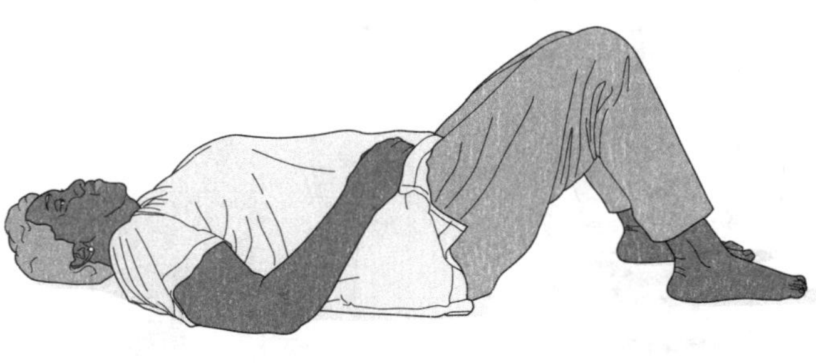

Relax and repeat the pelvic tilt. Keep breathing. Count the seconds out loud. Once you've mastered the pelvic tilt lying down, practice it sitting, standing, and walking.

7. Back Lift

This exercise improves flexibility along your spine and helps you lift your chest for easier breathing. Lie on your stomach and raise your upper body up onto your forearms. Keep your back relaxed and keep your stomach and hips down. If this is comfortable, straighten your elbows so that your upper trunk is raised higher. Breathe naturally and relax for at least 10 seconds. If you have moderate to severe low-back pain, do not do this exercise unless it has been specifically prescribed for you.

To strengthen back muscles, lie on your stomach with your arms at your side or extended overhead. Lift your head, shoulders, and arms off the floor. Do not look up. Keep looking down with your chin tucked into that double-chin position. Count out loud as you hold for a count of 10. Relax. You can also lift your legs, instead of your head and shoulders, off the floor.

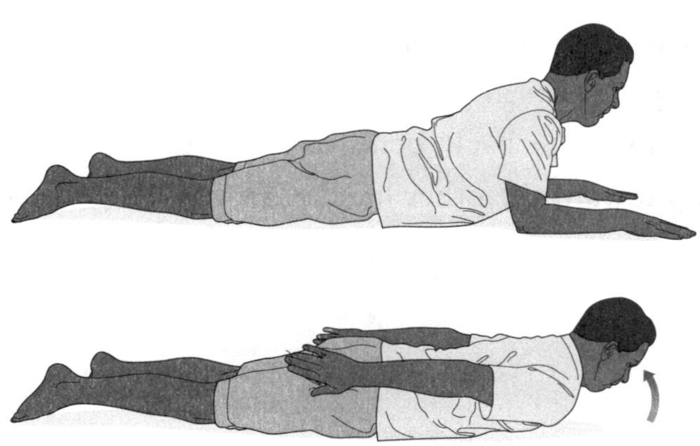

Note that lifting both ends of your body at once is a fairly strenuous exercise. It might not be helpful for a person with back pain.

8. Low-Back Rock and Roll

Lie on your back and pull your knees up to your chest. You can keep holding onto your legs with your hands on your shins or stretch your arms out to your sides to lie on the floor at shoulder level. Rest in this position for 10 seconds, and then gently roll your hips and knees to one side and then the other. Rest and relax as you roll to each side. Keep your upper back and shoulders flat on the ground.

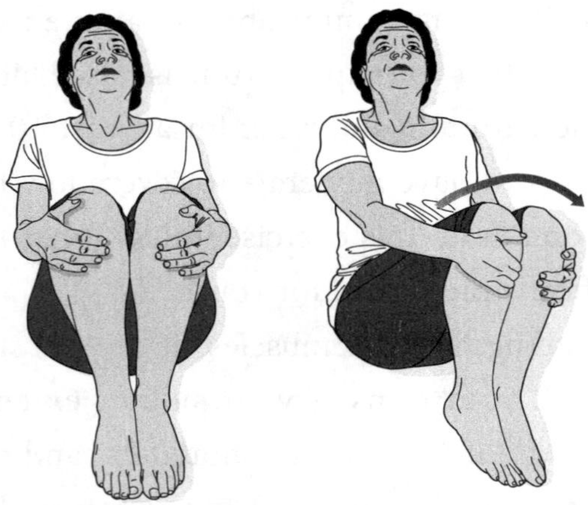

Arm and Leg Flexibility

9. Pat and Reach

This double-duty exercise increases both flexibility and strength for shoulders. Raise one arm up over your head and bend your elbow to pat yourself on the back. Move your other arm to your back, bend your elbow, and reach up toward the other hand. Can your fingertips touch? Relax and switch arm positions. Can you touch on that side? For most people, one position will work better than the other. Do not worry if you cannot touch. Many people cannot touch, but you will improve as you practice. If you wish, you can use a towel as if you were drying your back. This can provide you with feedback and assist in the motion.

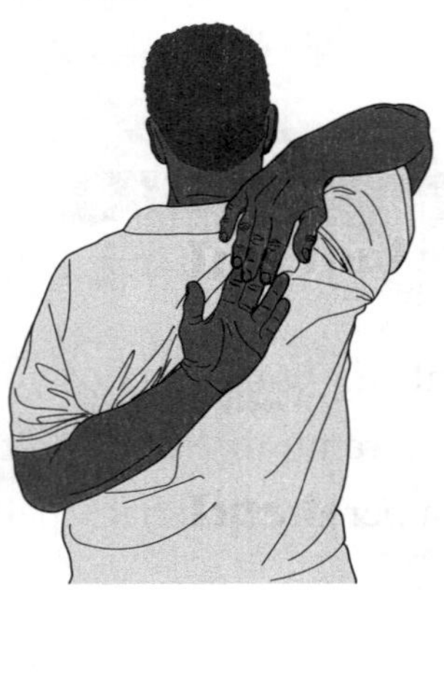

10. Shoulder Shape-Up

In heads-up position (Exercise 2), slowly raise the shoulders to the ears. Hold the position and then drop your shoulders. Next, raise the shoulders again to the ears and then begin to slowly rotate them backward by pinching the shoulder blades together. Bring the shoulders down and forward to complete a circle. Return to the heads-up position. Reverse the direction of the shoulder circles. This is a good exercise if the neck stretch (Exercise 3) is difficult for you.

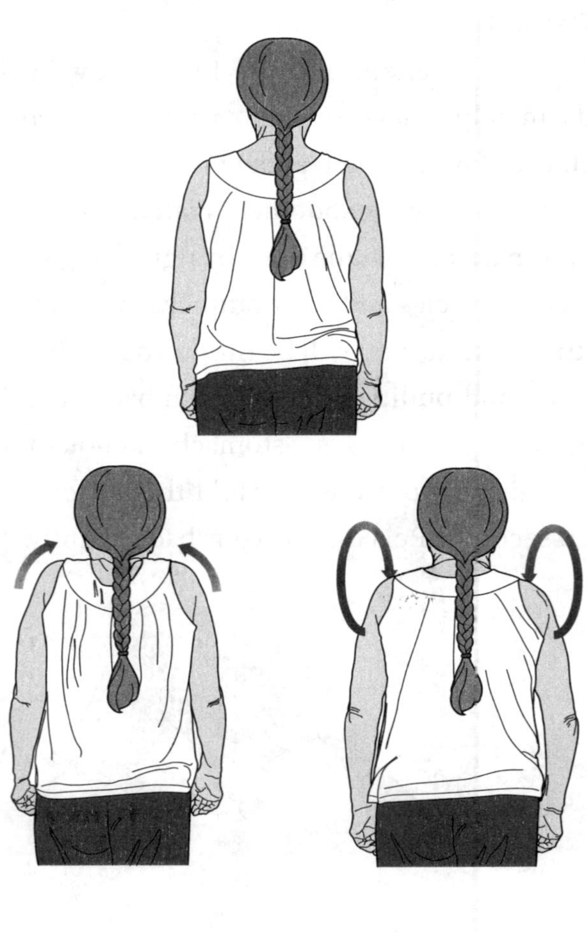

11. Good Morning

This exercise can be done seated or standing. Start with hands in gentle fists, palms down, and wrists crossed. Breathe in and stretch out your fingers while you uncross your arms and reach up for the sky. Straighten your elbows as much as you can as you reach up. Bend your elbows to touch your fingers to your shoulders and then reach up to the ceiling again. Breathe out as you stretch your arms and relax.

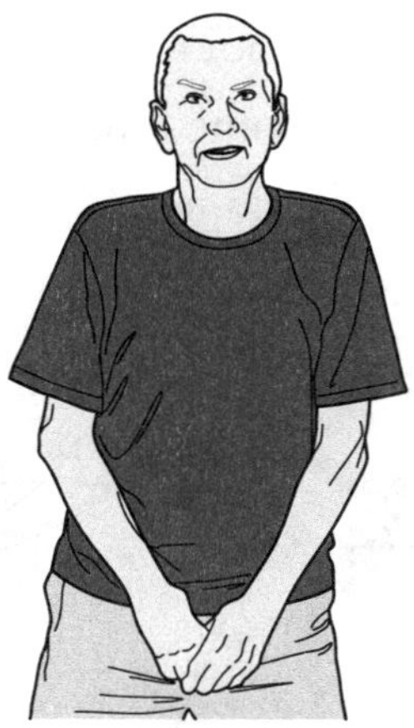

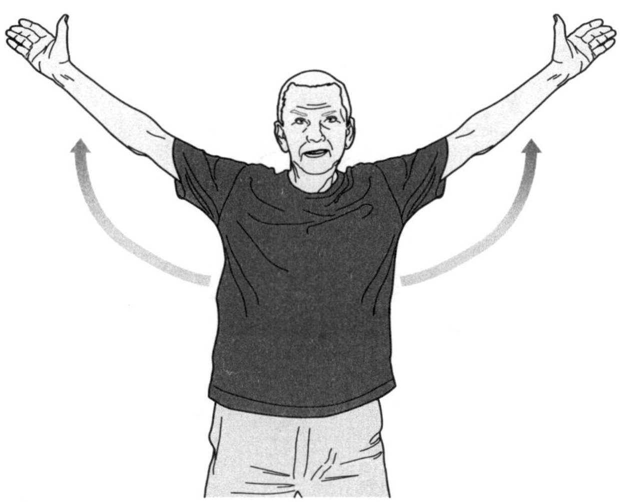

Maintaining the same position, stretch your wrists as described in the following instructions. The purpose of the wrist stretches is to fully extend the muscles that attach to the elbow on the top and the bottom of your forearm. Repetitive tasks can make these muscles stay in a tight and shortened position resulting in forearm or elbow pain. Stretching them often helps prevent this.

Wrist Stretch Down

Start with your elbow straight and palm facing down toward the floor. Make a fist with your hand and bend at the wrist to lower your knuckles down until you feel a stretch in your forearm or elbow. Hold for five seconds. Repeat several times.

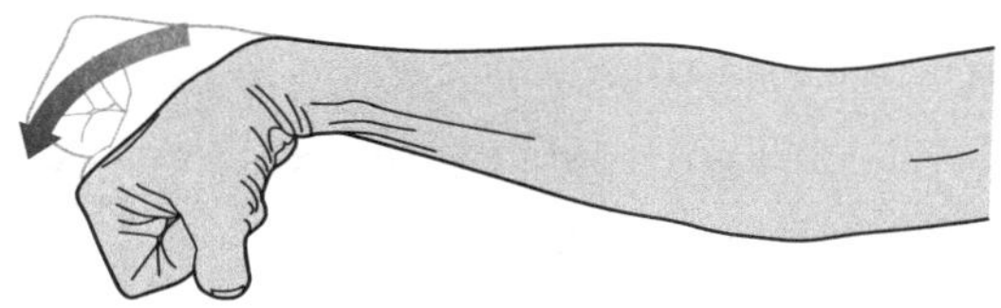

Wrist Stretch Up

Start with your elbow straight and palm facing away from you. Put your opposite hand over the away-facing palm. Gently stretch your palm toward you until you feel a stretch on the underside of your forearm near the elbow. Hold for five seconds. Repeat several times.

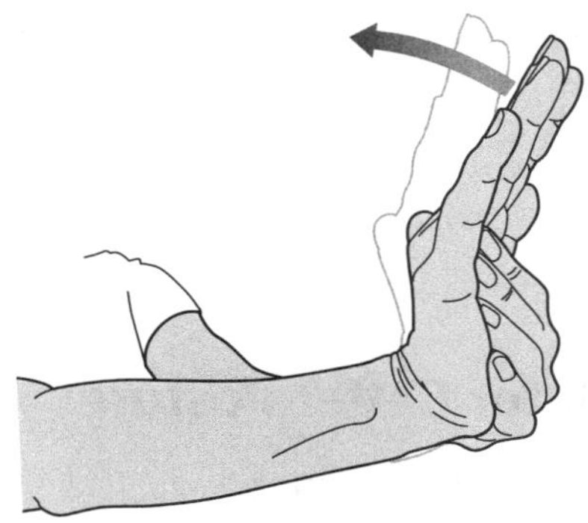

12. Hamstring Stretch

Lie on your back, knees bent, feet flat on the floor. Grasp one leg at a time behind the thigh. Holding the leg out at arm's length, slowly straighten the knee and extend the leg. Hold the

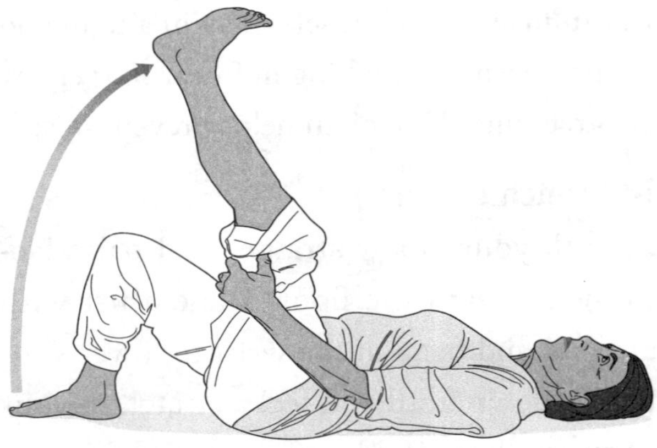

leg as straight as you can as you count to 10. You should feel a slight stretch at the back of your knee and thigh.

Be careful with this exercise. It's easy to overstretch and end up sore.

13. Achilles Stretch

Stand at a counter or against a wall. Place one foot in front of the other, toes pointing forward and heels on the ground. Lean forward, bend the knee of the forward leg, and keep the back knee straight, heel down. You will feel a good stretch in the calf. Hold the stretch for 10 seconds. Do not bounce. You can adjust this exercise to also stretch the other large calf muscle by slightly bending your back knee while you stretch.

This exercise helps maintain flexibility in the Achilles tendon, the large tendon at the back of your ankle. Good flexibility helps reduce the risk of injury, calf discomfort, and heel pain. The Achilles stretch is especially helpful for cooling down after walking or cycling and for people who get cramps in the calf muscles. If you have trouble with standing, balance, or spasticity (muscle jerks), you can do a seated version of this exercise. Sit in a chair with feet flat on the floor. Keep your heel on the floor and slowly slide your foot (one foot at a time) back to bend your ankle and feel some tension on the back of your calf (lower leg).

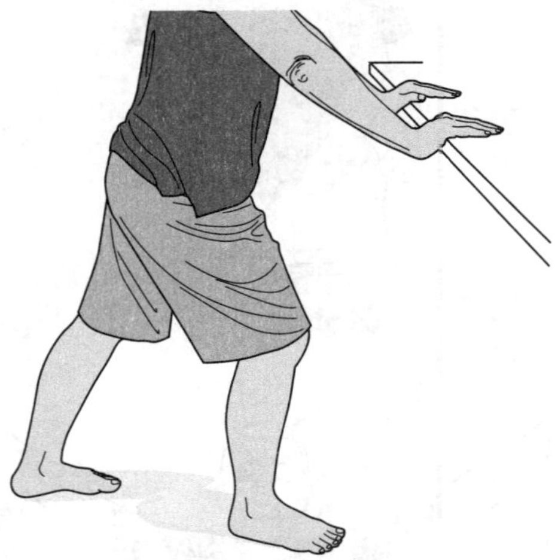

Strength Exercises

Strength for Better Posture

14. Shoulder-Blade Pinch

This is a good exercise to strengthen the middle and upper back and to stretch the chest. It can be an especially good exercise if you have breathing problems. Sit or stand with your head in heads-up position (Exercise 2) and your shoulders relaxed. Raise your arms out to the sides at shoulder height with elbows bent and forearms up. Pinch your shoulder blades together by moving your elbows as far back as you can. Hold briefly, and then slowly move your arms

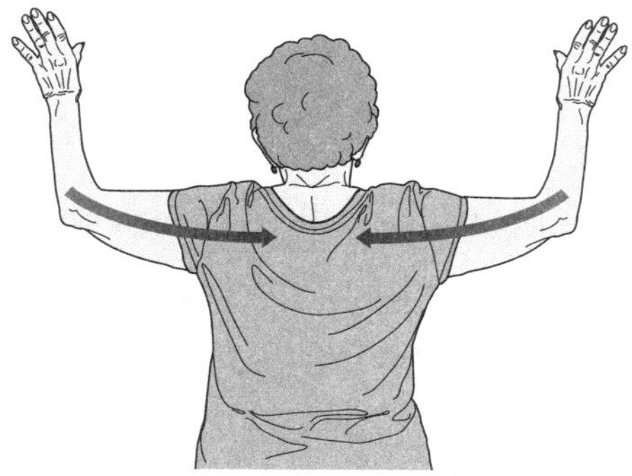

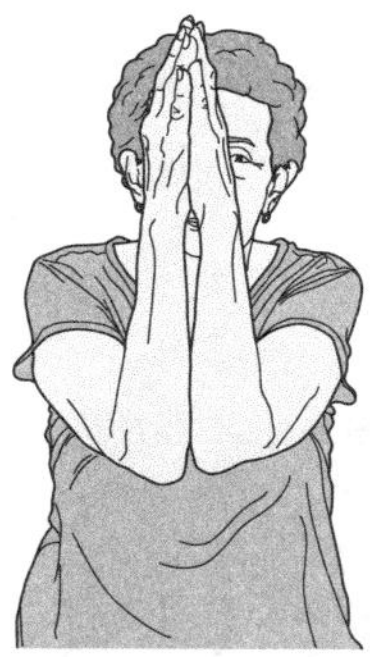

forward to touch your elbows together. If this position is uncomfortable, lower your arms or rest your hands on your shoulders.

15. Curl-Up

A curl-up is a good way to strengthen stomach muscles. Lie on your back, knees bent, feet flat. Do the pelvic tilt (Exercise 6). Slowly curl up in segments. Tuck your chin as you roll your head up and begin to lift your shoulders off the floor. Slowly uncurl back down or hold for 10 seconds and slowly lower. Breathe out as you curl up and breathe in as you uncurl back down. Do not hold your breath. If you have neck problems or

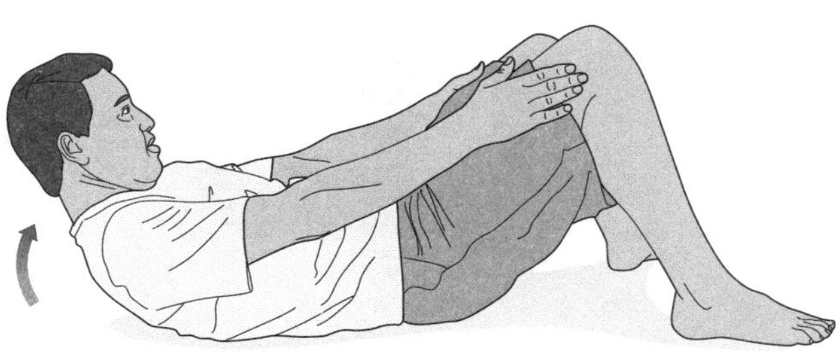

if your neck hurts when you do this exercise, try the roll-out (Exercise 16) instead. Never tuck your feet under a chair or have someone hold your feet!

16. Roll-Out

This is another good stomach strengthener and it is easy on the neck. Use it instead of the curl-up (Exercise 15) if you have neck pain. If neck pain is not a problem, do both exercises.

Lie on your back with knees bent and feet flat. Do the pelvic tilt (Exercise 6) and hold your lower back firmly against the floor.

Slowly and carefully, move one leg away from your chest as you straighten your knee. Move your leg out until you feel your lower back start to arch. When this happens, tuck your knee back to your chest. Reset your pelvic tilt and roll your leg out again. Breathe out as your leg rolls out. Do not hold your breath. Repeat with the other leg.

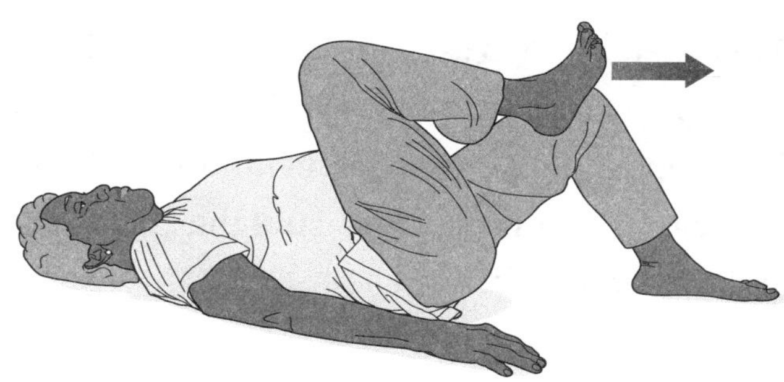

You are strengthening your abdominal muscles by holding your pelvic tilt against the weight of your leg. As you get stronger, you'll be able to straighten your legs out farther and move both legs together.

Leg Strength

17. Straight-Leg Raises

This exercise strengthens the muscles that bend the hip and straighten the knee. Lie on your back, knees bent, feet flat on the floor. Straighten one leg. Tighten the muscle on the upper surface of that thigh and straighten the knee as much as possible. Keeping the knee straight, raise your leg a foot or two (up to 50 centimetres) off the ground. Do not arch your back. Hold your leg up and count out loud for 10 seconds. Relax. Repeat with the other leg.

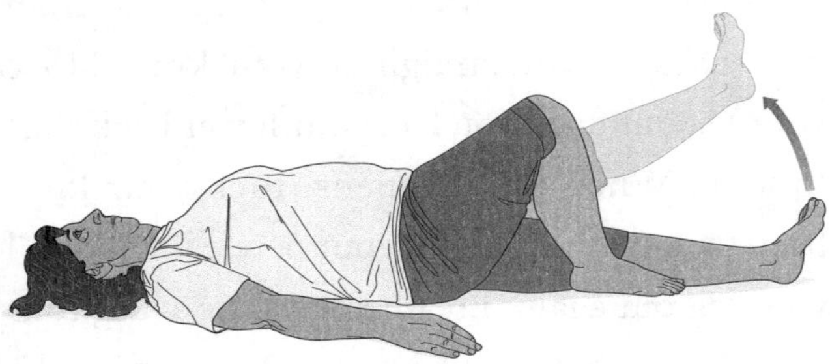

18. Back Kick

This exercise increases the backward mobility and strength of your hip. Hold onto a counter for support. Raise your leg behind you. Move the leg up and back, knee straight. Stand tall and do not lean forward.

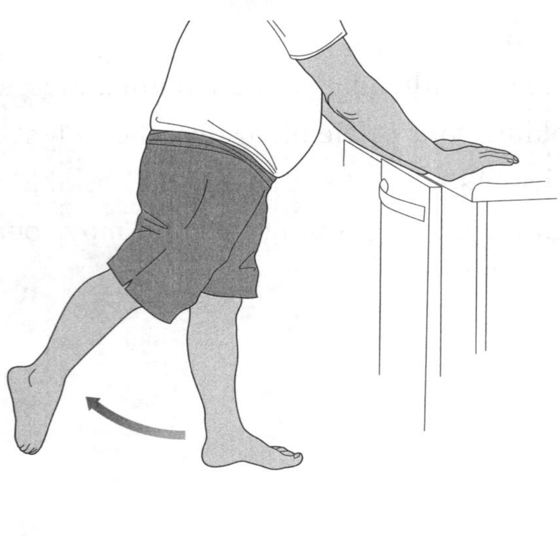

19. Hip Hooray

This exercise can be done standing or lying on your back. If you lie down, spread your legs as far apart as possible. Roll your legs and feet out like a duck, then in to be pigeon-toed. Then move your legs back together. If you are standing, move one leg out to your side as far as you can. Lead out with the heel and in with the toes. Hold onto a counter for support. You can make the muscles work harder while you are standing by adding a weight to your ankle.

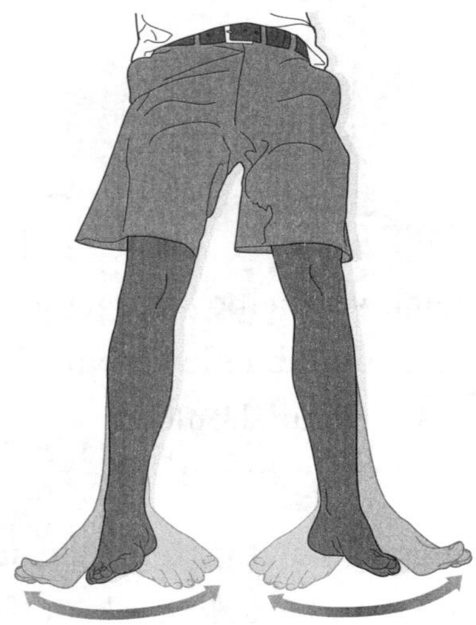

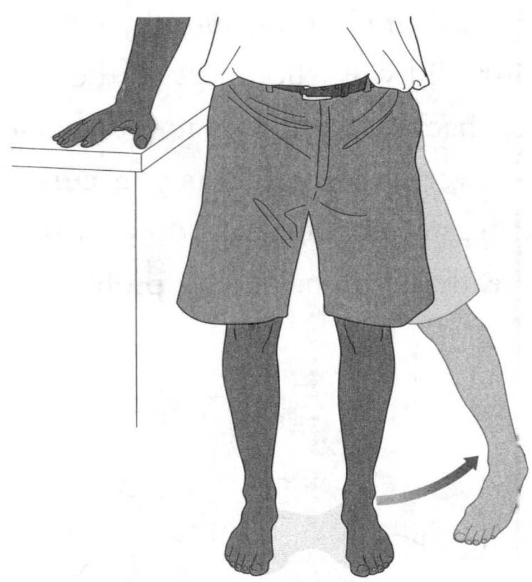

20. Knee Strengthener

Strong knees are important for walking and standing comfortably. This exercise strengthens the knee. Sitting in a chair, extend your leg and straighten your knee by tightening up the muscle on the upper surface of your thigh. Place your hand on your thigh and feel the muscle work. If you wish, make circles with your toes. As your knees strengthen, see if you can build up to holding each leg out for 30 seconds. Count out loud. Do not hold your breath.

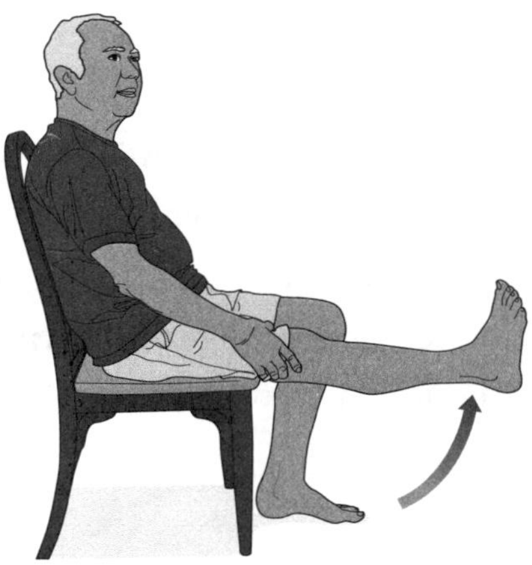

21. Power Knees

This exercise strengthens the muscles that bend and straighten your knees. Sit in a chair and cross your legs at the ankles. You can bend your knees as much as you like but keep your feet touching the floor. Try several positions to find one that works for you. Push forward with your back leg and press backward with your front leg. Exert pressure evenly so that your legs do not move. Hold and count out loud for 10 seconds. Relax. Switch leg positions. Be sure to keep breathing. Repeat.

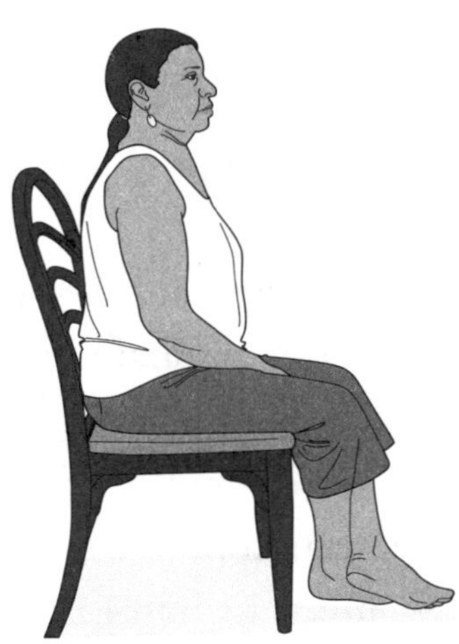

22. Ready-Go

Stand with one leg slightly in front of the other with the heel of the front leg on the floor, as if ready to take a step with the front foot. Now tighten the muscles on the front of the thigh on your front leg, making your front knee firm and straight. Hold for a count of 10. Relax. Switch positions and repeat with the other leg.

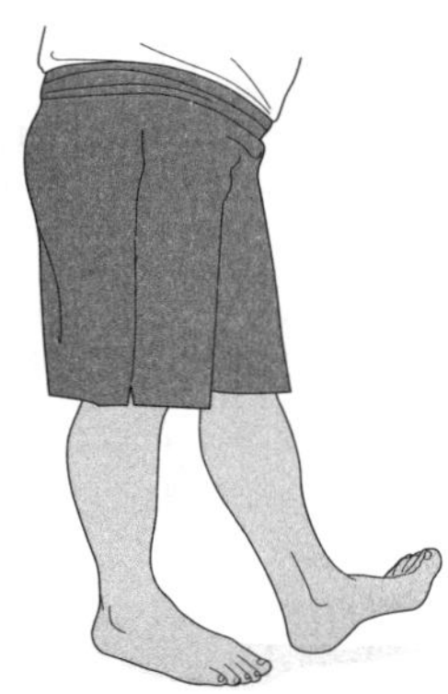

23. Tiptoes

This exercise strengthens your calf (lower leg) muscles and makes walking, climbing stairs, and standing less tiring. It can also improve your balance. Hold onto a counter or table for support and rise up on your tiptoes. Hold for 10 seconds. Lower slowly. How high you go is not as important as keeping your balance and controlling your ankles. It is easier to do both legs at the same time. If your feet are too sore to do this standing, do it while sitting until you are strong enough to do it standing. If this exercise

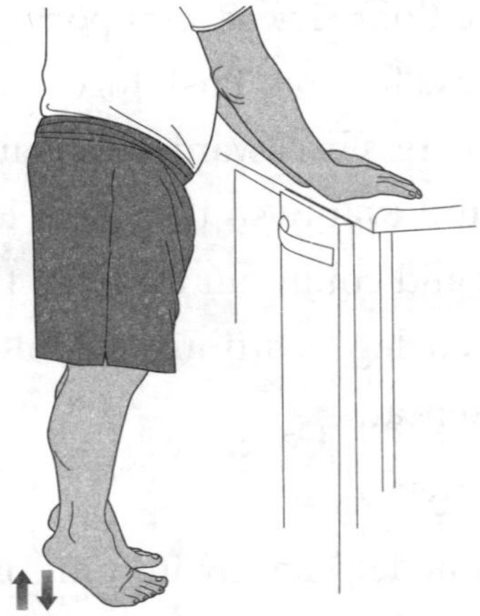

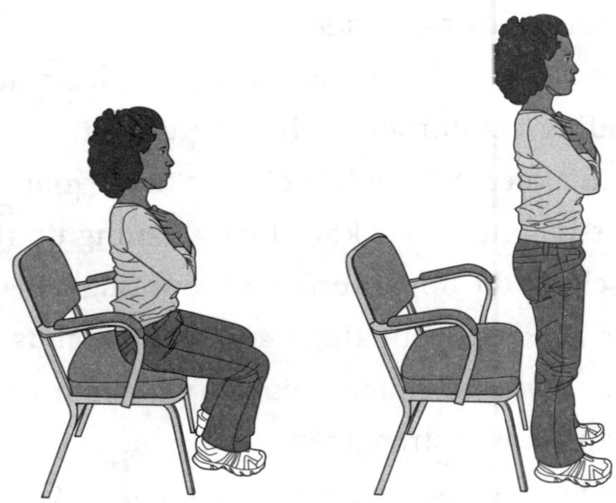

makes your ankle jerk, stop doing it and talk to your physical therapist about other ways to strengthen these calf muscles if needed.

24. Sit-to-Stand

Sit toward the front edge of a straight-backed chair with arms and a firm seat. Bend your knees so that your feet are flat on the floor and behind your knees. Lean a bit forward and stand up. Practice going from sitting to standing using your arms as little as possible. Work on standing up without using your arms. At first you may need your arms to push up. Stand up five times. Rest a bit and do five more. Little by little, as your hips and legs get stronger, you will be able to stand without using your arms.

Balance Exercises

Sometimes people decide that the best way not to fall is to spend more time sitting. At first you might think that if you and your care partner are not up walking around, you won't be at risk for falling. However, inactivity causes weakness, stiffness, and slower reflexes. All of these decrease your ability to balance and increase the risk of falling. Poor balance makes even simple things, such as getting up or sitting down in a chair, more risky. Physical conditions such as weakness, dizziness, stiffness, poor eyesight, loss of feeling in feet, or inner ear problems can put you at risk for falls, as can the side effects of medications. Falls can also happen because of your surroundings: poor lighting, uneven ground, rugs, and cluttered floors. To avoid falls, reduce all these risks and keep yourself strong, flexible, and coordinated. Research shows that people who have strong legs and ankles, are flexible, and do things that require them to balance have less fear of falling and fall less. Chapter 8, Preventing Injuries, has more specific information and tips to help you reduce the risk of falling.

If you or your care partner have fallen or you are afraid that one of you might fall, talk with your health care providers and get your balance checked to make sure there are no vision, inner ear, or medication problems that need to be fixed. Make sure your home is safe. (Learn more about keeping your home safe in Chapter 8, Preventing Injuries.)

The exercises in this section are designed to let you or your care partner improve your balance in a safe and progressive way. The exercises **are presented in order of difficulty.** Start with the first exercises and work up to the more difficult ones as your strength and balance improve. If you feel that your balance is particularly poor, exercise with someone else close by who can give you a supporting hand if needed. Always practice by a counter or stable chair that you can hold onto when necessary. You will know your balance is improving when you are able to hold a position longer or without extra support or you can do an exercise or hold a position with your eyes closed.

There might be some balance exercise classes in your community or you can find online programs to help continue your progress. Resources to find safe and effective balance programs are listed at

www.bullpub.com/resources.

25. Beginning Balance

Stand quietly with your feet comfortably apart. Place your hands on your hips and turn your head and trunk as far to the left as possible and then to the right. Repeat five to 10 times.

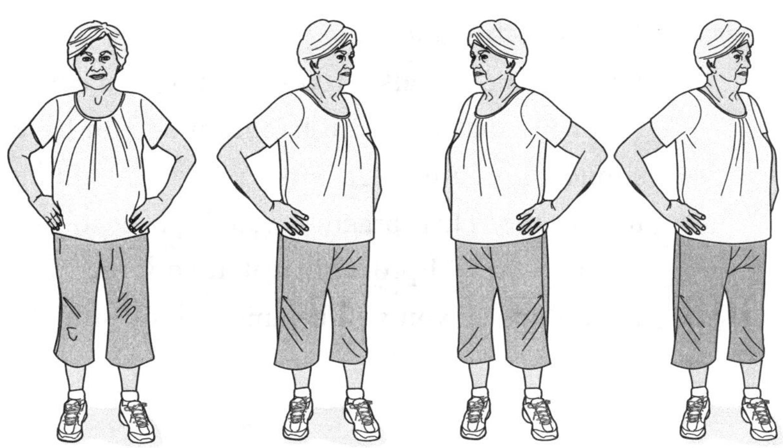

26. Swing and Sway

Using a counter or the back of a stable chair for support, rock back on your heels and then rise up on your toes. Do each five to 10 times.

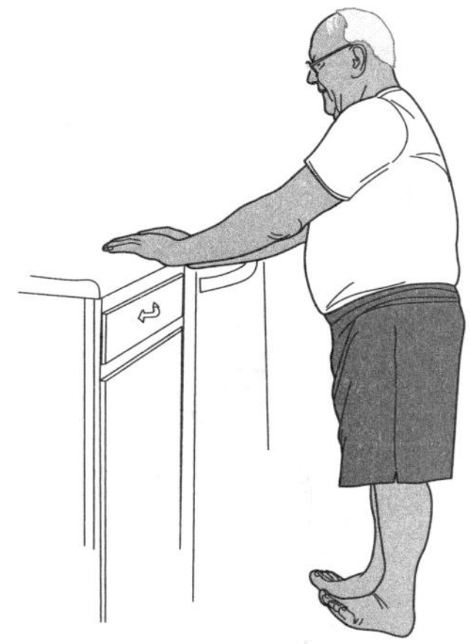

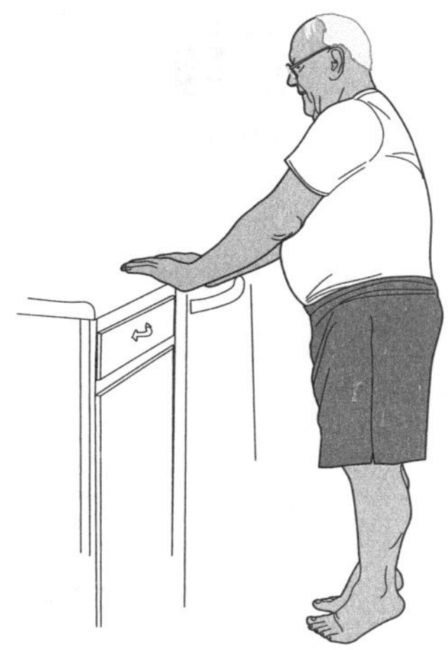

27. Toe Walk

This exercise increases ankle strength and gives you practice balancing on a small base of support while moving. Stay close to a counter for support. Rise up on your toes and walk back and forth next to the counter. Once you are comfortable walking on your toes and feel stronger, you will need less support.

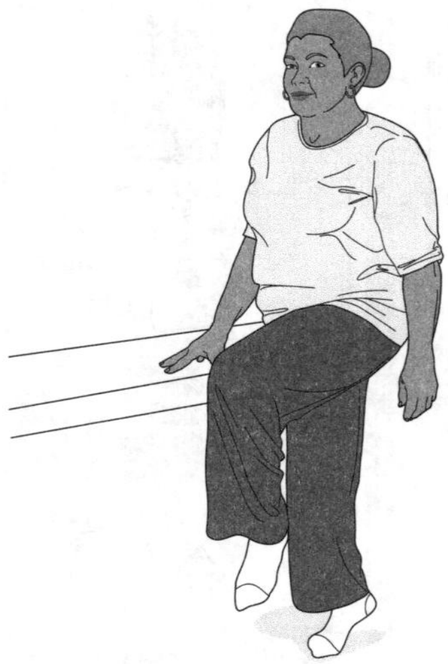

28. Heel Walk

This exercise increases your lower leg strength and gives you practice moving on a small base of support. Stay close to a counter for support. Raise your toes and forefoot and walk back and forth next to the counter on your heels. Once you are comfortable walking on your heels and feel stronger, you will find you need less support.

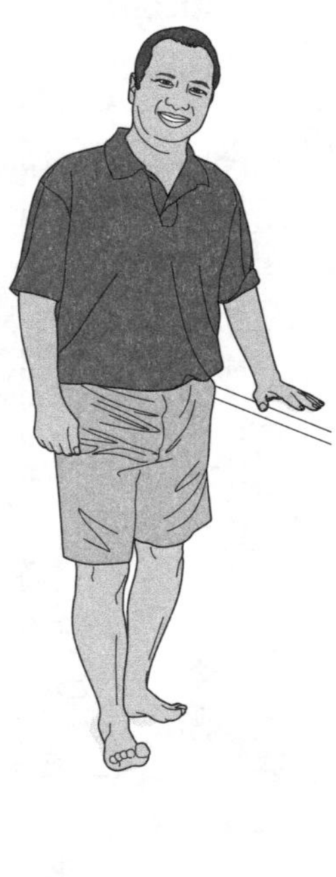

If you are not ready to walk, you can modify the toe and heel walk to practice standing in place.

29. One-Legged Stand

Holding onto a counter or chair, lift one foot completely off the ground and stand on one foot. Once you are balanced, lift the hand that is not holding onto the support. The goal is to hold the position for 10 seconds. Once you can do this for 10 seconds without holding on, practice it with your eyes closed. Repeat for the other leg.

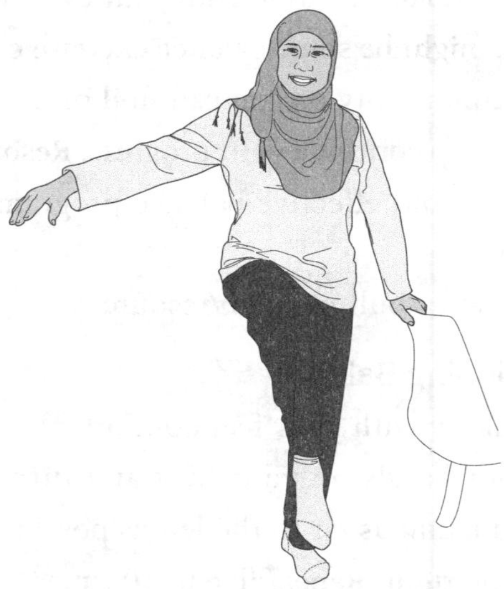

30. Walk-the-Line

Find a place to walk a few steps next to a counter or in a hallway with handrails so you have support if you need it. First, practice standing heel to toe. Then practice walking heel-to-toe. At first you will probably watch your feet, but with practice, you will be able to look straight ahead.

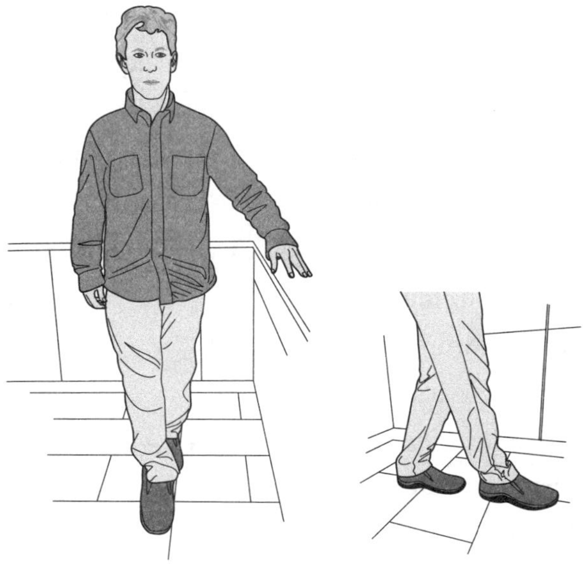

Endurance Exercises

Having good endurance means you can do your daily tasks without tiring quickly or feeling "worn out" all the time. Health guidelines recommend that adults exercise at a moderate intensity for at least 150 minutes each week in activities spread throughout the week. There are many ways to work endurance exercise into your day. The most important thing to remember is that some activity is better than none. If you start off doing what is comfortable and increase your efforts gradually, it is likely that you will build a healthy, lifelong habit. You will learn how to stay active and how to return to being active even when changes in your life or responsibilities may slow you down or derail your exercise efforts for a while. It is better to begin your program by underdoing rather than overdoing and to add more activity as you get stronger and more comfortable with exercise. Endurance exercise can also be an opportunity to spend time with others. You may want to find an exercise partner, join a class, or include your care partner in an activity that can help you both feel stronger and more energetic.

Flexibility and strengthening exercises are described by how many repetitions you do at a time. Endurance exercise is described by how often you do it (frequency), how long you exercise at a time (duration), and how hard you work (intensity).

- **Frequency (how often).** Most guidelines suggest doing at least some exercise most days of the week. Exercising four to five times a week is a good choice.
- **Duration (how much time).** According to the guidelines, it is best if you can exercise at least 10 minutes at a time. You can add up your 10-minute exercise periods to meet the weekly 150-minute recommended amount. For example, taking three 10-minute walks each day for five days gets you to 150 minutes for the week. If 10 minutes is too much at first, start with what you can do and work toward 10 minutes.

- **Intensity (how hard you work).** Aerobic or endurance exercise is safe and effective at a moderate intensity. When you exercise at moderate intensity, you feel somewhat warmer, you breathe more deeply and faster than usual, and your heart beats faster than normal. Exercise intensity is relative to your fitness. For an athlete, running a mile in 10 minutes is probably low-intensity exercise. For a person who hasn't exercised in a long time, a 10-minute walk at a constant pace may be moderate- to high-intensity exercise. For someone with severe physical limitations, a slow walk might be high-intensity exercise.

  There are a couple of simple ways to figure out what is moderate intensity for you.

- **Talk test.** When exercising, talk to another person or to yourself out loud. Moderate-intensity exercise allows you to speak comfortably. If you can't carry on a conversation because you are breathing too hard or are short of breath, you're working at a high intensity. Slow down. The talk test is an easy and quick way to recognize your effort and regulate intensity. If you exercise with your care partner, the talk test is an easy way to keep track of your care partner's intensity and make adjustments if needed. If you or your care partner have lung disease, the talk test might not work for you. If that is the case, try using the perceived-exertion scale.

- **Perceived exertion.** Another way to monitor intensity is to rate how hard you're working on a scale of perceived exertion. On a 0-to-10 scale, 0, at the low end of the scale, is sitting or lying down, doing no work at all. Ten is equivalent to working as hard as possible—very hard work that you couldn't do for more than a few seconds. A good level for moderate aerobic exercise on the perceived-exertion scale is between 4 and 5.

There are several kinds of exercise that you can use to improve your endurance. Walking, bicycling, swimming, water exercise, or low-impact aerobics classes are good choices and let you start comfortably and at your own pace.

Walking

Walking is easy, inexpensive, and safe. It can be done almost anywhere. You can walk inside or outside, by yourself or with company. Walking is something you might be able to do with your care partner. Walking is safer than jogging or running and puts less stress on the body. It's an especially good choice if you have been sedentary or have joint or balance problems.

If you walk to shop, visit friends, and do household chores, then you can probably walk for exercise. Using a cane or walker need not stop you from getting into a walking routine. Be careful the first two weeks of walking. If you haven't been doing much for a while, five or 10 minutes might be enough. Alternate brisk walks and slow walks to build up your endurance. Each week, increase the brisk walking interval by no more than five minutes until you are up to 20 or 30 minutes of brisk walking at a time.

Remember that a good goal is to walk most days of the week at moderate intensity and to build your time to get up to at least 10 minutes each time you walk. You are in charge of your walking. You control the frequency, duration, and intensity. The following walking tips can help you be safe and successful:

- **Choose your ground.** Walk on a flat, level surface. Walking on hills, uneven ground, soft earth, sand, or gravel is hard work and often leads to hip, knee, or foot pain. Fitness trails, shopping malls, school tracks, streets with sidewalks, and quiet neighborhoods are good places.
- **Always warm up and cool down with a stroll.** Walk slowly for five minutes to prepare your circulation and muscles for a brisker walk. Finish up with the same slow walk to let your body calm down gradually. Experienced walkers know they can avoid shin and foot discomfort if they begin and end with a slow stroll.
- **Set your own pace.** It takes practice to find the right walking speed. To find your speed, start walking slowly for a few minutes, then increase your speed to a pace that is slightly faster than normal for you. After five minutes, check your exercise intensity with the perceived-exertion or talk test (see page 168). If you are working too hard or feel out of breath, slow down. If your exertion is below moderate intensity, try walking a little faster. Walk another five minutes and check your intensity again. If you are still below your target intensity, keep walking at a comfortable speed and simply check your intensity in the middle and at the end of each walk.
- **Use a walking or hiking stick.** You can learn more about walking sticks in Table 8.3 in Chapter 8, Preventing Injuries (see pages 141–144).

Choosing Shoes

Choose shoes of the correct length and width with shock-absorbing soles and insoles. Make sure they're big enough in the toe area. There should be a thumb width between the end of your longest toe and the end of the shoe. You shouldn't feel uncomfortable pressure on the sides or tops of your toes. The back of the shoe should hold your heel firmly in the shoe when you walk. Be sure your shoes are in not too worn down.

Wear shoes with a continuous sole. Avoid shoes that have very thick, rubbery, or sticky soles that may create a tripping hazard. Shoes with laces or Velcro let you adjust width as needed and give more support than slip-ons. If you have problems tying laces, consider Velcro closures or elastic shoelaces. Shoes with leather soles and a separate heel don't absorb shock as well as athletic and casual shoes. Good shoes do not need to be expensive. Any shoes that meet the criteria we have just described will serve your purposes.

Many people like shoes with removable insoles that can be exchanged for more shock-absorbing insoles purchased separately. You can find insoles in sporting goods stores and shoe stores. When you shop for insoles, take your walking shoes with you. Try on the shoe with the insole inserted to make sure there's enough room for your foot to be comfortable with the insoles in place. Insoles come in different sizes and can be trimmed with scissors for a custom fit. If your toes take up extra room, try the three-quarter insoles that stop just short of your toes. If you have prescribed inserts in your shoes already, ask a professional about insoles.

Preventing Possible Problems

If you have pain around your shins or leg cramps when you walk, you might not be spending enough time warming up or you could be walking too fast. Start your walk at a slow pace. Stick to this pace for at least five minutes. Keep your feet and toes relaxed. Sore knees are another common problem. Take care of your knees by starting with a slower warm-up walk and walk on smooth and even surfaces (for example, on a sidewalk, mall trail, or track). If you are exercising with your care partner, watch out for these problems for both of you.

Exercising in the Water

When you exercise in the water, the buoyancy of the water lets you move your joints through their full range of motion. You can strengthen your muscles and cardiovascular system with less stress than on land. For most people, swimming is excellent exercise. It uses the whole body. If you haven't been swimming for a while, consider a refresher course. For swimming to be an aerobic exercise, you eventually need to swim continuously for 10 minutes. Try different strokes, changing strokes after each lap or two. This lets you exercise all joints and muscles without overtiring any one area. Water exercise classes are a good way to exercise with a leader and other people. Although water exercise can be an excellent aerobic exercise, you also will need to do other standing and walking exercise to improve balance and bone strength. You need to do weight-bearing exercise such as walking, jogging, lifting weights, or dancing to stress bones enough to get stronger.

Stationary Bicycling

Stationary bicycles offer the fitness benefits of bicycling without the outdoor hazards. Indoor use of a stationary bicycle may be preferable to outdoor bicycling for people who live in cold or hilly areas or in areas with lots of car traffic or limited bike lanes or paths. If you have your own equipment, stationary bicycling allows you to exercise without leaving home when you need to be present for caretaking. You can choose between the traditional upright or recumbent bicycle style. Make sure the bike is steady and you can get on and off safely.

The most common complaint about riding a stationary bike is that it's boring. Watching television, reading, or listening to music helps the time go by faster. Penny keeps her indoor cycling interesting by mapping out tours of places she would like to visit and then charts her progress on a map as she rolls off the miles. Henry uses an app to talk him through an interesting ride. Many people spend their bicycle time watching a half hour of a favorite series or listening to a radio program or podcast. There are videos of exotic bike tours. Book racks that clip onto the handlebars make reading easy. Use earbuds and your phone to take your music or podcast of choice along with you.

The following cycling tips can help you be safe and successful:

- **Remember that stationary bicycling uses different muscles than walking.** Until your leg muscles get used to pedaling, you might be able to ride for only a few minutes. Start off with no resistance. Increase resistance slightly as riding gets easier. Increasing resistance has the same effect as bicycling up hills.

- **Pedal at a comfortable speed.** For most people, 50 to 70 revolutions per minute (rpm) is a good starting pace. As you get used to bicycling, you can increase your speed. However, faster is not necessarily better. Listening to music at the right tempo makes it easier to pedal at an enjoyable and consistent speed.

Experience will tell you the best combination of speed and resistance.

- **A good target goal is 20 to 30 minutes of pedaling at a comfortable speed.** Build up your time by alternating intervals of brisk pedaling with periods of less exertion. If you get out of breath, slow down.
- **Keep a record of the times and distances of your bike trips.** You'll be amazed at how much you can do.

Exercise Classes

For many people, an exercise class is a good choice for building endurance and spending time with others. One advantage of joining a class is that you benefit from the experience and knowledge of a teacher and class members. You can take an exercise class in your community or find a class on television, online, or on DVD. With these, you can exercise at home, choose your time, and stop and start when you want. You can also do the class with your care partner. A community class adds social time and a change of scenery to your daily routine. There are many types of classes, including aerobic dance, ballroom and square dance, yoga, tai chi, and water exercise—all with different benefits.

Your local YMCA, senior center, or community recreation center are good places to look for classes. Talk to friends and family about what they do. Visit and observe classes. Choose a place, time, and class that feels comfortable and works for your needs and schedule. Talk with the instructor and take a trial class before signing up for a long-term commitment. Look for an instructor who encourages everyone to go at their own pace and a class where people are friendly and having fun. Check with the facility to find out if your insurance covers the cost of membership. There are some suggestions for classes listed at www.bullpub.com/resources, including programs that may be available in your community and others that are available online, on DVD, or on television.

Exercising with Your Care Partner

Many exercises and activities can be adapted in ways to let people with different needs and abilities take part. If your care partner is physically limited, for example, there are exercises that can be done sitting or lying down instead of standing. The good morning exercise (Exercise 11, page 159) and the shoulder-blade pinch (Exercise 14, pages 160–161) can be done standing, sitting, or lying down. The toe walk and the heel walk (Exercises 27 and 28, page 166) are described as standing and moving exercises, but they can also be done seated. The exercises shown lying down are best done on the floor or a firm mat but could be done in bed too.

When you choose exercises for yourself, discuss the exercises with care partners and explore what they might want to do. Try a couple types of exercises. Try to find a time during the day to exercise together. You don't need to do the same things, just be active together. You might also ask your care partner to count or keep time for you as you exercise, like a coach or cheerleader. When you are active together, you are encouraging and supporting each other in a healthy habit, and it is a pleasant way to spend time together.

Anuj and Leila do stretches and balance exercises for 10 minutes each morning after breakfast before it is time to get ready for the day. Anuj's favorite exercise is good morning stretch (Exercise 11, page 159). When the weather permits, on Monday, Wednesday, and Friday afternoons, they walk to the park, which is 20 minutes away. Leila also takes a yoga class at the local Y that meets three times a week while Anuj's sister visits with Anuj.

Overcoming Exercise Barriers

Health and fitness make sense. Yet when faced with being more physically active, people often come up with many excuses, concerns, and worries. These can prevent you from taking the first step. Here are some common barriers and possible solutions:

- **"I don't have enough time."** When you are a caregiver, you have many tasks to complete every day that require time and energy. Becoming stronger and more energetic can make the rest of your day better. Exercise doesn't take a lot of time. Ten minutes at a time two or three times a day can make a big difference in how you feel. Get your steps in first thing by making a morning stretch or several short walks part of your daily routine. For example, get your exercise in by doing a morning stretch and taking several short walks throughout your day. Try adding some exercise to things you already do. Stretch while you watch TV. Walk to visit your friend down the block. Sometimes on-demand classes are easier to fit in to a busy day. Take an exercise class via a virtual platform such as Zoom.
- **"I'm too tired."** When you're a full-time caregiver, stressed out, out of shape, or depressed, you might feel tired. You need to break out of the "too tired" cycle. Try an experiment: Next time you are too tired, do a few of stretching exercises in this chapter or take a short walk (five minutes or even just two!). You may be surprised how this changes your outlook and gives you energy. As you become more active, you will recognize the difference between feeling listless and feeling physically tired.

- **"I'm too old."** You're never too old for physical activity. No matter what your level of fitness or your age, you can always find ways to increase your activity, energy, and sense of well-being. Fitness is especially important as people age.
- **"I get enough exercise."** This might be true, but for most people, their jobs and daily activities do not provide enough sustained exercise at a moderate level to keep them fit and energetic. An interesting and often surprising way to really find out how active you are is to use a step counter. There are a variety of choices—some that you can wear on your wrist and some that hang on a belt or you carry in a pocket. There are step-counting apps for most smartphones as well as smart watches that count and record steps.
- **"Exercise is boring."** You can make exercise interesting and fun. Exercise with other people. Entertain yourself with headphones or earphones. Listen to a podcast or music. Vary your activities and your walking routes. Think of exercise time as a good opportunity to think and problem solve.
- **"Exercise is painful."** The old saying "no pain, no gain" is simply wrong. Health benefits come from regular moderate-intensity physical activity. Choose exercises that are comfortable and do not cause pain.
- **"I'm afraid I might fall."** Choose places to exercise that are safe (good lighting, well-maintained parking lots and walkways, handrails, and uncluttered floors). Choose exercises that feel safe. For example, chair exercise, water exercise, beginning yoga, or recumbent bicycling provide a lot of support as you get started. Remember, having good posture and balance and staying active reduces the risks of falls.
- **"I'm afraid I'll have a heart attack."** In most cases, the risk of a heart attack is greater for people who are not physically active than for those who exercise regularly. If you are worried about this, check with your doctor.
- **"I'm afraid I won't be able to do it right or won't be successful."** Many people don't start a new project because they are frightened they will fail. If you feel this way, remember two things. First, whatever exercise activities you are able to do—no matter how short or "easy"—will be much better than doing nothing. Be proud of what you have done, not guilty about what you haven't done. Second, new projects often seem overwhelming until you get started and learn to enjoy each day's adventures and successes.

Perhaps you have some other barriers. Be honest with yourself about your worries. Talk to yourself and others to develop positive thoughts about exercise. If you get stuck, ask others for suggestions, or try some of the positive thinking suggestions in Chapter 5, Using Your Mind to Manage Stress.

Getting in the Habit of Healthy Exercise and Keeping It Up

If you haven't exercised recently, you may experience some new feelings and frustrations when you first start exercising. Don't be surprised by setbacks. There will be interruptions. You might get off track for a while. Don't be discouraged. You may need a rest, a different schedule, or different activities. If you get derailed, take a short break. When you are ready, start again. Begin at a lower, gentler level. It can take you the same amount of time to get back into shape as you were out. For instance, if you missed three weeks, it might take at least that long to get back to your previous level. Go slowly. Be kind to yourself. You're in this for the long haul. Remember, it is regular moving that matters.

With exercise experience, you develop a sense of control over yourself and your schedule. You learn how to choose your activity to fit your needs. You know when to do less and when to do more. When there are interruptions, you know it isn't a disaster. You know you have the tools to get back on track. Give yourself a chance to succeed. Sticking with it and doing it your way makes you a sure winner.

For most people who are not already active, starting an exercise routine means getting into a new habit. This means making time on most days of the week to exercise. Exercise is part of good self-care and relaxation. Think of your head as the coach and your body as your team. For success, all parts of the team need attention. Be a good coach. Encourage and praise yourself. Design "plays" you feel your team will like. Choose places that you like and are safe. Good coaches know their teams, set good goals, and help the team succeed and get more confident. A good coach is loyal. A good coach does not belittle, nag, or make anyone feel guilty. Be a good coach to yourself.

Besides a good coach, everyone needs a good cheerleader or two. Of course, you can be your own cheerleader, but being both coach and cheerleader is a lot. Successful exercisers usually have at least one family member or friend who encourages them. Sometimes cheerleaders pop up by themselves, but don't be bashful about asking for a hand. Your cheerleader can exercise with you, help you get other chores done so you can exercise, praise you, or just consider your exercise time when making plans. Your care partner can be a good cheerleader and remind you and encourage you to take time for yourself to exercise. They can also participate in exercise with you.

We hope this chapter helps you learn to use exercise to feel better and stay healthy. Start by knowing your own needs and limits and respect your body. Talk to other people like you who exercise. You are likely to find other caregivers. Talk with your doctor and other health professionals. Always pay attention to your own experience. You will learn to know your own body and make wise choices.

There are many websites for finding online and local exercise resources. For a complete list, please see: www.bullpub.com/resources. Read the descriptions, looking for the research that has been done and the experience and certifications of the instructor. Programs that have been proven safe and effective in scientific studies are often referred to as "evidence-based."

- **National Council on Aging (https://www.ncoa.org/evidence-based-programs).** This site lists and provides links to many evidence-based exercise programs. Some are available online and some are in-person community classes. It is a good place to search for safe and effective programs.
- **OTAGA Exercise Programs.** These online exercise programs are evidence-based and come from OTAGA University in New Zealand. They can be accessed through the NCOA site listed above or directly through YouTube.
- **SilverSneakers (https://www.silversneakers.com).** This evidence-based program is taught in many communities by trained leaders. Some insurance plans provide it as a benefit. Many of the Silver Sneakers classes are also available for online participation. Links are on their website.
- **Sit and Be Fit (https://sitandbefit.org).** This program offers classes through public television, streaming, YouTube, and DVDs.
- **Moving Easy and Exercises for Chronic Conditions (https://www.bullpub.com).** These are audio programs that talk you through gentle exercise sessions.

For a complete list of suggested further readings, useful websites, and other helpful resources, please see www.bullpub.com/resources.

Special thanks to Ann Constance, MA, RDN, CDE, FAADE, Bonnie Bruce, DrPH, MPH, RD, Cindy Tran, MPH, Robin Edelman, MS, RDN, CDE, and Yvonne Mullan, MSc, RD, CDE for their contributions to this chapter.

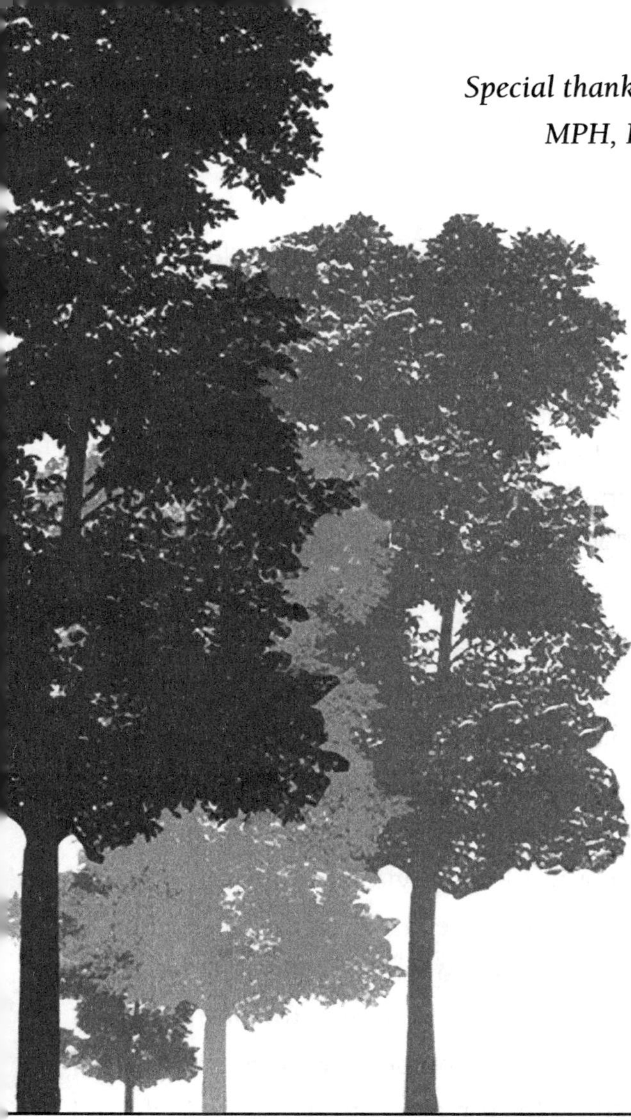

CHAPTER 10

Healthy Eating

WE ALL HAVE PERSONAL PREFERENCES about the food we eat. Your likes and dislikes have been shaped by your culture, family, religion, and health needs, as well as the media and society. What was once considered healthy when you were a child may not be so today. As scientists and nutritionists learn more about the body and nutrition, this will continue to change.

Healthy eating means making healthful food and drink choices most of the time. It also includes finding new or different ways to prepare meals and snacks to make them tasty and appealing. If you or your care partner have certain health conditions, you may need to be choosier about what and how much you eat. Eating healthier does not mean you have to be inflexible or perfect, depriving yourself all the time, or never enjoying your favorite foods. Sometimes, you can eat less-healthy foods in moderation.

About This Chapter

To write this chapter, we referenced the latest scientific research and the USDA Dietary Guidelines, as well as information from the Centers for Disease Control and Prevention, the Academy of Nutrition and Dietetics, the American Heart Association, and the American Diabetes Association.

For Canadian information, we referenced Canada's Dietary Guidelines and information from the Public Health Agency of Canada, Dietitians of Canada, Heart and Stroke Foundation of Canada, and Diabetes Canada. (Please note that most Canadian-specific content is shaded throughout the book.) The overall focus is on scientific, evidence-based, nationally established nutrition guidelines.

In this chapter, we give you some science-based information about nutrition and guidelines for healthier eating, but we do not tell you what or how to eat. This is something you decide. Remember, no matter what the media or your friends may say, there is no one best way of eating for everyone. There is no perfect food or perfect way to eat. There are different roads to healthier eating, and only you will know the best ways to do this for yourself and your care partner. We offer suggestions that are working for other people and are based on research by nutrition experts. On pages 197–203 you will find information for individuals with the most common long-term health conditions. Eating can be a source of joy or stress, especially when you must navigate the choices for your care partner as well as for yourself. We hope that this chapter will help to make eating a more joyful experience and not another cause of stress.

Why Is Healthy Eating So Important?

The human body is a marvelous machine. Much like a car, the human body needs the proper mix of fuel (food) to run well. Your body will not function well and may even stop working if you have the wrong type of fuel or are running on empty. Healthy eating is important to every part of your life and your care partner's life. It is linked to how well you move, think, and sleep; how much energy you have; and even how you enjoy life. What you eat helps prevent illness and promotes healing. This is also true for your care partner. When you give your bodies the right nourishment, you:

- have more energy and feel less tired.
- increase the chances of preventing or lessening further problems from health conditions such as heart disease, diabetes, kidney disease, and cancer.
- feed the brain, which can help you better handle life's challenges.
- may sleep better.

Guidelines for Healthy Eating

Healthy eating depends on the choices you make daily. Some people may need to be more aware of the foods they eat. For example, people with diabetes need to watch their carbohydrate intake to manage their blood sugar levels. They do best by planning which and the amount of carbohydrate foods (such as milk, fruit, breads, beans, cereals, and rice) they will eat daily. Others, who have heart disease or are at risk for heart disease, watch the amount and kinds of fat they eat to help control their blood cholesterol levels. Those with high blood pressure can help lower their blood pressure by eating lots of fruits, vegetables, low-fat dairy foods and by cutting back on salt. Those who want to lose or gain weight need to pay attention to how many calories they eat.

Here are some general guidelines for healthier eating for everyone including you and your care partner:

- Follow a healthy eating pattern no matter what your age, health conditions, or current weight. If you are trying to improve your eating, shift gradually to healthier food and drink choices.
- Eat a variety of whole, unprocessed, or less-processed foods, especially fruits, vegetables, and whole grains that are rich in vitamins, minerals, and other nutrients (substances that are essential for growth and maintenance of life).
- Use the USDA MyPlate (Canada's Food Guide Plate) to help you choose the right amounts of foods to include in your healthy meals or snacks. Learn more about the plate method on pages 195–196.
- Limit added sugars, saturated and trans fats, and sodium (salt). Choose healthier fats (see page 188) and salt-free seasonings, such as citrus, herbs, and spices.
- Eat a variety of lean protein foods, including seafood, lean meats and poultry, and legumes (dried beans, lentils, and split peas).
- Quench your thirst with water and/or beverages you enjoy, but choose beverages without extra calories from sugar, such as unsweetened water, coffee, or tea.
- If you drink alcohol, limit the amount to no more than one drink a day for women and two drinks a day for men. One alcoholic drink is 5 ounces (148 mL) of wine, 12 ounces (355 mL) of beer, or 1.5 ounces (44 mL) of rum, vodka, whiskey, or other liquor. Please note that the US Surgeon General has also issued a warning connecting alcohol use with cancer.

> Canada's Guidance on Alcohol and Health states that research shows that no amount or kind of alcohol is good for your health. It doesn't matter what kind of alcohol it is—wine, beer, cider, or spirits. Drinking alcohol, even a small amount, is damaging to everyone, regardless of age, sex, gender, ethnicity, tolerance for alcohol, or lifestyle.

That's why if you drink, it's better to drink less. If you are going to drink, don't exceed two drinks on any day. (Please note that most Canadian-specific content is shaded throughout the book.)

- Allow yourself small occasional treats even if they are not the healthiest choices.

The real concern is the consumption of less nutritious foods that people eat in place of healthier foods. People may choose these because less nutritious foods often cost less, are more available, are easy to fix, and taste good. About 75 percent of North Americans do not eat enough vegetables, fruits, and dairy. At the same time, many North Americans eat too many foods that are high in added sugars and sodium (salt); trans fats like stick margarine and hydrogenated oil; saturated fats, meats, and coconut and palm oils; and high-fat dairy products, such as butter, ice cream, and cheese. People in the United States and Canada also eat a lot of food made from white flour and other refined grains. These foods and added sugars, fats, and salt are linked to health problems such as obesity, high blood pressure, diabetes, heart disease, and chronic pain.

The best scientific studies and evidence suggest that healthy eating that is focused on plant-based foods is best for general health. The Mediterranean diet is a good example of this. We are not suggesting you change everything you eat overnight. Rather, use this information to help you make better food choices gradually.

Eating the Mediterranean Way

The Mediterranean-style eating pattern is based on the traditional diet of Italy, Spain, and Greece. Consider the pyramid with four layers in Figure 10.1.

The base of the pyramid shows the foods that should be the basis of every meal. Most people benefit from eating more of these foods more of the time. They include:

- fruits
- vegetables
- dried beans and other legumes, such as lentils, navy beans, pinto beans, and split peas

A Special Note for Caregivers

It may be that your care partner is nearing the end of life or that eating is one of their few pleasurable activities. While healthy eating is important, making perfect food choices might not be as important during this time. For example, it could be fine for your care partner to have dessert first, not eat all their greens, or have ice cream every night. If you are concerned about your care partner's nutrition, talk with a health care professional.

- nuts and seeds
- whole-grain breads, cereals, rice, and pasta
- plant-based oils, such as olive oil
- herbs and spices without added salt

The next layer in the pyramid is fish and seafood. These foods are okay to eat in moderate amounts often, at least twice a week.

The third layer is poultry, eggs, cheese, and yogurt. These foods can be eaten daily to weekly in moderate portion sizes.

At the very tip of the pyramid are red meats and sweets. Eat moderate portions of these foods no more than a few times a month.

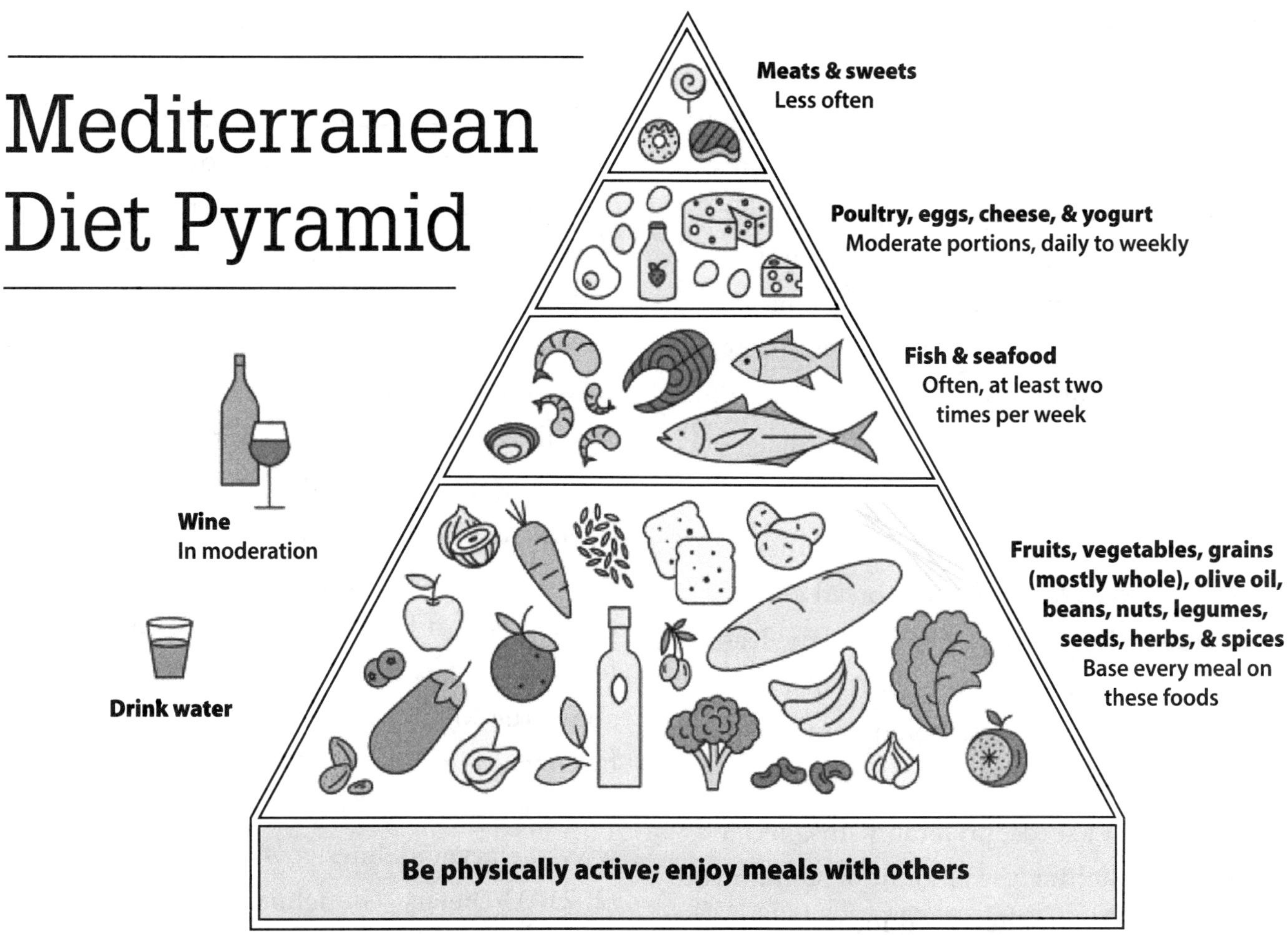

Figure 10.1 **Mediterranean Diet Pyramid**

Healthy Vegetarian Eating

The healthy vegetarian dietary pattern is very similar to the Mediterranean-style dietary pattern. In place of meat or fish, the vegetarian pattern suggests eggs, legumes (dried peas and beans), soy products, and nuts and seeds. You can learn more about this plan by consulting Table A3-4 on the Dietary Guidelines for Americans 2020–2025 website (https://www.dietaryguidelines.gov/sites/default/files/2021-03/Dietary_Guidelines_for_Americans-2020-2025.pdf).

Finally, the pyramid suggests drinking plenty of water and, if you drink wine or alcohol, do so in moderation.

The Mediterranean plan also advises you to:

- Work toward eating ten servings of plant-based food a day. At least five of these servings should come from vegetables and fruits. (A serving of fruits or vegetables is 4 to 6 ounces, or 112 to 168 g—for more information on serving sizes, see page 185.)
- Eat fish and other seafood at least twice a week.
- Instead of butter, use olive oil or other plant-based oils for dipping bread and cooking. (Extra-virgin olive oil—the least refined oil—helps prevent heart disease, avoid blood clots, lower blood pressure, and reduce inflammation.)
- Eat nuts and seeds, preferably unsalted if you are watching the amount of sodium you eat. Not only are they good for you, but they also help fill you up. Eat small amounts, such as one serving (1/3 cup or 75 mL), a few times a week.
- Eat red meat less often (no more than a few times a month), and when you eat meat, choose small portions. Avoid fatty processed meats, such as bacon and sausage. Choose poultry, eggs, and cheese more often than red meat on a daily to weekly basis.
- When you eat or drink dairy products and milk, choose low-fat options.

The Mediterranean diet may look quite different from how you eat now. Remember this motto: "Go for the real, not the ideal." You will be surprised at how small, gradual changes can lead to big health gains. You can learn more about the Mediterranean-style dietary pattern by consulting Table A3-5 on the Dietary Guidelines for Americans 2020–2025 website (https://www.dietaryguidelines.gov/sites/default/files/2021-03/Dietary_Guidelines_for_Americans-2020-2025.pdf).

Knowing What and How Much to Eat

It is easy to say that you and your care partner should eat the amount that your bodies need and not more or less, but this can be difficult to put into action. Eating well means knowing

Your Intestines and Your Health

Trillions of *microorganisms*, including helpful bacteria and yeast, live in your gut, which is also called a *microbiome*. These microorganisms play an essential role in your health. Your microbiome helps you digest food and protects you from harmful bacteria.

Each person has a unique microbiome, and people's microbiomes differ in both the kinds and number of organisms they include. The foods you eat affect your microbiome. Some foods contain healthy living microorganisms called *probiotics*. Fermented foods are the best sources of probiotics. Fermented foods or beverages have been transformed by age or by the addition of a bacterial or yeast culture. Fermented foods include yogurt, sauerkraut, and kombucha. Other foods contain *prebiotics*, which are a type of fiber that feeds the friendly bacteria in the gut. Prebiotics are healthy food for the gut microbiome. They allow healthy bacteria and yeast to thrive. Sources of prebiotics include whole grains, onion, leek, asparagus, banana, garlic, honey, yogurt, and legumes (such as beans, peas, and peanuts).

Scientists are not exactly sure how the microbiome works to help prevent and treat illness. But they believe healthier eating—as described in this chapter—promotes a healthier gut which, in turn, helps reduce the discomfort from different health conditions.

something about what you and your care partner eat as well as being mindful of how much you eat. The following tips can help:

- **Create a healthy microbiome/gut** (your digestive tract, which includes the mouth, esophagus, stomach, and intestines). Recently, scientists have discovered that the millions of micro (very small) organisms in your gut are very important. These organisms help people digest food. Scientists also now know that the organisms called *probiotics* also protect people from harmful bacteria and can affect many health conditions.
- **Stop eating when you first feel full.** This can prevent overeating. Pay attention to your body to learn what this feels like. Like all new skills, it takes practice. To stop eating when you begin to feel full, remove your plate or get up from the table.
- **Eat slowly.** This allows you to enjoy your food more and helps keep you from overeating. Make your meals or snacks last at least 15 to 20 minutes. It takes this much time for the brain to catch up and tell your stomach that it is getting full. If you finish quickly, wait at least 15 minutes before getting more food.
- **Pay attention to how much you eat.** Be mindful of how much you eat. It is easy to eat too much food without even knowing it. This happens easily when we are socializing with friends, reading, using the computer, or watching television. In these situations, measure out and take only the portion you want to eat before you sit down. Keep food out of reach or out of sight.
- **Know the difference between a portion and a serving.** A portion is how much

you eat. An easy way to remember this is that *portion* starts with the letter *p*, and a portion is what you put on your *plate*. A *serving* is the amount of food on a Nutrition Facts label or in food guides and charts. A serving may be a different amount than the portion size you usually eat. For example, a serving might be 1/2 cup or 4 ounces (118 mL) of a food. If the portion you eat is more than a serving, for example, 1 cup or 8 ounces (236 mL), you need to use math to figure out how many nutrients and calories you are eating. In this example, you are eating two servings and therefore you are eating two times the amount of nutrients and calories. Serving sizes also differ from one food product to another. Read the following section about Nutrition Facts label to learn more about the serving sizes of common foods.

- **Make your food attractive.** We really do eat with our eyes! Compare a monotone plate of white fish, white rice, and white cauliflower with the colorful mouth-watering appeal of one with golden-brown chicken, grilled sweet potato, and bright green spinach. Which of these two meals is more appetizing?

The Nutrition Facts Label

Knowing what you and your care partner are eating means knowing what nutrients are in foods. On pages 185–195, you can find a discussion of specific nutrients. There are several ways to find out what nutrients you and your care partner are eating. You can read the Nutrition Facts labels on food packaging, which is the approach we discuss in this section of the chapter. In Canada, these labels are referred to as Nutrition Facts tables.You can also use the plate method for healthy eating explained on pages 186–195. And you can use the information found in the "Recommendations for a Healthy Eating Plan" box starting on page 197. Or you can look up general guidelines provided by governmental agencies online and follow those. You may want to use one or more of these ways and mix and match as you choose. There are many different ways to help you make healthier food choices.

Labels such as the one shown in Figure 10.2, along with the ingredients list, can help you learn more about what is in the packaged foods you eat. The Nutrition Facts and ingredients list are two key parts of food packaging. They tell you more about what you are eating and help you make informed choices.

Some US labels are in both English and Spanish, such as the one in Figure 10.2. In this section, we explain the information provided on the label in detail.

> The Canadian Nutrition Facts table in Figure 10.3 differs slightly from the US Nutrition Facts label. In the next section, we present the US label and discuss the key differences in the Canadian table.

Nutrition Facts/Datos de Nutrición	
8 servings per container/8 raciónes por envase	
Serving size/Tomaño por reción	**2/3 cup/2/3 taza (55 g)**
Amount per serving/Contidad por reción	
Calories/Calorias	**230**
	% Daily value*/Valor Diario*
Total Fat/Grasa Total 8g	**10%**
Saturated Fat/Grasa Saturada 1g	**5%**
Trans Fat/Grasa *Trans* 0g	
Cholestero/Colestero 0mg	**0%**
Sodium/Sodio 160mg	**7%**
Total Carbohydrate/Carbohidrato Total 37g	**13%**
Dietary Fiber/Fibra Dietetica 4g	**14%**
Total Sugars/Azúcares Total 12g	
Includes10g Added Sugars/Incluye 10g azúcares añadidos	**20%**
Protein/Proeínas 3g	
Vitamin D/Vitamina D 2mcg	18%
Calcium/Calcio 260mg	20%
Iron/Hierro 8mg	45%
Potassium/Potasio 235mg	6%

*The % Daily Value (DV) tells you how much a nutrient in a serving of foods contributes to a daily diet. 2,000 calories a day is used for general nutrition advice

*El % Valor Diario (VD) le indic cuánto un nutriente en una porción de alimentos contribuye a una dieta diaria. 2,000 calorías al dia se utiliza para asesoramiento de nutrición general.

Figure 10.2 **U.S. Nutrition Facts Label**

Nutrition Facts Valeur nutritive Per 1 cup (250 mL) pour 1 tasse (250 mL)	
Calories 110	**% Daily Value*** **% valeur quotidienne***
Fat / Lipides 0 g	0 %
Saturated / saturés 0 g + Trans / trans 0 g	0 %
Carbohydrate / Glucides 26 g	
Fibre / fibres 0 g	0 %
Sugers / sucres 22 g	22 %
Protein / Protéines 2 g	
Cholesterol / Cholestérol 0 mg	
Sodium 0 mg	0 %
Potassium 450 mg	10 %
Calcium 30 mg	2 %
Iron / Fer 0 mg	0 %

*5% or less is **a little**, 15% or more is **a lot**
*5% ou moins c'est **peu**, 15% ou plue c'est **beaucoup**

Figure 10.3 **Canadian Nutrition Facts Table**

Servings per Container and Serving Size

Serving information is at the very top of the label. All the other information on the label is based on this serving size. As we noted before, a serving may be more or less than what you usually eat, which is a portion. So, you must compare the serving size to what you are actually eating. If you eat a cup (250 mL) of cooked rice and the serving size is 1/2 cup (125 mL), you have eaten two servings. This is neither good nor bad, but it does mean that when you look at calories, carbohydrates, fats, and sodium, you must remember to double the amounts shown on that label. If the label says 15 grams of carbohydrates per serving and you eat two servings, then you have eaten 30 grams of carbohydrates.

Calories

Total calories are listed for the stated serving size. Calories are a measure of energy. Your body weight depends on the number of calories you eat and the number of calories you burn. When a person eats more calories than their body needs, the extra energy is stored as fat, which leads to weight gain. The number of calories you need per day depends on your body size as well as your activities. Eating an average of 1,400 to 2,000 calories a day results in a steady weight for many people. However, it depends on how active a person is. The calories you need for your body weight goals may be different from those of another person. If you are very active you may need more calories, or if you are very inactive you may need fewer calories.

Percent (%) Daily Value

There are daily recommendations for some nutrients on the label. The % Daily Value tells you what percentage of that nutrient is in each serving. This percentage is based on a 2,000-calorie-a-day diet. Even if you don't eat 2,000 calories each day, this information can still help you make decisions. The percentage indicates if there is a smaller or a larger amount of that nutrient in the food. In general, 5 percent or lower daily value means that the food is low in that nutrient. A daily value of 20 percent or higher means that the food is high in that nutrient. Please note that there are no percent daily values for trans fats and proteins. It is best to eat little or no trans fats.

> In Canada, the percent daily value is calculated the same way as in the US, although Health Canada uses the terms "a little" or "a lot." A food with a daily value of 15 percent or higher has "a lot" of that nutrient.

Total Fat

Fat, by weight, has twice as many calories as protein and carbohydrate. An ounce of flour (which is mostly carbohydrate) has about 100 calories, while an ounce of butter (which is all fat) has about 200 calories. An ounce of chocolate chip cookie (about a three-inch cookie) has about 140 calories. Part of the ounce of cookie is fat and part is carbohydrate with a little protein. Ounce for ounce, foods with fat have more calories than foods with little or no fat.

The total fat number listed on the nutrition label includes the healthier fats (polyunsaturated and monounsaturated) and the less healthy fats (saturated and trans). Note that saturated and trans fats are listed separately on the food label. Some people think that all fat is bad. This is not true. For your body to work well, you need some fat—about a tablespoon (15mL) per day. Although all fats have the same number of calories, some fats are more healthful than others, and some can be harmful when we eat too much. Research indicates it is better to eat healthier fats.

The healthier fats (also called unsaturated fats) are usually liquid at room temperature. These fats help keep our cells healthy, and some can help reduce blood cholesterol. Healthier fats include olive, canola, soybean, safflower, corn, peanut, and sunflower oils. Foods rich in healthier fat include nuts, seeds, olives, and avocados.

There is another group of healthier fats called omega-3s. These can be helpful for some people in reducing the risk of heart disease and may help with inflammation and chronic pain symptoms. Omega-3s are found in fatty deep-water fish, such as salmon, mackerel, trout, sardines, and tuna. Other sources of omega-3s include some oils (canola and soybean), chia seeds, flaxseed, and walnuts. However, studies indicate that the body might not be able to use omega-3s from plants as well as it uses the omega-3s from fish.

The unhealthier fats (saturated and trans fats) are usually solid at room temperature. Shortening, butter, lard, and bacon grease are unhealthier saturated fats. Consuming these saturated fats can increase blood cholesterol and the risk of heart disease. Most saturated fats are found in animal foods, such as butter, beef fat (tallow, suet), chicken fat, and pork fat (lard). Other foods high in saturated fat include stick margarines, red meat, ground meat, processed meats (sausage, bacon, luncheon, and deli meats), poultry skin, and whole- and low-fat milk and cheeses, including cream cheese and sour cream. Palm kernel oil, coconut oil, and cocoa butter are also high in saturated fat.

The unhealthiest fats are the trans fats. Trans fats raise blood cholesterol and risk of heart disease more than saturated fats. Trans fats are found mostly in processed foods, including pastries, cakes, cookies, crackers, icing, margarine, and most microwave popcorn.

Be warned! Food companies can legally claim "no" or "0 grams" trans fats on the label even when the food has up to half a gram (0.5 g) per serving. You can tell if a food contains trans fats if the words *hydrogenated* or *partially hydrogenated oils* are in the ingredients list. Eat as few trans fats as possible. Again, notice that the food label lists saturated and trans fats separately.

There is no specific daily recommendation for how much fat you should eat. Most people get more than enough daily. The best recommendation is to eat less saturated and trans fats and replace them with the healthier unsaturated fats. When making this change, do not increase the overall amount of fat you eat.

> In Canada, they list "Fat" and not "Total Fat" in the Nutrition Facts table. Also note that, in Canada, if a food has less than 0.2 grams of trans fat, it can be labeled as trans-fat free.

Cholesterol

Cholesterol is an important part of all our cells. The body makes cholesterol to build healthy cells, but cholesterol is also in foods. Too much cholesterol is a problem because it can clog the blood vessels and cause heart attacks and strokes. Most cholesterol in your blood is made by your body. However, some cholesterol comes from the foods you eat. Cholesterol is only in foods from animals, including shellfish, meat, eggs, milk, and cheese. Plant foods do not contain cholesterol. Foods highest in cholesterol are often also highest in saturated fat.

To tell if a specific food is high or low in cholesterol, look at the % Daily Value column on the food label. Any food with a value of 20 percent cholesterol or more is high in cholesterol. If you want to eat less cholesterol, or if you tend to eat more than one serving of a food, choose foods with cholesterol values of 5 percent or lower.

Tips for Choosing Healthier Fats

When Choosing Foods

- Eat portions of cooked meat, fish, and poultry that are 3 to 5 ounces (85 to 140 g). This portion is about the size of a deck of cards or the palm of your hand.
- Eat poultry without skin. (The skin contains saturated fat.)
- Eat more cold-water fatty fish, such as salmon, tuna, and mackerel.
- Choose leaner cuts of meat, such as lean ground beef, round, sirloin, or flank cuts.
- Trim all the fat you can see from meat before cooking.
- Choose lower-fat or fat-free milk and dairy products, such as cheese, sour cream, cottage cheese, yogurt, and ice cream.
- Choose fats from plant-based whole foods, including olives, nuts, nut butters, seeds, and avocados.

When Preparing Foods

- Cook in a nonstick pan or a pan with small amounts of sprayed cooking oil or broth.
- Broil, barbecue, or grill meats.
- Avoid frying or deep-frying foods.
- Skim the fat from stews and soups. (If you refrigerate them overnight, the solid fat lifts off easily.)
- Eat less butter, gravies, meat-based and cream sauces, spreads, and creamy pasta sauces and salad dressings.
- Consider using extra-virgin olive oil or grapeseed oil in place of butter on vegetables and in spreads, sauces, and salad dressings.
- When cooking and baking, use oil, such as olive or canola oil, and plant-based margarines, such as olive oil, flax, or soy, instead of shortening, lard, butter, or stick margarine.
- Use avocado, canola, peanut, and olive oil when cooking at medium or high heat. Extra-virgin olive oil is best for cooking at low heat or using uncooked, such as on a salad.

Sodium

An average adult needs only about 500 milligrams (mg) a day of sodium. This amount of sodium is less than a fifth of a teaspoon of table salt. Most people in the US and Canada eat more than six times that much. Most of the sodium (salt) in people's diets comes from processed and refined foods rather than the saltshaker at the table. Too much sodium can raise blood pressure, and high blood pressure can lead to heart disease, stroke, and kidney failure. Cutting back on sodium can help lower blood pressure. Adults should limit sodium to 2,300 mg a day (about 1 teaspoon of table salt). Some people benefit from even lower levels of sodium (1,500 mg a day).

> In Canada, the recommendations for sodium are 1,500 to 2,300 mg per day. Foods labeled as "low in sodium or salt," "low sodium," and "low source of sodium or salt" contain less than 140 mg of sodium per serving.

You get sodium from the foods you eat—from tiny amounts in some plant foods to higher amounts in some animal foods (red meat, chicken, fish, eggs, and dairy products). You do not have to worry about sodium in foods that you eat in their natural unprocessed form. To control sodium intake, limit eating processed foods. Processed foods often have different forms of sodium added to them and contain high amounts of sodium.

A love of sodium comes from eating salty foods. When trying to eat foods with less salt, your taste needs to adjust. It can take time to learn to like food with less salt and enjoy the natural flavors of less salty food. Here are some tips to help reduce your sodium intake:

- **Always taste your food before salting it.** It may already taste good without adding more salt.
- **Cut down on the salt in recipes when cooking.** Add one half of the salt called for in the recipe, and instead season food using spices, herbs, pepper, garlic, onion, lemon, or lime.
- **Choose minimally processed fresh or frozen poultry, fish, and lean meat instead of canned, breaded, or pre-prepared processed and packaged food.**
- **Choose foods labeled "low" or "reduced" sodium or those with 140 mg or less per serving.** Check the Nutrition Facts label for this information.
- **Save high-sodium food for special occasions.** Eat the following only occasionally rather than every day: canned soups, packaged mixes, bacon, luncheon or deli meats, salted snacks (such as chips, nuts, and pretzels), and pepperoni or sausage pizza.
- **In restaurants, ask that your food not be salted.** Sauces; breading; rice, pasta, or potato dishes; stuffing; and foods containing ham, sausage, or bacon are often high in sodium. Soups and salad dressings can also be high in sodium. Ask for sauces and dressings on the side.

Total Carbohydrate

Carbohydrates are the body's main source of fuel. Your body breaks down carbohydrates (except for fiber) into glucose (sugar). Glucose is the energy source for your brain and the rest of your body. Carbohydrates—more than protein or fat—largely determine your blood glucose (sugar) level. They also do much more. Carbohydrates are the building blocks of nearly every part of your body.

There are two types of carbohydrates: sugars and starches. Carbohydrates are found in plant foods (grains, fruits, vegetables), as well as milk and yogurt.

Sugars occur naturally in foods, including fruits (fructose) and milk/yogurt (lactose). Other packaged and processed foods, such as soda, candy, and crackers, often have added sugar. The added sugar adds extra calories. Also, it is common that these processed and packaged products are missing healthful nutrients.

Vegetables such as green peas, potatoes, winter squash, dried beans, and peas contain starchy carbohydrates. Lentils and other legumes and grains, such as rice, corn, and wheat, also have starchy carbohydrates. Pasta, bread, tortillas, and baked goods that are made from those grains are also high in carbohydrates.

Some grain-based foods are more processed and refined than others. While processing does not change the amount of carbohydrates in grain-based foods, it does remove healthful nutrients such as vitamins, minerals, and fiber. This is why it is better to eat brown rice and whole grain than white rice and other processed grains. Whole grains are more nutritious and include more fiber. The body changes some carbohydrates to glucose more quickly than others. The carbohydrates in most high-fiber foods get converted into glucose more slowly than those in low-fiber foods. The health benefits of fiber are presented in the next section.

If you have diabetes, your body has trouble using all the carbohydrates you eat and higher levels of glucose build up in the blood. If left untreated, this causes many problems.

> In some countries, including Canada, diabetes education materials refer to glycemic index (GI), which measures how quickly different carbohydrates are absorbed into the blood and glycemic load (GL), which estimates approximately how much a food will raise blood glucose. To learn more about GI and GL, see the resources available at https://www.diabetes.ca/DiabetesCanadaWebsite/media/Managing-My-Diabetes/Tools%20and%20Resources/glycemic-index-food-guide.pdf?ext=.pdf and www.bullpub.com/resources.

Dietary Fiber

Fiber is a carbohydrate that is not absorbed into the body. Fiber occurs naturally in whole and minimally processed plant foods with skins, seeds, and strings, such as those found in celery and string beans. Whole grains, dried beans, peas, lentils, fruits, vegetables, nuts, and seeds all have fiber. Some foods have added fiber (such as when pulp is added to juice). Animal foods (red meat, chicken, fish, eggs, and dairy products) and refined foods (white flour, bread, many baked and snack foods) have little or no fiber unless the manufacturer adds it.

Even though it is not absorbed by the body, fiber helps the body. There are two types of fiber: soluble and insoluble. Most plants contain both soluble and insoluble fiber in different amounts. Insoluble fiber, such as the fiber in wheat bran, some fruits and vegetables, and whole grains, act as "nature's broom." These foods keep your digestive system moving and help prevent constipation. The soluble fiber, such as the fiber in oat bran, barley, nuts, seeds, beans, apples, citrus fruits, carrots, and psyllium seed, can help regulate your blood sugar. The soluble form of fiber slows the amount of time it takes for sugar to get into the bloodstream. Foods that contain soluble fiber can help lower blood cholesterol. High fiber diets may also help reduce the risk of rectal and colon cancers. The US daily recommendation for fiber for adults ranges from 22 to

Tips for Choosing Healthier Carbohydrates and Eating More Fiber

- Fill at least half of your plate with whole fresh or frozen vegetables and fruits.
- At least half of the grains you eat should be whole grains (brown rice, whole-grain breads and rolls, whole-grain pasta, and corn tortillas).
- Choose foods that list whole wheat or a whole grain, such as oats, first on the ingredients list.
- Choose dried beans, split peas, and lentils instead of meat or as side dishes at least a few times a week. Add cooked dried beans to your vegetable salads and pasta dishes.
- Choose whole fruit rather than fruit juice. Whole fruit contains fiber, takes longer to eat, fills you up better than juice, and may help keep you from overeating.
- Limit added sugars, especially sugar-sweetened beverages. (Learn more about added sugars below on this page.)
- Choose higher-fiber breakfast cereals, such as All-Bran® or oatmeal.
- Eat higher-fiber crackers, such as whole-rye or multigrain crackers and whole-grain flatbread.
- Snack on whole fruit, raw vegetables, and whole-grain crackers rather than chips, sweets, or ice cream.
- When you add high-fiber foods to your diet, do it gradually over a period of a few weeks.
- Drink plenty of water to prevent constipation.

34 grams, generally more for men than women and less for older adults than younger adults. If you are eating the recommended amounts of whole, plant-based foods you likely are getting enough of both types of fiber.

> In Canada, the fiber recommendation is 25 grams for women and 38 grams for men.

Total Sugars and Added Sugars

The Total Sugars information on the Nutrition Facts label lists the amount of sugar in one serving of the food. Many foods, such as fruit, contain natural sugar. In many other cases, such as carbonated drinks, sugar is added by the manufacturer during processing.

Are natural sugars and added sugars different? No, your body uses natural sugars and added sugars the same way. They both have the same number of calories for the same weight (grams, ounces, etc.). However processed foods tend to have more added sugars. A sugar—whether it is natural or added—is sugar, but foods with natural sugar usually also contain healthy ingredients in addition to sugar.

Added sugar gives us extra calories. If you are trying to lose weight or lower your blood glucose, eat as little added sugar as possible. A 12-ounce (355 mL) can of cola has almost 10 teaspoons (nearly 40 grams) of added sugar and no beneficial nutrients. Twelve ounces (355 mL) of orange juice with no added sugar has 9½ teaspoons (33 grams) of natural sugar but also lots of vitamins and other nutrients. Juice is a better choice than cola. An even better choice is a fresh medium orange. An orange has about 12 grams of carbohydrate, and it provides healthy nutrients and fiber. To quench your thirst, choose water, coffee, and tea more often. These drinks have no added sugar and no carbohydrates.

Both US and Canadian recommendations suggest limiting added sugar to no more that 10 percent of your total daily calories. For example, if you consume 2,000 calories in a day, your added sugar intake should not exceed 200 calories or 50 grams. In the United States, this is equivalent to 12½ teaspoons. The American Heart Association takes this public health message further and recommends that women not exceed 6 teaspoons (24 grams, 96 calories) of added sugar per day and men not exceed 9 teaspoons (36 grams, 144 calories) per day. This may seem like a lot, but it is surprising to learn how much sugar is in foods and drinks. This is why food label reading is so important.

Protein

Protein is part of every cell in your body and helps control the way your body works. Protein helps your immune system fight infection. Your body also uses protein to build tissues, including muscles and bones, and repair damaged tissues. Protein provides a feeling of comfortable fullness after you eat. It satisfies your appetite and prevents you from getting hungry again too soon after you have eaten. Most people eat more than enough protein. However, many people get most of their protein from meat, which tends to be high in saturated fats. Eating protein mainly from plant foods, along with small amounts of lean meat, poultry, or fish, is better for your health.

There are two types of proteins: complete and incomplete. Your body uses complete proteins just as they are. *Complete proteins* are found in fish and animal foods (meat, poultry, eggs, milk, and other dairy products), as well as in foods made from soybeans, such as tofu and tempeh.

Incomplete proteins do not contain one or more parts of a complete protein. These are found in plant foods such as grains, dried beans and peas, lentils, nuts, and seeds. Nearly all plant proteins are incomplete proteins. (Most fruits and nonstarchy vegetables have little, if any, protein.)

Even though plant proteins are incomplete, they are at the heart of eating healthy. Scientists once thought that we had to eat two or more incomplete plant proteins at the same meal to get the complete protein we need every day. But now we know that our bodies store a supply of spare protein parts, and these parts are available to transform incomplete plant proteins after we eat them. In addition, we now know that by eating a small amount of an animal protein, such as chicken, with a plant protein, such as lentils or black beans, you get all the benefits of a complete protein. Casseroles and stir-fries are tasty ways to do this. Common incomplete proteins that pair up to form a complete protein when eaten together include rice with beans and peanut butter with bread.

In addition to containing protein, some plant foods, such as nuts and seeds, are sources of healthy fats. Many plant foods are also sources of fiber and other nutrients. Plant foods have no cholesterol and little to no unhealthy fats.

For these reasons, plant foods are often the best choice for healthy eating.

Vitamins and Minerals: Vitamin D, Calcium, Iron, and Potassium

Vitamins and minerals keep your body functioning properly and are needed for survival and health. Most people can get all the vitamins and minerals they need from eating healthy foods. In this section, we discuss only a few of the key ones that are important to health: vitamin D, calcium, potassium, and iron.

Vitamin D

Vitamin D and four minerals—sodium (see information on sodium on pages 188–189), potassium, calcium, and iron—are listed on Nutrition Facts labels. You will find information about other vitamins and minerals on a food's packaging only if these are added or a health claim about vitamins and minerals is made on the package. The four minerals that are always listed are linked to current health problems. Many of us eat too much (sodium) and/or too little (calcium, iron, and potassium) of these nutrients.

Potassium

The mineral potassium helps regulate the heartbeat and can lower blood pressure. Many kinds of vegetables and fruits are good potassium sources. These include broccoli, peas, dried beans (white, adzuki, and pinto), tomatoes, potatoes, sweet potatoes, avocados, winter squash (acorn, delicata, and butternut), citrus fruits, plantains, bananas, prunes, apricots, and nuts. Some fish (salmon, tuna, mackerel, and halibut), milk, and yogurt are also good sources of potassium.

> In Canada in 2024, a standardized Supplemented Food Facts table has replaced the nutrition facts table on all supplemented foods. Full implementation is required by December 31, 2025. Supplemented foods are prepackaged items with specific ingredients, such as vitamins, minerals, amino acids, or caffeine, added for purposes beyond basic nutrition. The new supplemental table is being mandated because certain supplemented foods contain supplemental ingredients that can pose a risk to health if too much of them are consumed or they are consumed by people who are pregnant, breastfeeding, under the age of 14, or sensitive to caffeine.

Calcium

Many people know that calcium helps build bones, but did you know that it is also needed for blood clotting and blood pressure regulation? It may also protect against colon cancer, kidney stones, and breast cancer.

Unfortunately, some people, especially older women and young children, may not get enough calcium in their diets. Most women under 60 should get the amount of calcium found in three cups (750 mL) of milk every day. Good sources of calcium are yogurt, cheese, and kefir (a fermented beverage similar to yogurt); calcium-fortified soy, rice, oat, and almond milks and orange juice; calcium-fortified cereal and breads; and canned salmon and sardines with bones. Brussels sprouts, kohlrabi, and leafy greens (bok choy, kale, collards, beet greens, turnip greens, and spinach) have calcium, but our bodies cannot use some of it because these

More Is Not Better

When it comes to vitamins and minerals, some people think that if a little is good, then more is better. This is not true. Too much of a good thing can cause harm. This is because everything in your body must be in balance. Too much of anything throws off the balance. Think of baking. If you put too much of almost any ingredient into cookies, cakes, or pies, they do not come out right. If you stick to eating mostly whole foods and limit processed food, you will likely consume vitamins and minerals in the quantities your body needs.

plant foods also contain natural chemicals that partially block calcium absorption. Most fruits are low in calcium. The exceptions are dried figs (there's not much in fig cookies, though) and tropical cherimoya (custard apple). Note that salt can cause your body to lose calcium, so this is another reason to eat less salt.

If you do not get enough calcium from what you eat and drink, talk to your health care provider about calcium supplements (pills).

Iron

Iron is a mineral that helps your body use oxygen. If you do not have enough iron in your diet, you can feel tired, weak, dizzy, and generally unwell. Iron is found in both plant and animal foods. In the US and Canada, grain products such as breads, pasta, and cereals have iron added to them. Iron from animal foods is easier for our bodies to use than from plants. Eating foods with vitamin C at the same time we eat plant foods with iron allows our bodies to better absorb the iron from plants. Excellent sources of vitamin C include citrus fruits (grapefruit, orange, lemon, and lime), sweet red peppers, and broccoli.

Water

Water, which makes up more than half of our bodies, is the most important nutrient. Water fills the spaces in and between body cells. All the natural chemical reactions in our bodies require water. Water keeps our kidneys working, helps prevent constipation, and helps us eat less by making us feel full. Drinking water can also help prevent medication side effects.

Most adults lose about 10 cups of water a day through urine, sweat, and breathing. However, people usually have no problem getting enough water. The exact amount you need differs depending on the weather, your activity, and your weight. To determine if you are drinking enough water, check the color of your urine. If it is light colored, you are fine. If it is darker, you probably need more water. When you feel thirsty, your body needs more water. Milk and many fruits and vegetables are good sources of water. Coffee, tea, and other drinks with caffeine are also good sources of water. Alcohol is not a good source of water. Do not depend on alcohol to meet your need for water.

If you have kidney disease, congestive heart failure, or are taking special medications, you may need to drink less water. Talk to a registered dietitian or your health care provider.

Word about Vitamin D

Everyone needs some vitamin D to keep their bones healthy. The body cannot use calcium without vitamin D. Beyond this, there is a lot of controversy about how helpful vitamin D is and its role in preventing heart disease and cancer. The National Academy of Medicine suggests people under 70 get 600 IUs (international units) daily and people over 70 get 800 IUs. If you do not get much sunlight or are dark-skinned or overweight, you may need a vitamin D supplement. This is especially true if you have a family history of osteoporosis. If you are not already taking a supplement recommended by your doctor, talk with your health care provider or a registered dietitian.

Health Canada recommends that men and women over 50 take a daily vitamin D supplement of 400 IU. It is generally considered safe to take a supplement that provides 1,000 or 2,000 IUs. The recommendation is to stay below 4,000 IUs per day.

The Ingredients List

An ingredients list is usually found on food labels under the Nutrition Facts, but it may be elsewhere on food packaging. It lists all the ingredients in the food package starting with the most abundant or heaviest ingredient. The last ingredients listed are those that are present in the smallest amounts in the food. The ingredients list uses the common names of the ingredients and gives you more detailed information about what you are eating. This list is especially important if you are trying to avoid certain items, such as soy or gluten.

A Simplified Way to Make Healthy Food Choices: The Plate Method

Nutrition Facts labels and ingredient lists inform you about what and how much you and your care partner are eating and how what you eat compares to a healthy diet. However, not all foods have labels, and sometimes you need an easier way to eat healthier. The plate method is another way of deciding what and how much to eat.

MyPlate, shown in Figure 10.4, is a visual guide produced by the US Department of Agriculture (USDA) to help you make good food choices. This guide encourages you to cover one-half of the plate with vegetables and fruit, one-fourth with protein (lean meat, fish, poultry, or, better yet, plant foods such as tofu, cooked dry beans, or lentils), and the remaining one-fourth with grains (preferably at least half from whole grains) or other starches such as potatoes, sweet potatoes, yams, corn, peas, or winter squash. Finish off your meal with calcium-rich foods, such as milk or foods made from milk (preferably fat-free or low-fat),

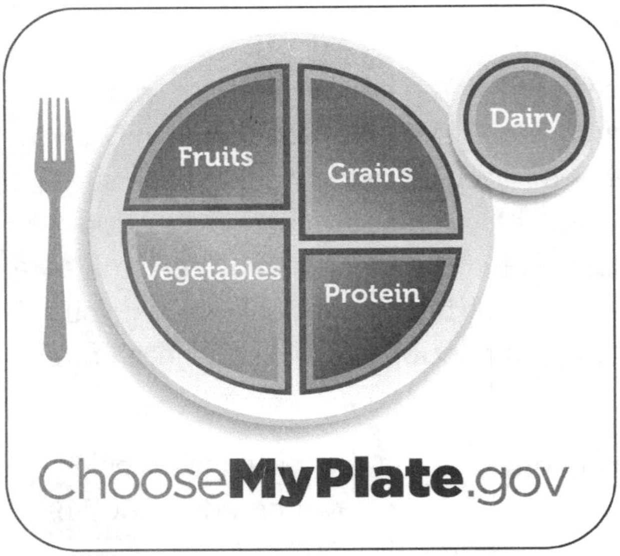

Figure 10.4 **MyPlate: A Map for Healthy Eating** (http://www.chooseMyPlate.gov) from the USDA. For people with diabetes, the American Diabetes Association recommends a similar plate (see page 199).

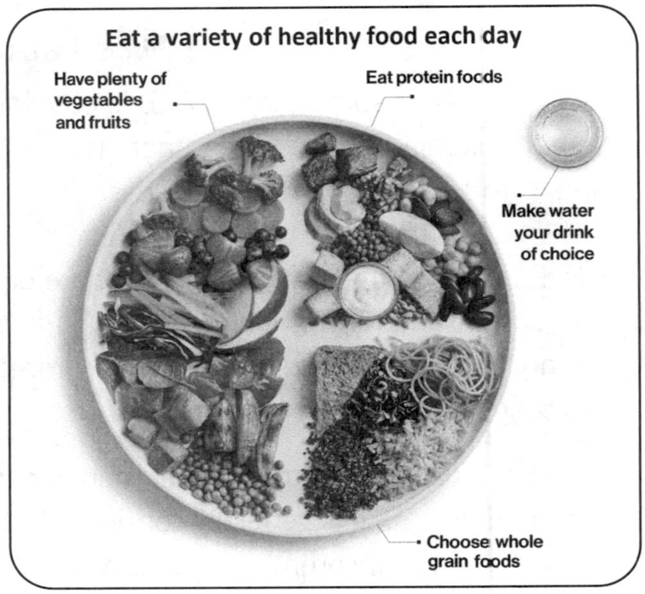

Figure 10.5 **Eat Well Plate from the Canadian Government**

The graphic can be found at https://food-guide.canada.ca/en/

including cheese, yogurt, frozen yogurt, or calcium-fortified foods like soy milk. Of course, your food choices and amounts should depend on what you like and need. A small amount of healthier unsaturated fat (see pages 186–188) is healthy at each meal. This may come from oil you use while cooking the food, dressing a salad, or seasoning food. It could also come from nuts mixed in with a grain such as brown rice. Read more about suggestions for choosing healthy fats and seasonings on page 188.

With the plate method, as with any eating guidelines, the amounts of food you eat are important. Plate sizes have grown over the years, causing people to get more calories than needed. A plate that measures 9 inches (22.5 centimeters) across the center is a good size. The box "Recommendations for a Healthy Eating Plan" on page 197 can help you plan healthy meals. It lists some examples of serving sizes based on Choose MyPlate. Note that these amounts may be different if you have special dietary needs. If you have questions about how much you should eat, check with your health care provider or a registered dietitian.

Canada's Food Guide Plate

The Canadian government's recommendations for the Food Guide Plate are very similar to the US plate, with minor differences. As you can see in the Canadian Eat Well Plate, shown in Figure 10.5, Canada's Food Guide recommends water as your drink of choice. It also suggests that you choose proteins that come from plants more often than animal proteins. To find more about Canadian food guidelines, please see: www.bullpub.com/resources.

Recommendations for a Healthy Eating Plan

Here are some recommendations for daily healthy eating for people eating 2,000 calories a day.

Notice that we refer to cup or ounce/gram equivalents in the lists of recommended foods. A cup holds about 250 mL. Within a food group, foods can come in many forms and are not created equal in terms of what counts as a cup or an ounce. Some foods are more concentrated. Some are airier or contain more water. Cup and ounce equivalents identify the amounts of foods from each food group with similar nutritional content.

We offer the following to get started. If you want more information, please talk to your health care provider or a registered dietitian.

- Vegetables: 2½ cup/91 mL equivalent per day. Each week this can be broken down into:
- Dark green vegetables: 11/2 cup/355 mL equivalent
- Red and orange vegetables: 51/2 cup/1301 mL equivalent
- Beans and peas: 1½ cup/355 mL equivalent
- Starchy vegetables: 5 cup/1183 mL equivalent
- Other vegetables: 4 cup/946 mL equivalent
- Fruit: 2½ cup/591 mL equivalent per day
- Grains: 6 ounce/168 g equivalents **per day** with as much of this as possible being whole grains
- Dairy: 2 cup equivalent a day
- Protein: 5½ ounce/162 g equivalent **per day.** Each week this can be broken down into:
  - Seafood: 15 ounce/425 g equivalent
  - Meat, poultry, eggs: 26 ounce/737 g equivalent
  - Nuts, seed, soy products: 5 ounce/140 g equivalent
- Oils: a little less than 1 ounce/30 mL equivalent per day (1 ounce of oil equals 2 tablespoons)
- Limit calories from other foods such as cookies, ice cream, and chips to 260 calories **a day.** You can find the calories on food labels, which are discussed in this chapter on pages 184–195.

Healthy Eating for Specific Long-Term Conditions*

The recommendations for healthy eating listed above will help create a general plan that works for most caregivers as well as for care partners. However, some people have different needs and likes that depend on age, sex, body size, activity level, health, and even availability and affordability of food. In the following sections, we present some general eating considerations for selected long-term health issues. If you have any of these conditions, it is important to talk to your health care provider or a registered dietitian about how to eat healthfully.

Healthy Food Choices and Diabetes

When a person eats a meal, the body breaks down the carbohydrates into glucose, the basic fuel for the body's cells. Glucose is then absorbed into the bloodstream. (Protein and fat usually contribute little to the body's blood sugar.) The hormone insulin takes glucose (blood sugar) into the cells. In people with diabetes, the cells do not absorb or use glucose very well. That means that glucose builds up in the bloodstream and leads to other serious health problems. Managing blood sugar levels is one of the prime goals in diabetes care and involves many different things, including taking medication, exercising, and keeping a careful eye on what and how much a person eats.

In the past, people with diabetes were told that they could not eat sweets and that they could only eat certain types of carbohydrates. More current research indicates that people with diabetes should eat to meet their individual needs as long as they watch what and how much they eat, especially the carbohydrates. The American Diabetes Association (ADA) recommends that people with diabetes eat fewer foods that are high in sugar and processed foods like white rice or those made with white flour. They should eat carbohydrates from vegetables, beans, fruits, milk, yogurt, and foods made with whole grains. The ADA strongly discourages drinking sugar-sweetened beverages, such as soft drinks (soda pop), and other drinks, such as energy drinks and many juice products, and eating foods with high amounts of processed grains and added sugar, such as breads, pastry, and some cereals. Because people with diabetes are at higher risk of heart disease, the type of fat they eat is also especially important. They should choose unsaturated fats and avoid saturated and trans fats. Eat little to no trans fats.

Unfortunately, heart disease is the number one complication of diabetes so people with diabetes should follow the recommendations for both diabetes and heart disease. If you have diabetes, please also read the section on heart disease on page 200.

The American Diabetes Association (ADA) encourages the use of the Create Your Plate to plan meals (Figure 10.6). Diabetes Canada uses the same Canada's Food Guide Plate and also recommends that people with diabetes focus more on vegetables and less on fruit, which contains more sugar. To create your plate, divide your 9-inch diameter plate in half. Then take one of those halves and divide it in half again. You should now have three sections. Use the following guidelines to add food to your plate to create a healthy and balanced meal:

- Fill half of your plate with nonstarchy vegetables, such as salad greens, spinach, cabbage, broccoli, green beans, tomatoes, cauliflower, cucumber, okra, peppers, mushrooms, beets, or turnips.
- Fill one quarter of your plate with foods higher in carbohydrates (starchy foods). Opt for whole grains, such as whole grain breads, cereals, brown rice, pasta, corn tortillas, dal, oatmeal, hominy grits; cooked beans; starchy vegetables, such as potatoes, sweet potatoes, corn, lima beans, and green peas; fruit; and yogurt or a cup of milk.
- Fill the remaining quarter of your plate with a lean protein, such as chicken or turkey (without the skin), fish, lean cuts of beef or pork, eggs, or tofu.

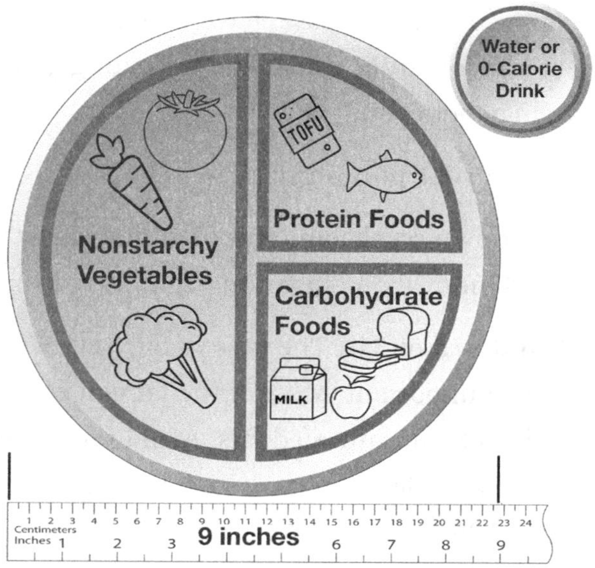

Figure 10.6 **Diabetes Plate (US)**

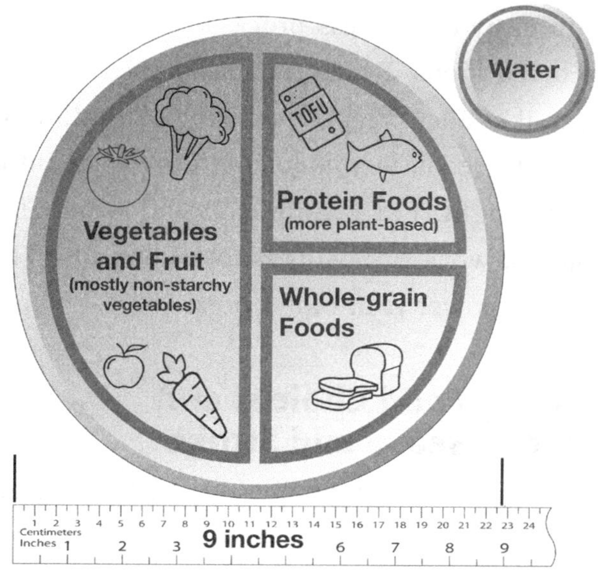

Diabetes Plate (Canada)

- Choose water or a low-calorie drink such as unsweetened iced tea as a beverage.

The following are some additional general suggestions for healthy eating, if you or your care partner have diabetes:

- Use the Create Your Plate method (see Figure 10.6) to plan your meals.
- Start each day with something to eat. Eating something in the morning is "breaking the fast." Breakfast fuels the body after a long night of foodless resting. It provides energy to start the day's activities.
- Space out your meals and snacks regularly throughout the day. Don't skip meals. Eating regularly at similar, planned times gives your body the chance to produce and use its insulin. Eating regularly scheduled meals also gives your medication time to keep up your energy level. The number of meals you eat and the time between your meals varies depending on your personal health and lifestyle. You might eat three meals a day, but some people prefer or need to eat smaller meals more frequently.
- Eat the same amount of food at each meal, including snacks. This helps you maintain an even energy flow and blood sugar level throughout the day. Skipping meals or alternating large meals with small meals can throw off your energy level. It can also lead to overeating or making less healthy food choices. This can, in turn, cause swings in your blood sugar and result in symptoms such as irritability, shakiness, poor sleep, mood swings, or pain or difficulty breathing resulting from stomach bloating, heartburn, and indigestion.

Because people with diabetes are at increased risk for heart disease and stroke, they should eat less saturated and trans fats (see page 186). Replace saturated fats (such as butter and bacon) with unsaturated fats (such as olive and canola oils), but don't add to your overall fat intake. In addition, eat more plant foods and consume less sodium by eating less processed, takeout, and prepared foods. Reach for the salt shaker sparingly, if at all. If you are carrying extra pounds, the ADA recommends losing 5 to 7 percent of your weight. For example, if you weigh 150 pounds, work on losing 8 to 10 pounds. This can help lower your blood sugar.

Healthy Food Choices and Heart Disease and Stroke

Healthy eating for people with heart disease and for those who have had a stroke involves the following: lowering weight if overweight, lowering blood pressure, and lowering cholesterol so the arteries do not harden or become clogged. Losing just a little weight often makes it easier for the heart to work and lowers blood pressure. The Mediterranean diet discussed on page 181 is good for people with heart conditions. Watch the amount of food, the types of fats, and the amount of sodium you eat, as well as the amount of alcohol you drink. Drinking more than two drinks in one sitting raises blood pressure. If you drink more than that and want to cut back, do so slowly over a one- to two-week period. Stopping drinking suddenly can also raise blood pressure. The definition of heavy drinking is having five or more drinks (four or more for women) over a short period of time (two hours) on five or more days in the last month. Moderate drinking is no more than one drink with alcohol per day for women and up to two drinks per day for men.

> As noted earlier in the chapter, Canada's Guidance on Alcohol and Health states that if you are going to drink, you should not exceed two drinks on any day.

If you have heart disease, have had a stroke, or are at risk for stroke, the following eating guidelines may help you:

- Watch your portion sizes.
- **Cut down on the amount of added sugar.** Read more about sugar on pages 191–192.
- **Cut down on fat.** The type of fat you eat is also important. Most of the fat you eat should be unsaturated fats. Avoid saturated fats. Eat little to no trans fats. See pages 186–188 for suggestions for ways to make healthy fat choices.
- **Increase the amount of fiber you eat.** Fiber—especially from oats, barley, dried beans and peas, lentils, apples, citrus fruits, carrots, and psyllium seed—can be helpful in managing high blood cholesterol, a major risk factor for heart disease. See pages 190–191 for suggestions for ways to eat more fiber.
- **Eat less sodium to help prevent or control high blood pressure.** Try to limit the daily total amount of sodium you get to no more than that found in 1 teaspoon of table salt (about 2,300 mg). Some people may need to eat less than 2,300 mg of sodium. Read Nutrition Facts labels to learn how much sodium is in the processed food you eat. Instead of salt, use herbs, spices, lemon, and vinegar for flavor.
- **Maintain a healthy lifestyle to control high blood pressure.** Weight loss, limiting alcohol, being physically active, and following a healthy eating plan are also important for controlling high blood pressure. If medication is needed, taking it as directed is also

important for controlling cholesterol, blood pressure, and blood sugar.

Healthy Food Choices and Lung Disease

If you or your care partner have lung disease, such as emphysema and COPD, it is important to eat a balanced diet that includes fruits and vegetables. Sometimes it may be recommended that you increase the amount of protein you eat. This helps increase energy, strength, and the ability to fight lung infections. When it is hard for you or your care partner to eat enough food, such as when you have little or no appetite, try eating higher-calorie foods—fruit nectars instead of juice, dried fruit instead of fresh fruit, sweet potato instead of white potato—or try nibbling on a small handful of nuts over the course of the day.

If you have specific concerns about what you or your care partner should eat, talk to a registered dietitian. These professionals can tell you what's best for you as well as help you fit our general recommendations to any unique health needs.

Here are some tips to help you or your care partner eat a balanced diet with lung disease:

- **Limit salt in meals and drink plenty of liquids.**
- **Avoid carbonated beverages.**
- **Don't fill up on drinks like coffee and tea.** If you have trouble getting enough calories in your diet, try sipping on a smoothie or a high-calorie liquid supplement.
- **For some, eating several smaller meals per day and waiting until the end of the meal to drink liquids** may help with breathing.
- **Try eating higher-calorie foods throughout the day such as dried fruit and nuts** if it is hard to eat enough food (when there is little or no appetite).
- **Keep healthy, easy-to-eat food nearby and available in the kitchen.**
- **If you or your care partner often don't feel like eating, talk with your doctor** to find out if there is some other problem, such as depression.
- **Although not a part of healthy eating, avoid smoking and secondhand smoke.**
- **Participating in a pulmonary rehab program can be helpful to learn about healthy eating as well as exercise and breathing.**

Lung disease can cause problems resulting in weight gain, such as from steroid medicines that have this side effect. You will find some tips for losing, maintaining, and gaining weight starting on pages 204–207. A registered dietitian can help you and your care partner with concerns about weight gain or loss.

Healthy Food Choices and Osteoporosis

Osteoporosis makes bones brittle. It has been called a silent disease because its first symptom can be a bone fracture, especially in the spine, hip, or wrist. If you or your care partner have osteoporosis, include enough calcium and vitamin D in your eating plan. Do muscle-strengthening and weight-bearing exercise regularly (for example, walking; see Chapter 9, Exercising for Health and Wellness). And follow your health care provider's recommendations, such as taking prescribed medications for bone loss.

It is never too late to help slow the progress of osteoporosis. Osteoporosis is not a calcium-deficiency disease, and after bone has been lost, getting more calcium will not fix it. However, getting vitamin D along with enough calcium can help the body better absorb calcium and slow bone loss. Everybody needs some calcium every day. The best sources are milk and foods made from milk. But some people avoid milk products because they don't like them, do not eat animal products, or have problems digesting milk sugar due to lactose intolerance. You can still get enough calcium from your diet even if you have problems with milk. Many people can enjoy milk products if they eat them in small amounts or eat other foods at the same time. Consider eating cereal with nonfat milk or nonfat Greek yogurt with berries. If you are lactose intolerant, you can take lactase tablets to better digest the lactose. You can also eat foods that are lower in lactose such as kefir. Non-dairy alternatives, such as soy and almond products, are also good options, as long as they are fortified with calcium.

Some fruits and vegetables are high in calcium, including kale, collard greens, bok choy, and broccoli. However, the calcium in fruits and vegetables is not as well absorbed by the body as calcium from animal (dairy) sources. Some foods and beverages have calcium added such as tofu and orange juice. Calcium and vitamin D supplements are available without a prescription (over the counter). If you think you or your care partner may not be getting enough calcium, talk to your health care provider or a registered dietitian about your diet and whether calcium and vitamin D supplements (pills) are needed. It is best, though, to try and meet your calcium needs through your eating plan first.

Healthy Food Choices and Kidney Disease

Kidneys are organs that rid the body of waste. If the kidneys are not functioning well, it is difficult for the body to remove waste. There are different stages of kidney disease. Depending on what stage of kidney disease you or your care partner are experiencing, there are different suggestions for what is best to eat and drink. You may need to limit foods and fluids that are high in potassium, phosphorus, and sodium. Also, you may need to change the amount and type of fluids you drink. Your health care provider or registered dietitian can help you follow the right guidelines.

It can be tricky identifying the potassium, phosphorus, and sodium in foods and fluids. For example, some salt substitutes are very high in potassium. But this is often overlooked as a source of potassium in the diet. It is important to read all food labels and ingredient lists to identify potassium and sodium. Recall that Nutrition Facts labels list potassium and sodium (see page 184).

Identifying phosphorus is more difficult because phosphorus is not listed on food labels, and phosphorus occurs naturally in many foods. Foods that are high in phosphorus include whole-grain bread, bran cereals, oatmeal, nuts, and sunflower seeds. Dark soft drinks such as colas are also high in phosphorus. To identify other ingredients that contain phosphorus, find ingredients that include PHOS in their names. Because it is in so many common foods, it may be difficult to reduce the amount of phosphorus in your diet. Your health care provider may recommend a medication that "binds" to the phosphorus in food and helps the body prevent phosphorus from building up. Ask your doctor or pharmacist for more information about medication options to avoid having to restrict your food intake too much.

Most people with kidney disease can drink water and other fluids as desired. However, depending on the stage of kidney disease, fluids may need to be limited, as well as foods that are high in water such as soup, ice cream, gelatin, and watermelon. If you limit fluids and foods like these, you may feel thirsty. If thirst is a problem, chewing gum or sucking on hard candy may help.

Some people with kidney disease may also need calcium and vitamin D supplements. Managing kidney disease is different for each person. Working with a registered dietitian with special training in kidney disease will help you design an eating plan that works for you or your care partner. Your health care provider can help you find the right professional to guide you and your care partner through changes in your kidney disease.

More Tips for Healthy Eating

This section contains more information for making choices to support your and your care partner's healthy eating habits.

Tips for Choosing Foods

- **Choose foods that are close to the way nature made them.** Shop in the perimeter (outer) areas in your local grocery store. These areas are where you find fresh fruits, vegetables, meat, seafood, and dairy. Buy fewer items in the middle aisles that contain junk foods, snacks, and other ultra-processed foods. To make processed foods, manufacturers add something (often sugar, salt, or fat) or remove something (often fiber and healthful nutrients).
- **Eat foods high in phytochemicals.** The prefix *phyto-* means plant. Plant foods such as fruits, vegetables, whole grains, nuts, and seeds have naturally occurring healthy phytochemicals that fight disease. When manufacturers refine or process food, phytochemicals are lost.
- **Eat a wide variety of colorful unprocessed foods.** The more variety in your food, the better. The more colors on your plate from vegetables and fruits, the better.
- **Eat foods that are minimally processed.** Choose grilled chicken breast instead of fried breaded chicken nuggets. Choose a baked potato (with skin) rather than French fries. And opt for whole grains, such as whole-grain bread, whole-wheat pasta, and brown rice.
- **Get your nutrients from food, not supplements.** Dietary supplements cannot make up for unhealthy eating. Foods in the form that nature made them have the right nutrient amount and combinations for our bodies. Nutrients that are not naturally found in foods may be present in amounts that are not healthy, or they may not work the way they should. They may even have harmful side effects.

- **There is a place for supplements in some diets.** Sometimes we cannot get all the nutrients we need from food. For example, older people need a larger amount of calcium to help prevent or slow osteoporosis. If you or your care partner are thinking of taking a supplement, talk to your health care professional or a registered dietitian first. It is important to know how supplements will interact with medications.
- **Eat at regular, preferably evenly spaced, times during the day.** This prevents you from getting overly hungry and maintains and balances your blood sugar level. Eating regularly means different things for different people. It can mean three regular-size meals, or five small meals, or whatever works for you and your health conditions.
- **Eat the amount of food that your body needs (not more or less).** This is easy to say but more difficult to put into action. How much you should eat depends on the following:
    - your age. (We need fewer calories as we get older.)
    - if you are a man or woman. (Men usually need more calories than women.)
    - your body size and shape. (In general, if you are taller or have more muscle, you may need to eat more.)
    - your health needs. (Some conditions affect how the body uses calories.)
    - your activity level. (The more you move or exercise, the more calories you can eat without gaining weight.)

Tips for Losing Weight

The following are some tips to help you or your care partner lose weight:

- **Set small, gradual weight loss goals.** Break the total amount of weight to lose into small, reachable goals. For most people, losing 1 to 2 pounds (0.5 to 1 km) a week is realistic and doable, especially in the first several weeks. After a while, a smaller goal (such as 1/2 pound or 1/4 kilogram per week) may be more doable. Once you have lost weight, you may also consider yourself successful if you hold your lower weight steady without gaining any pounds back.
- **Identify your specific actions to lose weight.** For example, plan to walk 20 minutes a day five days a week, not eat between meals, and eat more slowly. Review the information about action planning in Chapter 2, Becoming a Better Caregiver: The Basics.
- **Pay attention to what you eat.** Overeating is common when people are with friends, using the computer, or watching television. Set out the portion you want to eat and keep the other food out of sight. By focusing on what you are eating and not what you are doing, such as watching television, you will be more satisfied and will eat less.
- **Know the serving size when you see one and choose appropriate portions.** A 3/4-cup (175 mL) serving is the size of a tennis ball or a small, closed fist. A 3-ounce (84 g) serving of cooked meat, fish, or poultry is the size of a deck of playing cards or a checkbook. The end of your thumb to the first joint is about 1 tablespoon (15 mL). Using a

measuring cup or a food scale is a great way to learn about serving size. Especially when starting to make changes, measure your portions—and do this frequently over time. It is amazing how easily 1/2 cup (125 mL) of rice can "grow" to a 1-cup (250 mL) serving. Foods that come prepackaged as single servings can help you learn how much you eat. When eating out, select appetizers or first courses over main entrées or order a child's meal. This will help you eat fewer calories. Another trick is to order a carryout box with your food and put half of your meal in the box before you start to eat. Don't eat family style by putting serving dishes on the table. Put your meal on a plate and leave everything else in the kitchen. Put leftovers away as soon as you have finished eating or after you have dished out your meal.

- **Watch out for supersizing and portion inflation.** Portion sizes have grown over the years. The typical cheeseburger used to have about 330 calories. Now it has 590 calories. Twenty years ago, an average cookie was about 1½ inches (3.8 cm) wide and had 55 calories. Now a cookie is 3½ inches (8.9 cm) wide and has 275 calories—*five times* the calories! Soda came in 6½-ounce (195 mL) bottles with 85 calories. Today a typical soda is 20 ounces (600 mL) with 250 calories. Pay attention to the Nutrition Facts label (Nutrition Facts Table in Canada) to see if you are eating one or more servings from the portion size you choose when eating at home. Ask for calorie information about menu choices when eating out.
- **Do not skip meals.** Eat three meals per day, including breakfast. If you skip a meal, you may feel hungrier later and end up eating more than you need to satisfy your larger appetite.
- **Eat slowly.** If you take less than 15 or 20 minutes to eat a meal, you are probably eating too fast. Give your brain time to catch up with your stomach. If you find it hard to slow down how fast you eat, try putting your fork down on the table between bites, and pick it up only after you have swallowed the food. Make it a game not to be the first person at the table to be finished eating.
- **Clock yourself.** Get in the habit of waiting about 15 minutes before either taking another portion or starting to eat dessert or a snack. You'll often find that this is enough time for the urge to eat or to continue eating to go away.
- **Keep on top of what is happening.** Check your weight on a schedule that works for you. You may not need to check it every day. If you check your weight at the same time of day (usually first thing in the morning), it is easier to note changes.
- **Make sure you are drinking enough water.** Sometimes people think they are hungry when they are actually thirsty.
- **Join a support group (either in person or online) and stay with it for at least four to six months.** Look for a group that does the following:
  - Emphasizes healthy eating.
  - Emphasizes lifelong changes in eating habits and lifestyle patterns.

- Gives support in the form of ongoing meetings or long-term follow-up.
- Does not make miraculous claims or guarantees. (Remember, if something sounds too good to be true, it probably is not true.)
- Does not rely on special meals or supplements.

- **Talk to your physician if you are considering weight-loss medications.** In the past few years, several prescription weight-loss medications have been approved and are on the market. These medications are not for everyone. Some people who take them experience side effects and many people regain weight when they stop taking them, so the medications may have to be used long term. Researchers know little about the long-term effects of these medications. These weight-loss drugs are also expensive and may or may not be paid for by insurance. It is best to discuss this topic with your health care provider.

Tips for Keeping Weight Off

If you or your care partner begin to lose weight, make sure to keep weight loss within healthy guidelines. If you or your care partner are feeling well, have good blood sugar and cholesterol levels, and are managing other health issues well, you may not need to lose more weight. Maintaining weight loss also requires effort. The following are some tips to move from weight loss to keeping the weight off:

- **Instead of focusing on weight loss,** focus on staying at the same weight and not gaining any weight for a few weeks; then reconsider your weight loss plan.
- **Plan to be active on most days.** Once you have lost some weight, exercising most days of the week improves your chances of keeping the weight off.
- **Plan your meals ahead.** Dinner is usually the largest meal. Dinner planning helps you make sure you have the ingredients you need when you want them. Take time once per week to plan meals for the week and make a grocery list. This can help you plan more healthy meals as well as reduce food waste and save money.
- **Log what you are eating in a food diary periodically to keep on track with making good choices.**
- **Try different fruits to end your meals with something sweet but light and refreshing.**
- **Allow yourself an occasional treat so you don't feel deprived.** A treat is a higher-calorie food you don't usually eat. Be sure to eat only a small portion of your treat food.
- **Think positively.** Remind yourself of what you have already done. Write positive comments to yourself on sticky notes and post them where you will see them.
- **Set a personal weight gain "upper limit."** Decide on a weight you don't want to exceed. Knowing your upper limit can help you take action, if needed. Weigh yourself regularly and if you regain, say, 3 pounds (1.4 kg), get back into eating less or moving more. If you hit this mark, go back on your weight loss program. The sooner you start, the faster the newly added pounds will come off.

- **If something big is happening in your life**, weight management may need to take a back seat for a while. Set a date when you will restart your weight management program.
- **If you have not already done so, join a support group.** Some of these are specifically for people using weight loss medications. Most health care facilities have a nutritionist and you might call them for a referral.

Tips for Gaining Weight

- **Eat dried fruit in place of some fresh fruit** or drink nectars instead of regular fruit juice.
- **Choose whole milk** instead of lower-fat dairy products.
- **Add extra whole milk** or milk powder to sauces, gravies, cereals, soups, and casseroles.
- **Drink liquid supplements or smoothies** with or between meals.
- **Drink high-calorie beverages** such as shakes, malts, fruit whips, smoothies, and eggnogs.
- **Top salads, soups, and casseroles** with shredded cheese, nuts, dried fruits, or seeds.
- **Eat smaller meals** several times a day.
- **Try waiting to drink beverages** 30 minutes after a meal so you have more room to eat food with higher calories. Or **sip high-calorie drinks with your meal** if you are thirsty. Try both options to find what works best for you.
- **Leave some nuts or dried fruit out** and eat a few pieces each time you pass the bowl.
- **Eat the highest-calorie foods first**, saving lower-calorie foods for later (for example, eat buttered bread before cooked spinach).
- **Add melted cheese** to vegetables and other dishes.
- **Use butter, margarine, or sour cream** as toppings. Add a flavored plant-based oil as a heart-healthy topping.
- **Keep a snack at your bedside** so that you can eat something if you wake in the middle of the night. Dried fruit and nuts are healthy snacks.

Tips for Mindful Eating

Go for the real, not the ideal. Healthy eating is not all or nothing. Healthy eating is making small changes.

- **Be mindful while you eat.** Notice what you eat, how much you eat, and how you are enjoying it. Practice mindful eating without distraction, such as friends, video games, or television. When you eat, concentrate on eating. When something tastes good, savor the flavor.
- **Replace thoughts like *never, always,* and *avoid*.** Instead, tell yourself that you can enjoy things occasionally, "but a healthier choice is better for me most of the time."
- **Retrain your taste buds.** Making healthier choices can help you on the road to healthier eating. This is especially true when cutting back on salt. Your taste buds eventually adjust to less salty flavors and learn to enjoy them.

- **Try a relaxation exercise** before eating. Pause to take a few deep breaths during eating.
- **Keep a food-mood diary.** Every day, list what, how much, and when you eat. Note how you feel (your mood or emotions) when you have the urge to eat. Try to spot patterns so you can anticipate when you will want to eat without being overly hungry. Use what you learn to make small changes.
- **When you are bored** and thinking about eating, ask yourself, "Am I really hungry?" If the answer is no, make yourself do something else for a few minutes. Keep your mind and hands busy.
- **Write down action plans for when challenging situations arise.** Sometimes it is easier to refer to the written word than to remember what you said you would do.

Tips for Enjoying Cooking and Eating

- **Cook something new.** Take a cooking class or watch videos on television or on YouTube. If you have odds and ends or leftovers, search the internet for recipes to figure out how to use them.
- **Illness, medicines, and surgery can change how food tastes.** Here are some things you might try if the lack of taste is keeping you or your care partner from eating enough.
  - Ask the doctor about possible medication changes.
  - Avoid smoking and limit alcohol.
  - Practice good oral care. Ask the dentist or doctor about treatment for dry mouth, if that is a problem.
  - Use herbs, such as basil, oregano, or tarragon, and spices, such as cinnamon, cumin, curry, ginger, or nutmeg.
  - Squirt fresh lemon juice on foods.
  - Use a small amount of vinegar in or on foods. There are many flavored vinegars. Try different ones.
  - Add healthy ingredients, such as carrots or barley to soup or dried fruits and nuts to salads, to make them tastier.
  - Chew your food slowly and well to release more flavor.
- **If fatigue gets in the way of cooking or eating, here are some hints.**
  - Cook enough for two or three meals and freeze for the future.
  - Exchange meals with friends or family.
  - Break your food preparation into steps, resting in between.
  - Ask for help, especially for big holiday meals or family gatherings.
  - Use a meal delivery service such as Meals on Wheels or many of the new food delivery services you can find on the internet.
- **If eating causes discomfort or shortness of breath for you or your care partner, try these tips.**
  - Eat four to six small meals a day.
  - Avoid foods that produce gas or are bloating, such as cabbage, broccoli, brussels sprouts, onions, and beans.

- Eat slowly, take small bites, and chew food well. Pause occasionally. Eating quickly to avoid shortness of breath can cause shortness of breath.
- Choose easy-to-eat foods such as yogurt, puddings, shakes, or fruit smoothies.

For a complete list of suggested further readings, useful websites, and other helpful resources, please see: www.bullpub.com/resources.

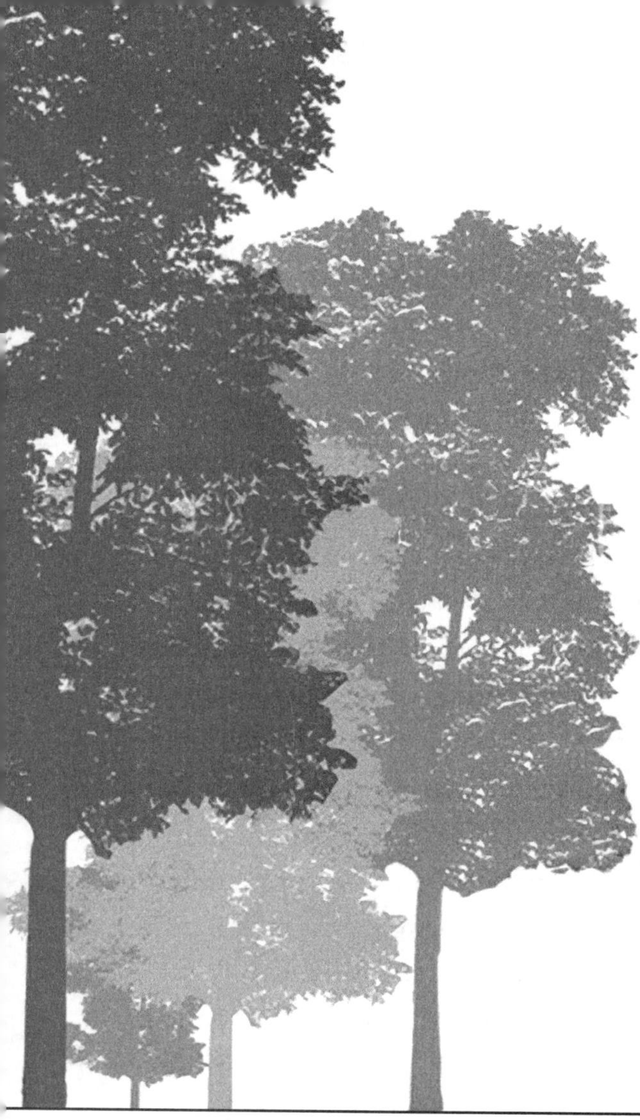

CHAPTER 11

Understanding Your Care Partner's Brain

In this chapter, we discuss some common conditions that can cause people to need a caregiver. There are many reasons a person needs care. You may be caring for someone with a mental health disorder, such as schizophrenia, or maybe your care partner has a spinal cord injury, ALS, or some other physical condition. Unfortunately, we cannot address every condition in detail in this book. If you need information about a condition that is not covered in this chapter, we suggest you contact an organization that serves the population with that condition. Even if your care partner's problem is not mentioned specifically in this chapter, the content you find here and in the rest of this book can be useful to you and your care partner.

Understanding Dementia

Dementia is a group of brain diseases. Early signs of dementia include memory problems, personality changes, and difficulty in understanding or remembering words. People with dementia can also have problems with activities such as driving, using the phone, handling their finances, and shopping. Over time, dementia gets worse. The course of the disease can take a year or two or up to 15 or 20 years. In the later stages of dementia, people can have hallucinations (seeing or hearing things that are not real) or paranoia (thinking that people are listening to or watching them). They can also have problems with bathing, dressing, toileting, transferring, and eating. At these later stages, people with dementia usually need care 24 hours a day.

Most people with dementia also have other chronic conditions such as high blood pressure, diabetes, or heart disease. Poor control of these conditions can cause the dementia to progress more rapidly. For this reason, it is important to treat the whole person, not just the dementia. As a caregiver, your job is to understand all your partner's medical conditions and determine the best course of care. Your health care provider can help you in determining which lifestyle strategies and medications can be helpful. Organizations, such as the Alzheimer's Association and the Parkinson's Foundation, can also help you learn about your partner's specific disease. More importantly, these groups can connect you to people like you who are living the caregiving experience. For a complete list of useful websites and other helpful resources, see www.bullpub.com/resources. Learning from the experiences of others and from experts can help with the many caregiver tasks.

People with dementia may or may not be able to participate in their own care. There are at least two possible issues that can interfere with a person who has dementia from making their own decisions about care. The person might deny there is problem, or they might not be capable of understanding or remembering what they need to do to care for themselves. As a caregiver, your job is to create a structured means of helping your care partner. It might help to remember that what you see as very difficult behaviors are not your care partner's fault. The behaviors are the fault of the disease.

Unfortunately, all dementias get worse over time. As we write, there are no cures. Because of this, as a caregiver, you have one more thing to think about: Do you want to make health care decisions based on your care partner's quality of life or length of life? For example, should your care partner have regular breast imaging exams or colonoscopies or other tests to find early cancers? The question you must answer is: If a tumor or growth is found, would it be in your care partner's best interest to treat them with chemotherapy or surgery or not? If the answer is no, then there is probably not a reason to have the test. Your health care provider can help with these decisions. We bring this up to point out that the health care decisions for someone with dementia may be different than for someone without dementia. As you will find in the rest of this book, there are many things you can address to make your life less stressful and your care partner's life easier. Sometimes these things are the same things you would do for someone without dementia. For example, hearing loss and poor eyesight can contribute to worsening any dementia. Therefore, hearing aids or eyeglasses and even cataract surgery can help with both you and your care partner's quality of life. But there may also be times when you decide against medical care when it prolongs life but may hurt quality of life.

Types of Dementia

Before we discuss specific diseases, we want to note that it is not always easy to diagnose different types of dementias. Often, but not always, the treatments are similar. Sometimes getting a diagnosis takes time and there can be a combination of two types of dementia. For example, vascular dementia may also be accompanied by Alzheimer's disease. This is not uncommon, and a definite diagnosis often cannot be made. However, many kinds of dementia and their treatments are similar to Alzheimer's.

Alzheimer's Disease

Greta was always very involved. As she got older, she did lots of volunteer work, played cards with her friends, and still managed to cook for her husband and babysit her grandchildren from time to time. Her daughter first became concerned one day after Greta had been babysitting. When Greta's daughter returned home after work, her children were very hungry and out of sorts. That had never happened before. When her daughter investigated, she found out that Greta had given the children lunch at 9:30 in the morning and then taken them to the park for the rest the day. Greta's daughter talked with her father who said that lately Greta seemed to be confused when driving, even when going to places that they had gone to for the last 20 years. Greta's daughter and husband decided to watch her more closely. They noticed that she was often angry—a very new and unusual development—and sometimes was forgetting words. They urged her to see a doctor. Greta was eventually diagnosed with early Alzheimer's disease.

For older adults, Alzheimer's disease is the most common source of dementia. More than 6 million Americans, most of them age 65 or older, may have Alzheimer's. In Alzheimer's disease, the brain develops abnormal clumps of protein called *amyloid plaques* and tangled bundles of fibers called *neurofibrillary* or *tau tangles*. The medical community believes that these changes take place 10 years before there are any changes in behavior or memory. There is a new test using a PET scan that can differentiate Alzheimer's from other types of dementia. It is quite expensive but can be useful when a patient is being considered for a treatment targeting amyloid (discussed on page 217).

Lewy Body Dementia (LBD)

Lewy body dementia (LBD) is the second most common reason for dementia after Alzheimer's. LBD affects 1.4 million Americans. The symptoms of Lewy body dementia are similar to those of Alzheimer's but may also include symptoms such as ridged muscles, slow movements, and tremors. Often people with Lewy body dementia have complex visual hallucinations that are well formed and detailed. They might also have fixed beliefs that events have happened that have not been seen or reported by others.

Lewy body dementia is caused by deposits of proteins (Lewy bodies) in the parts of the brain that control memory and movement. It affects the part of the brain that produces dopamine, a chemical produced in the brain that affects physical movement. The changes in dopamine production in individuals with LBD cause symptoms similar to Parkinson's disease, such as slowness, muscle rigidity, and tremors. Medications for Parkinson's disease are often prescribed to treat these symptoms in people with LBD. Unfortunately, these drugs can cause side effects such as hallucinations, confusion, and delusions. Before your care partner starts these drugs, it is important to have a discussion with their provider. As with all drugs, it is important to watch for and report side effects.

It might take a few years to obtain the right diagnosis but doing so is key as LBD is often treated with specific drugs that are not effective for Alzheimer's. These drugs help improve your care partner's quality of life. There are also some drugs that cause bad reactions for people with LBD. People with LBD should avoid antipsychotic medication and medications with anticholinergic properties (including some antidepressants and some antihistamines) if possible. It is important that all health care providers know that your care partner has LBD before they prescribe any medications.

HIV-Associated Dementia or AIDs Dementia

Because human immunodeficiency virus (HIV) can cross into the central nervous system, it can cause dementia. This usually occurs in cases of advanced HIV disease. The virus can damage a person's ability to think, impairing memory and the ability to function. HIV-associated dementia can usually be prevented with early diagnosis and treatment of HIV disease. Thankfully, with better treatment, this disease is less common. It is important to note that older people with HIV can get other types of dementias just like anyone else.

Frontotemporal Dementia (FTD)

Frontotemporal dementia (FTD) has a wide range of symptoms and progresses slowly. Commonly the disease starts in people in their 50s and 60s, but it can occur in people who are younger and in people up into their 80s. FTD first causes progressive damage to the frontal and/or temporal lobes of the brain. It often starts with a gradual decline in behavior and language but no memory loss. As the disease continues, a person with FTD loses the ability to plan or organize activities, behave appropriately, interact with others, and care for themself. FTD is often misdiagnosed as a psychiatric disorder or a different form of dementia. Sometimes, a full specialized neurological evaluation, called a neuropsychological test, is done to determine the difference between FTD and a psychiatric disease.

Vascular Dementia

Vascular dementia results when the brain does not get enough blood. Vascular dementia may come on suddenly with a stroke (and be followed by further stepwise decline) but can also progress in slow steady fashion.

Dementia Treatment

All the types of dementia we just introduced have three stages (mild, moderate, and severe). Treatment for all dementias is aimed at improving your care partner's quality of life and making your life as a caregiver easier.

Rena and Morris were both aware that Morris was becoming more forgetful. After much discussion, Morris went to the doctor and allowed Rena to come along. The diagnosis of dementia was devastating. The doctor suggested that they go home and come back in a week with questions and concerns. During the week, Rena and Morris talked about the diagnosis. Morris said he wanted to remain active and helpful to others if he could. He was also very clear that he did not want Rena to be a full-time caregiver nor did he want major medical treatment that would not improve his quality of life. Morris was especially concerned about driving. A week later, they talked with the doctor again. The doctor suggested that Morris start on medications and that both Morris and Rena attend a group at the Alzheimer's Association. The doctor thought it best for Morris to consider giving up driving. He recommended a driving evaluation be done at the local hospital to assess Morris's ability. The doctor also told Morris about a transportation program provided by the local senior center.

Morris and Rena found support in their community, Morris decided to give up driving and has become a speaker for the Alzheimer's Association. They both know that the disease will get worse but working with their doctor and others has helped them make realistic plans to address different things that might happen. By discussing the disease early, both Rena and Morris know what Morris wants. This can make it easier for Rena as the disease progresses.

With all dementias and brain disorders, work with your care partner's primary care provider to learn about treatment options. Seek out community resources to help you and your partner manage the challenges of the disease. For more useful information and help, see the link to caregiver resources at www.bullpub.com/resources as well as the information in Chapter 3, Dealing with Stress and Difficult Care Partner Behavior, on getting help.

Dementia Medications

Medications used to treat dementias do not keep dementia from getting worse. Only in very few rare cases, do medications possibly slightly slow decline. Instead, medications are prescribed to improve the function and quality of life of the person with dementia. For someone already taking many drugs to treat other conditions, the decision to add additional medications is made based on what combination of medications will result in the best quality of life.

In this part of the chapter, we discuss common drugs used for dementia. Two main classes of medications are typically prescribed to treat dementia currently. The first class is cholinesterase inhibitors and the second class is the

N-methyl-D-aspartate (NMDA) receptor antagonist. These medications are approved for treatment of Alzheimer's disease and dementia due to other causes including Lewy body dementia and vascular dementia. Please note that there are several new drugs under consideration. A new class of medications, called anti-amyloid antibodies, that have been developed specifically to treat Alzheimer's disease have recently been tested in people with Alzheimer's disease. The results of the studies are controversial and only two of these drugs (lecanamab and donanemab-azbt)) are approved by the Food and Drug Administration in the US. As of 2024, use of anti-amyloid antibodies is under review in Canada. (Please note that most Canadian-specific content is shaded throughout the book.) For the latest information on approved drugs in the US, search for FDA approved drugs for Alzheimer's and other causes of dementia at https://www.alz.org/getmedia/4f4ca289-a2c6-4df9-8cdf-390365bd477e/alzheimers-dementia-fda-approved-treatments-for-alzheimers-ts.pdf

Cholinesterase Inhibitors

Cholinesterase inhibitors boost the amount of acetylcholine in the brain by reducing the breakdown of acetylcholine. The three medications in this class are donepezil, rivastigmine, and galantamine. These medications may improve symptoms for some patients who are in the mild and moderate stages of Alzheimer's disease and other forms of dementia. Unfortunately, cholinesterase inhibitors have only a very limited impact on more advanced forms of dementia. Side effects vary among the three cholinesterase inhibitors but can include stomach upset, diarrhea, weight loss, tiredness, insomnia, unusual dreams, and dizziness. Severe side effects can include a low heart rate, which may cause fainting.

There is some evidence that cholinesterase inhibitors may improve cognition, behavior, and function for those with vascular dementia or mixed dementia. For people with Lewy body dementia, cholinesterase inhibitors may improve cognitive function as well as decrease hallucinations and other behavioral problems. In patients who have dementia associated with Parkinson's disease, the use of cholinesterase inhibitors might have some modest benefit in function. In addition, cholinesterase inhibitors could lessen some of the visual hallucinations.

Because of their limited impact, many health care providers prescribe cholinesterase inhibitors for a two- to three-month trial. They see if there is improvement based on the patient's or caregiver's observations or on testing. If there is no improvement, these medications are often stopped. Sometimes people get worse, in which case the medication is also stopped. Like all current medications for dementia, cholinesterase inhibitors are not a cure. They are given to help quality of life.

N-methyl-D-aspartate (NMDA) Receptor Antagonists

Memantine, the most common drug of the N-methyl-D-aspartate (NMDA) receptor antagonist class, works very differently than cholinesterase inhibitors. Memantine is used to treat people with moderate to severe Alzheimer's disease. People with mild Alzheimer's disease have not been shown to benefit. Those with vascular dementia also appear to benefit from memantine, but there is no clear benefit to treating people with Lewy body dementia with memantine.

There is some evidence that memantine may impact the progress of Alzheimer's disease even though it does not improve functioning. Memantine seems to have fewer side effects than the cholinesterase inhibitors. Dizziness is the most common side effect, but confusion as well as agitation and delusions might also occur. Some health care providers use memantine in combination with a cholinesterase inhibitor for patients with advanced dementia.

Anti-amyloid Antibodies

A number of new medications that remove amyloid from the brain have been developed as treatments specifically for Alzheimer's disease. These drugs are antibodies, proteins that the body normally makes to help fight off infections. In this case, the antibodies are made in a laboratory to attack amyloid. Anti-amyloid antibodies are very effective at removing amyloid from the brain but have only a small benefit in slowing progression of Alzheimer's disease. Lecanamab and donanemab are the only anti-amyloid antibody drugs available in the US and some other countries. Lecanamab and donanemab are given by injection in a vein and require frequent evaluations and brain scans. Lecanamab is given every two weeks and donanemab is given every four weeks. Both of these medications are only available to those who have a positive amyloid-PET scan, which is a test for amyloid accumulation discussed earlier in this section on page 213. Inflammation and bleeding in the brain are the most concerning side effects.

Antipsychotic Medications and Dementia

Antipsychotic medications are used to treat psychosis (a loss of contact with reality) and agitation. Unfortunately these medications are associated with a higher rate of death in people with dementia and should be used only when absolutely necessary. Most antipsychotics work by blocking receptors for dopamine. They can cause problems with movement that can resemble Parkinson's disease. Second generation (atypical) antipsychotic medications have less of this effect and are used to treat dementia-related agitation or psychosis. The American Psychiatric Association has outlined how to best use these medications, weighing the risks versus benefits. These medications are often used for a limited time and the health care team attempts to decrease and/or stop the medications several months after behaviors are no longer present. Brexpiprazole (Rexulti) is approved by the FDA for treatment of agitation associated with Alzheimer's disease. Other second-generation antipsychotics, including quetiapine, are often used to treat agitation and psychosis in Alzheimer's disease and other forms of dementia but are not specifically approved for use in those with dementia. As a caregiver, you play a central role in how these medications are used and on reporting how these medications impact your care partner.

Other Medications for Dementia

Many other potential dementia medications have been studied and have not been shown to be effective. These include estrogen replacement; nonsteroidal anti-inflammatory medications (or NSAIDs), such as ibuprofen, naproxen, and aspirin; ginkgo biloba; cholesterol-lowering medications, such as statins; and dietary supplements, such as B vitamins, vitamin E, and omega-3 fatty acids. Most medications have side effects. As a caregiver, you need to be on the lookout for side effects and report anything you think might be a medication side effect to your care partner's provider. (See Chapter 12, Managing Treatment Decisions and Medications.)

Understanding Stroke

Strokes (which are also called CVAs or cerebrovascular accidents) are brain injuries caused when the flow of blood to the brain is stopped. This blood flow stoppage causes brain cell death. There are two main types of stroke: ischemic and hemorrhagic. The less common type of stroke is a hemorrhagic stroke. During a hemorrhagic stroke, a blood vessel in the brain bleeds and damages the surrounding brain tissue. Eighty percent of strokes are ischemic stokes. During an ischemic stroke, an artery in the brain is blocked and the area of the brain served by that artery is damaged. There are two kinds of ischemic strokes: embolic and thrombotic. An embolic stroke occurs when a blood clot travels from another part of the body through the blood stream and lodges in the brain. The lodged clot stops blood flow, causing damage to the brain in an embolic ischemic stroke. One of the most common causes of this type of stroke is atrial fibrillation (an irregular heartbeat). Thrombotic ischemic strokes result from fatty deposits (plaques) lining the blood vessel. These deposits can break off and clog the blood vessel or get larger and block the artery.

The Effects of Strokes

A stroke almost always begins suddenly, but symptoms sometimes develop slowly over hours to days. Strokes can cause long-term disability and sometimes death. The location of the stroke in the brain determines the part of the body that is affected. The location also determines stroke patients' ability to speak, understand, or express themselves. Strokes can cause damage to the part of the brain that controls emotions. A person who has had a stroke may anger or cry very easily. This is not a character flaw and is not the fault of you, the caregiver. The changes in emotions are a result of the stroke.

Injury from a stroke might be temporary or permanent. Outcome depends on how much and which part of the brain is affected and how fast the stroke patient gets treatment. Treatment after the stroke is also important. Unfortunately, many stroke survivors are left with physical and/or cognitive (thinking) disabilities and might need supervision for the rest of their lives. This supervision may include medication management and lifestyle management, including help with eating, exercise, hygiene, emotions, and social support. Depending on the damage caused by the stroke, this supervision and help may be minimal or be very demanding. Treatment for strokes includes rehabilitation and medication. Rehabilitation can include physical, occupational, and/or speech therapy depending on your care partner's needs. It is best to start rehabilitation as soon as possible after a stroke, but your care partner may benefit even if rehabilitation is begun a year or more after a stroke. Some communities have community stroke rehabilitation programs. Be sure to ask your health care provider about these.

Stroke Treatment and Medications

In the first hours after the onset of an ischemic stroke, thrombolytic medications (tenecteplase or alteplase) that can dissolve clots may be helpful. In rare cases, a device can be used to directly remove the clot. This requires placing a catheter in a large artery in the leg and threading it up into the clogged artery in the brain. Treatment must start as soon as possible after the onset of a stroke and can only be given in a hospital. If you think you or your care partner is having a stroke, call 911 in the United States, Canada, and Mexico. In many other countries, the number to call is 112. The medications that are prescribed once the stroke occurs depend on the type of stroke as well as the type of damage that was done. For ischemic strokes caused by thrombosis or blood clots, medications are prescribed to prevent blood clots from reforming and causing another stroke. Stroke medications include those that help prevent blood clots, antihypertensive (high blood pressure) medications that lower blood pressure to help stop the damage high blood pressure causes to blood vessels, and cholesterol-lowering medications. Cholesterol can damage or block arteries.

Antiplatelet Medications (Platelet Inhibition Medications)

Antiplatelet medications (and anticoagulant medications) are prescribed to try to prevent future clots. Antiplatelet medications keep platelets (a part of your blood that helps it to clot) from sticking together and causing an unwanted blood clot. Aspirin is the most commonly used antiplatelet medication.

Anticoagulant Medications

Like antiplatelet medications, anticoagulant medications can prevent blood clots from forming. For anyone who has a heart condition that affects the rhythm of the heart, there is a danger of clots forming. People with these conditions may need to take an anticoagulant permanently.

While antiplatelet and anticoagulant medications help prevent a future stroke, they also can cause bleeding. There is a fine line between enough medication and too much medication, which can be harmful. All of these medications must be carefully monitored. These medications can also interact with other medications. An adjustment in dosage for all medications might be necessary whenever a new medication is started or an old medication is stopped. This is usually determined by blood tests. Finally, it is important to avoid falls, bumps, and accidents when a person is taking anticoagulant medications, since these medications slow blood clotting. If a person is taking an anticoagulant medication, there is a danger of bleeding too much. See Chapter 8, Preventing Injuries. As a caregiver, you need to be alert to bleeding and bruising. Do not hesitate to call your care partner's health care provider if you think that there could be a problem.

High Blood Pressure (Hypertension) Treatments and Medications

High blood pressure is a leading cause of stroke. High blood pressure damages the walls of blood vessels and can lead to smaller blood vessels becoming blocked by clots. This is why it is so important to keep blood pressure under control. A diet that is low in sodium (salt is the largest source of sodium in the human diet) can help control blood pressure and prevent further damage and strokes. While lifestyle choices such as exercising; eating a healthy, balanced diet; and not smoking can help, people with high blood pressure usually also need to take medications. There are many medications for high blood pressure, and sometimes people take more than one. People taking these medications must be monitored closely and it is important that the right medications and the right doses are being taken.

Statins

Statins are medications that help prevent and shrink plaque (the fatty deposit lining the blood vessels) that cause ischemic stroke. They work by lowering cholesterol, which causes plaque formation.

Diabetes Treatments and Medications

Diabetes is a leading cause of stroke. Like high blood pressure, diabetes damages the walls of blood vessels and can lead to smaller blood vessels becoming blocked by clots. This is why keeping diabetes under control is important. While lifestyle choices such as exercising; eating a healthy, balanced diet; and not smoking can help, people with diabetes may also need to take medications. There are many medications for diabetes and sometimes people take more than one. Again, care must be monitored closely and make sure the right medications and the right doses are being taken.

Antidepressant Medications and Stroke

Depression is common one to six months after a stroke. Be aware of this and seek treatment if needed. Antidepressant medications, such as selective serotonin reuptake inhibitors (SSRIs) can be helpful, but they can also interfere with some other medications taken after a stroke. Again, it is important that caregivers observe, monitor, and work with health care providers to find help for post-stroke depression.

Taking Stroke Medications

Medications cannot help if they are not taken. People who have had strokes or wish to prevent strokes often have to take several medications. Sometimes people do not want to take medication but do not tell their doctor that they are not taking it. Consider the following story of three people. All three go to the doctor with the exact same high blood pressure. In each case, the doctor asks if they have been taking their medication. Each patient answers, "Yes." Lourdes has been taking the medication but has seen little change in her blood pressure. The doctor orders a second medication to be added to the first. Her blood pressure goes down. Henrik has been taking the medication and his blood pressure has been going down but is not quite low enough yet. The doctor notes this and increases the dose of his current medication. His blood pressure goes down. Bonnie has not been taking her medication regularly but is embarrassed to say so. The doctor prescribes a second medication, which Bonnie also does not take. She eventually has a stroke. The moral of this story is that you have to be honest and work with a doctor to get good treatment. Doctors cannot read minds.

Understanding Parkinson's Disease (PD)

Parkinson's disease (PD) is a movement disorder with symptoms that continue to worsen over time. Unfortunately, the medical community does not know the cause or cure of Parkinson's disease. We do know that the symptoms result from a loss of brain cells in a part of the brain called the *substantia nigra*. This is the area of the brain where dopamine is made. Dopamine is a neurotransmitter (brain chemical) that affects movement. The loss of these brain cells decreases the amount of dopamine available. This, in turn, affects movement and coordination.

The Effects of Parkinson's Disease

People with PD are unable to control their movements. This lack of control can involve the hands, legs, arms, jaw, and feet. PD symptoms include tremors, rigidity, slowness of movement (bradykinesia), and impaired balance. There might also be changes in the voice, especially softening and decreased volume. Other symptoms may include psychosis, hallucinations, daytime sleepiness, pain, fatigue, depression, and dementia. As a caregiver, be aware of these symptoms and report changes to your health care team. Doing so will help ensure that your care partner gets the best treatment for the stage of the disease they are in.

Correct diagnosis is important. Other diseases might look like Parkinson's disease but progress differently and may or may not respond to PD treatments. These other diseases are known as Parkinson's-plus syndromes and feature classic symptoms of Parkinson's disease as well as additional symptoms that are different from common Parkinson's.

Parkinson's Disease Treatment and Medications

Parkinson's disease treatments include medications and implantable deep brain stimulators (DBS). Drug treatments for Parkinson's disease, like treatments for dementia, do not slow or reverse the natural history and progression of the disease. However, some medications can be very helpful for some symptoms. DBS is used for some patients who no longer respond enough to medications.

Parkinson's disease medications can interact with certain foods, other medications, vitamins, herbal supplements, over-the-counter (OTC) cold medications, and other remedies. The doctor and pharmacist must know everything your care partner is taking, including OTC drugs, vitamins, and supplements. Both you and your care partner must know exactly how medications should be taken and what foods or other medications should be avoided when taking these medications. For example, alcohol can change the action of some Parkinson's disease medications. Other Parkinson's disease medication must be taken on an empty stomach to ensure that they are fully absorbed and have maximum effect.

Levodopa and Carbidopa

Levodopa is the single most effective drug in Parkinson's disease management. As we noted earlier in this section, when a person has Parkinson's, less dopamine is produced. Levodopa helps replace the missing dopamine. Although levodopa might improve the function and decrease the symptoms, it does not decrease the progression of the disease. Levodopa is usually given in combination with the drug carbidopa. Carbidopa helps prevents the nausea caused by levodopa and enhances the action of levodopa.

Monoamine Oxidase B (MAO-B) Inhibitors

Selegiline, rasagiline, and safinamide are monoamine oxidase B (MAO-B) inhibitors, which are prescribed to help control Parkinson's disease symptoms. People taking these drugs often also take levodopa and carbidopa. These medications work by blocking the breakdown of dopamine which leads to an increase in the amount of dopamine in the brain. They can help people with Parkinson's disease by decreasing the amount of levodopa and carbidopa needed to control symptoms. They can also help lengthen the time that the levodopa/carbidopa combination is effective. A person should not stop taking these drugs without talking with a doctor. If the doctor advises that your care partner stop taking them, your care partner may need to wait at least 14 days before beginning to take certain other medications.

Dopamine Agonists

Dopamine agonist medications mimic the effects of dopamine in the brain. Dopamine agonists can be used effectively taken alone in early stages of Parkinson's disease or in combination with carbidopa and levodopa after the disease has progressed. These medications play a significant role in reducing tremors, allowing people with Parkinson's disease to carry out the activities of daily living, such as transferring, toileting, bathing, and walking.

Amantadine

Amantadine was initially developed as a flu treatment and was noted to benefit people with Parkinson's disease. It is often given in the early stages of Parkinson's disease with levodopa to treat tremors or problems with voluntary movement (movements such a picking up a fork or walking).

Catechol-O-Methyltransferase (COMT) Inhibitors

Catechol-O-methyltransferase (COMT) inhibitor drugs are only used with levodopa. When a person takes levodopa, an enzyme in the body called catechol-O-methyltransferase (COMT) converts a portion of the levodopa into a form that is useless. These drugs block the COMT enzyme from doing this, which makes more levodopa available in the body for reducing Parkinson's disease symptoms. People taking these drugs need to have a blood test to check their liver enzymes every six months.

Anticholinergics

Medications that block the effects of acetylcholine in the brain are sometimes used in younger individuals with Parkinson's disease who have a tremor as their most significant problem. Trihexyphenidyl and benztropine are two anticholinergic medications used to treat patients with Parkinson's disease. Because these medications can worsen problems with memory and thinking, they should be avoided in people with these problems and are generally not used in older individuals.

Parkinson's Disease Medications and Psychosis

As noted earlier, psychosis (visual hallucinations and delusions) are common for people with Parkinson's disease. Patients may also have paranoia. (When a person is paranoid, they believe without reason that others do not like them or are trying to harm them.) Psychosis and paranoia are most common as the disease progresses, but these symptoms can also be triggered by hospitalization. Management of these symptoms is dependent on identifying and treating the causes. Medications used for the treatment of Parkinson's disease are the most common cause. Sedatives, anxiety medications, and antidepressants are all medications that can cause psychosis. Be aware of this and if you see changes in your care partner's behavior, contact their health care provider. It might be necessary to change some of the medications they are taking. Do not try to adjust doses or medications yourself. If symptoms continue despite attempts at dose adjustments, they may need to take additional medications. Antipsychotic medications—the drugs most often used to treat psychosis—can make the problems with movement for people with Parkinson's disease worse. This is especially true of first-generation antipsychotic medications, such as haloperidol. Because of this, treatment options may be limited to low doses of second generation (atypical) antipsychotic medications such as quetiapine, olanzapine, clozapine, and pimavanserin.

As mentioned in the previous section on dementia (see pages 216–217), people with Parkinson's disease and dementia may also benefit from cholinesterase inhibitors. These may not be helpful in managing psychotic symptoms.

Understanding Traumatic Brain Injury (TBI)

Traumatic brain injury (TBI) occurs when a person suffers a jolt or a blow to the head and the brain is damaged and injured. Depending on the extent of the trauma, this can range from a mild to severe injury. No two TBIs are alike and every traumatic brain injury patient is different. Traumatic brain injury is very common, and each year an estimated 2.5 million people in the United States and 400,000 Canadians suffer TBIs. Men are more than twice as likely to suffer from traumatic brain injury as women. This is mainly due to sports and military injuries. Most people with traumatic brain injury seen in emergency rooms are the very young, but the highest hospitalization rates are for those over age 65. Many different types of injuries can lead to traumatic brain injury. Falls are the leading cause of TBI in older patients, followed by unintentional blunt trauma resulting from auto or bicycle accidents. Risk factors include alcohol and drug use and underlying mental health and cognitive disorders. TBI from combat and sports injuries also occurs in young people.

The Effects of Traumatic Brain Injury

Concussions are a mild injury that affects the way the brain functions. Concussions are the most common type of traumatic brain injury. Headaches, mild confusion, problems with memory, and dizziness can all be caused by a concussion. Anyone with a concussion should be evaluated by a health care provider. Even seemingly minor brain injuries can have major complications that can be devastating if the complications are not recognized and treated early. Concussions can be challenging for caregivers. The good news is that if they are treated, they usually improve in days to weeks.

More challenging are moderate and severe traumatic brain injuries. People who have experienced moderate and severe traumatic brain injury often have significant neurological (brain) damage. Depending on the part of the brain that is affected, moderate to severe TBIs can interfere with daily function. If a person has experienced a moderate to severe TBI, they might lose the ability to be independent (for example, to drive, bank, shop, or clean). They may also lose the ability to perform basic activities of daily living, such as dressing, bathing, transferring, eating, and toileting. Depending on the extent of the injury, these changes can be permanent. Because TBIs happen suddenly, sometimes family members become caregivers without warning.

Based on the cause of the traumatic brain injury, there are different treatments for TBI. Treatments are all aimed at dealing with the trauma (injury) and getting the best possible outcome. Once a care and treatment plan is started, the challenges for caregivers begin. Caregivers have to deal with and manage the physical needs of someone with a TBI, such as giving pills or using special equipment, as well as managing the functions and emotions of a care partner. Like other brain diseases and conditions, traumatic brain injury impacts the entire family and is stressful to all those involved in caring for the person with TBI. Understanding how stressful this condition can be for the whole family is critical in developing care plans that are effective and can help everyone adapt to a new normal.

Individuals suffering from traumatic brain injury typically face a lot of personal concerns and issues. They may feel they are a burden to the family. In addition, they are likely to develop depression, anxiety, post-traumatic stress disorder (PTSD), or anger about their TBI. Management of these mental health issues is important. Plan for this and talk over what is happening or might happen with your care partner's health care providers. Remaining socially engaged is a key part of treatment. Friends, family, and support groups are very important. As a caregiver, it is key to understand that care will be long term. Begin early to seek help and make plans.

Caring for someone with TBI is like running a marathon, requiring slow, steady, and persistent effort. As a caregiver, you should not try to do this alone. Look into some in-home assistance, such as personal care attendants or home health aides. (See Chapter 7, Getting Help.) This will give you a chance to relax and do some of the things you want and need to do. Seek out short-term counseling and longer-term support from brain injury support groups. In addition, having a family and friend support network is important. (See the discussion about family meetings on pages 100–102.) One last note, caregiving should never put you in danger. See Chapter 3, Dealing with Stress and Difficult Care Partner Behavior, for more discussion on this difficult situation.

Traumatic Brain Injury Treatment and Medications

Treatment of traumatic brain injuries involves managing medical and behavioral issues as well as physical and occupational therapy. Here we will only discuss medications.

Anticonvulsant Medications

Trauma to the brain from TBIs can cause areas of the brain to be hyperactive (overly active). This can trigger the nerve cells in the brain to cause a seizure. Anticonvulsant medications prevent seizures by suppressing this activity. Common side effects of anticonvulsant medications include confusion, hair loss, lethargy, poor coordination, loss of appetite, nausea, vomiting, tremors, and weight gain. Sometimes more than one drug may need to be tried to find out which works best. Caregivers play a key role in observing and reporting changes to the doctor.

Antidepressant Medications and TBI

Antidepressant medications treat anxiety, depression, insomnia, headaches, and pain. All of these symptoms can occur with traumatic brain injuries. It might seem strange that antidepressants can treat so many things. In the case of TBIs, many symptoms have very similar origins in the brain. Side effects of antidepressants can include dry mouth, dizziness, confusion, constipation, drowsiness, skin rash, seizures, tremors, and urinary retention (that is, problems urinating). Observe care partners who are taking these medications and report changes to the doctor.

Antipsychotic Medications and TBI

Antipsychotic medications are prescribed to treat some people with traumatic brain injuries who have severe mental or emotional issues or lose contact with reality (psychosis). In addition, antipsychotic medications are sometimes prescribed for severe sleep disturbances and aggressive or agitated behaviors. Common side effects of antipsychotic medications include blurred vision, dizziness, dry mouth, headache, low blood pressure, abnormal movements of the body, tremors, weight gain, and urinary retention. These side effects are more common in the first generation (typical) antipsychotic medications. If your care partner is taking antipsychotic medications, it is especially important that you observe and report changes as your care partner might not be an accurate reporter.

Understanding Post-Traumatic Stress Disorder (PTSD)

Post-traumatic stress disorder (PTSD) is a mental health disorder that develops after a person experiences or witnesses trauma. That trauma could be a life-threatening event, such as a natural disaster; an assault; military combat; some other violent experience; or involvement in an accident. Trauma can also be the result of sexual abuse. PTSD is often long-term and severely disabling. People with PTSD may have nightmares, flashbacks (sudden and disturbing vivid memories of events in the past), sleep disorders, or may be on edge. In addition, people with PTSD often are unable to take part in social, work, or family relationships. Another common symptom of PTSD is blaming problems on someone other than themselves.

Diagnosing Post-Traumatic Stress Disorder (PTSD)

PTSD can be diagnosed when symptoms continue for at least four weeks after the traumatic event. Unfortunately, it sometimes takes years to diagnose PTSD because health care professionals, family, friends, and the person with PTSD fail to recognize the symptoms and connect them with a traumatic event. Early identification and treatment of this condition may help PTSD from becoming long-term. As a caregiver, you have a central role. You may know your care partner better than anyone else. It is up to you to report symptoms and changes, tell health professionals about any trauma, and help your care partner find treatment.

In many instances, people with post-traumatic stress disorder are unaware for a long time that they have this condition. We know of one case of a World War II officer with PTSD who returned home and had a successful career and was not diagnosed until fifty years after the trauma occurred. If your care partner is violent, or if you experienced the same trauma as your care partner, you might also suffer from PTSD. If you think this might be possible, ask your health care provider for an assessment. We have said this before, but we will say it again: Being a caregiver should never expose you to physical harm. See Chapter 3, Dealing with Stress and Difficult Care Partner Behavior, to read more about this topic.

Post-Traumatic Stress Disorder (PTSD) Treatment

The first step to PTSD recovery is for the people who experience the trauma to recognize that they have been exposed to experiences that have altered their world views. This is often difficult, as people with PTSD are typically distrustful of others and unwilling to accept a diagnosis that brings with it an accompanying suggestion of weakness or mental instability. The most important step for people with PTSD is that they form trusting relationships with someone who can be an impartial advocate for them. Your care partner must find a person to talk to who does not disbelieve or judge your care partner's history in any way. Once individuals with PTSD have established trusting relationships, they are more open to observations and opinions.

People with PTSD typically are able to establish only one or two such trusting relationships and often disregard opinions of people whom they see as lacking traumatic life experiences. This could include you, the caregiver. Remember that this lack of trust comes from the condition. It is not your fault. Care partners might relate better to others who have experienced similar trauma than they do to their caregivers. In fact, your care partner may find your opinions, no matter how well intentioned, uninformed at best and patronizing at worst. People with PTSD are typically rigid in their thinking and easy to anger. Your care partner might see the world in black and white with very few shades of gray (in other words, either good or bad with nothing in between). If you suggest that you know how they feel, the person with PTSD may reject what you say. To combat this, listen to their story without adding your own ideas or assumptions. Just listen!

Many people with PTSD abuse drugs and/or alcohol as coping mechanisms. In these cases, drug or alcohol use must be treated at the same time as one is trying to come to terms with a PTSD diagnosis. The continued use of drugs or alcohol can get in the way of PTSD treatment and recovery. This is difficult, as traumatic events often encourage isolation, depression, distrust, and alienation. All of these can lead to further drug or alcohol abuse. If you do not believe this, just think how often you have heard someone say, "I have had a really hard day, so I need a drink." Unfortunately, alcohol and drugs are a common but not successful attempt to deal with stress.

PTSD treatment aims at getting rid of or decreasing the troubling symptoms as well as getting people to become aware of the triggers and what active steps they can take in preventing or eliminating symptoms. One of the common treatments for PTSD is cognitive behavioral therapy (CBT). Cognitive behavioral therapy can take place in individual therapy sessions or in groups and is effective in treating people with a variety of mental health issues. CBT helps people develop personal coping strategies. In CBT treatment, patients learn to develop action plans and new ways of dealing with problems. CBT is often recommended when medications for PTSD are prescribed. We discuss PTSD medications in the following section.

Post-Traumatic Stress Disorder (PTSD) Medications

Before we talk about specific medications, it is important to note a few things. Not everyone responds to every medication. Therefore, it may take several trials of medications until the right one is found. Of course, medications will never work if they are not taken. Unfortunately, many people with PTSD do not believe they need medications and do not ever begin taking their medications, take less or more than was prescribed, or stop taking their medications altogether. For this reason, medications are often prescribed as part of a treatment plan that includes therapy, such as cognitive behavioral therapy (CBT), so the patient can be regularly encouraged by a therapist to take their medications. It is very important that people with PTSD trust the health care providers who prescribe medications.

Sometimes people do not respond to medications. Medications are typically more effective in treating mood disorders, agitation, anger, anxiety, and depression and less effective in managing flashbacks and behavioral issues. The medical community knows less about PTSD in older people than about military-related PTSD in younger people.

Antidepressants and PTSD

The antidepressants known as selective serotonin reuptake inhibitors (SSRIs) have been widely studied for people with PTSD. The amount of medication (the dose) is low at first and is slowly increased until symptoms decrease. If nothing happens within two months, then the dose is tapered off and another medication is tried. Patients should not stop these medications suddenly without their doctor's approval. Serotonin-norepinephrine reuptake inhibitors (SNRIs) are similar to the SSRIs. Some older antidepressant medications, such as tricyclic antidepressants, and atypical antidepressants have not been shown to be effective for PTSD.

Second-Generation Antipsychotics and PTSD

If antidepressants and cognitive behavioral therapy are not working after multiple tries, second-generation antipsychotics may be prescribed for PTSD. Often these are prescribed if the person with PTSD has agitation and psychotic symptoms combined with depression. Unfortunately, these medications do not have a strong evidence base to support their use.

Other Medications and PTSD

Alpha-adrenergic receptor blockers have been used to reduce nightmares and improve sleep for PTSD patients. The alpha-adrenergic receptor drug most often used is prazosin, which is also used in the treatment of high blood pressure. Prazosin is used with SSRI medications and is usually given at a very low dose and then increased.

Sometimes people with PTSD are hypervigilant. This means that they are constantly searching for any sign of threat and are more aware of sights, sounds, and smells that many of us take for granted such as cars backfiring, children shouting at play, or planes flying overhead. They are very anxious, and this leads to mental and physical exhaustion. Although benzodiazepines are often used to treat these symptoms, they have a downside as they are easily abused. Thus, benzodiazepines should be avoided if possible. If prescribed, a medication contract and close monitoring is necessary. As a caregiver, you might be asked to monitor your care partner.

For a complete list of suggested further readings, useful websites, and other helpful resources, please see: www.bullpub.com/resources.

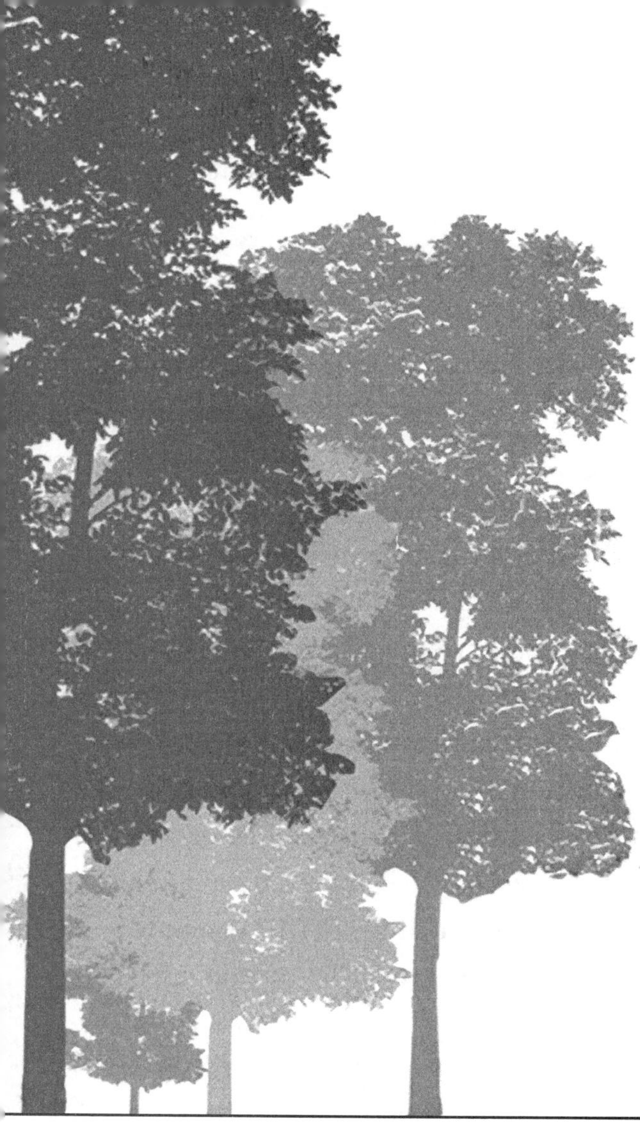

Chapter 12

Managing Treatment Decisions and Medications

You may often hear about new treatments, new drugs, nutritional supplements, and alternative treatments. Hardly a week goes by without some new treatment making the news. Websites, newspapers, magazines, television, and social media are full of ads for drugs and nutritional supplements. You may receive emails that promise new treatments and cures. Your health care providers, and even neighbors and friends, may recommend new procedures, medications, or other treatments. Drug companies spend billions of dollars advertising and marketing to physicians and patients. When you see drug ads on TV, have you noticed that they present the benefits in a slow, upbeat voice, while the side effects are recited very rapidly? The main message of drug advertising is that for every symptom, every ache and pain, and every problem, there is a medication solution. This is a problem because ads like this may keep you from managing your illness in less medication-centered ways. Imagine if such marketing power was behind promoting self-management skills. There might be far less chronic illness and even less need for medications, surgery, herbs, supplements, and alternative medicine offerings.

Evaluating Medical and Health Claims

When it comes to medical claims, what can you believe? How can you decide what might be worth a try? A big part of managing your own care and that of your care partner is being able to evaluate these claims or recommendations and make informed decisions about trying something new. This chapter provides information on how you can make informed decisions and manage your treatment and medications effectively. The following are some key questions you should ask yourself when making decisions about any treatment, whether it is a mainstream medical treatment or a complementary or alternative treatment.

Where did you learn about the treatment?

Was it reported in a scientific journal; a supermarket tabloid; an online, print, or television ad; a website; or a flyer you picked up somewhere? Did a friend, neighbor, or family member suggest it? Did your doctor recommend it? The source of the information is important. Results that are reported in a respected scientific journal are more believable than those you might see in a supermarket tabloid or in advertising. Results reported in scientific journals are usually from research studies. Scientists carefully review these studies before publication. Although bias, errors, and fraud can still occur in mainstream scientific publications, they are less likely and there is a formal process for correcting errors when they do occur. Many alternative treatments and nutritional supplements have not been studied scientifically. Claims may appear to be backed up by scientific investigation but the studies may be very weak, poorly designed, and even be falsely generated by artificial intelligence (AI) computer programs. Testimonials, anecdotes, unsupported claims, and opinions aren't the same as objective, evidence-based information from a reliable source. If it sounds too good to be true, it's probably not true.

Consider this example. A neighbor returns from a stay at a spa. She reports that her arthritis improved. She credits the special diet, herbs, and supplements. But could it be that the warm weather, daily exercise, relaxation, and pampering caused her improvement? It is common to take up a generally healthier lifestyle when starting a new treatment—could that be playing a part in the improvement? This example shows that it is important to look at everything that has changed since someone started a treatment.

In addition, the latest may not be the greatest. Some treatments are promoted as "breakthroughs." Only later is it shown that these treatments may be ineffective or that unanticipated side effects occur. Sometimes it is best to wait. If a new discovery is truly an effective treatment, time will often tell.

Does the treatment involve extreme diet changes or stopping other medications or treatments?

Are you considering trying a food or supplement that is being promoted in ads, news, or on a social media site? If you change your eating habits, be sure you don't sacrifice important nutrients. You may hear about alternative care regimes and not know exactly what the phrase alternative care means. *Alternative care* is used *in place of* conventional medicine. *Complementary care* is used *along* with conventional medicine. When you use complementary care, you may be getting treatment from your doctor while using additional therapies to manage the same condition. For example, you may be taking medication for arthritis and doing yoga. In this example, yoga is complementary care and as long as you are cleared for exercise, it may be a good add-on for your self-care. If, on the other hand, an alternative treatment requires you to stop taking prescribed medication or participating in other medical treatments, be cautious. Talk with your health care provider before stopping any treatment or making a change.

Is the treatment safe and effective?

All treatments have side effects and possible risks. Only you can decide if the potential problems are worth the possible benefit. Many people think that if something is natural or organic, it must be good for them. This is not always true. When something is strong enough to have an effect, it's also strong enough to have side effects. Natural isn't necessarily better or safer than a manufactured product just because it comes from a plant or animal. The heart medication digitalis comes from a plant, but it can be deadly if the dose is not right. Some natural treatments, herbs, or even vitamin supplements may be safe in small doses but dangerous in larger doses.

Just because many people use a product or practice, or it has been used for many years, also doesn't mean that it's safe or effective. Some practices, such as meditation, have proven health benefits and little or no risk. Other traditional methods may not be safe for certain people to use. And others simply don't work or haven't yet been proven.

The US Food and Drug Administration (FDA) regulates over-the-counter (OTC) and prescription drugs. It does *not* regulate herbs or other supplements sold in the US. In Canada, Health Canada's Health Products and Food Branch (HPFB) regulates, evaluates, and monitors the safety, quality, and effectiveness of therapeutic and diagnostic products available to Canadians. Herbs and supplements do not have to meet the same standards for safety, effectiveness, and manufacturing that over-the-counter and prescription drugs must meet. (Please note that most Canadian-specific content is shaded throughout the book.) Tests of some supplements have found striking differences between what's listed on the label and what's in the bottle. Some products have been found to not even contain the active ingredient they advertise. And some are contaminated with metals, unlabeled prescription drugs, pesticides, microorganisms, or other substances. Do some research about the company selling the product before you try it.

All prescription drugs and over-the-counter medications have the potential to interact or counteract with each other. Sometime safe and effective medications can cause real problems when taken with certain other drugs. The same is true for herbs and supplements. They may not get along with each other and they may also not get along with prescription or over-the-counter drugs. We know a caregiver who spent hundreds of dollars giving supplements and herbs advertised on TV to a care partner. The caregiver also took several supplements. Unfortunately, the caregiver had to go to urgent care and received months of treatment to reverse the effects of the supplements. The care partner had more energy and was able to participate more once most of the supplements were stopped. It is important to have all your medications, supplements, and herbs reviewed by your health care provider or pharmacist.

As a caregiver, you want what is best for your care partner. There are lots of products that claim to improve memory or slow dementia without sufficient evidence. Some are even touted on TV by real or make-believe health professionals. So far, there are no herbs or supplements that have been shown to improve memory or slow or stop dementia. Companies and advertisers know that people will buy and try almost anything to help a care partner. Sometimes people buy these for their own use as well. Unfortunately, most supplements you see on TV or read about in popular magazines will not help people with serious medical and mental health conditions. What these supplements might do is interfere with each other and cause more symptoms or cause prescribed medication to be less effective. In the best case, they will do nothing and cost you money. Before purchasing any herbs or supplements, research them and ask your health care provider about them.

What is the cost of the new treatment?

Do you have the money to spend on this treatment? What are the other costs that do not involve money? Is your health strong enough to handle any side effects? Will the effects put a strain on your ability to function at home or at work? How long will you have to wait until you see the promised improvement? Will the cost put a strain on your monthly or annual budget? Some of the newer medications available today are very effective but very costly. If you think you cannot afford a medication, ask your health care provider or health insurance company for suggestions. Many pharmaceutical companies offer discounts or even take care of copayments. To take advantage of these offers, you must contact their patient or consumer services group. In the US, keep up to date on Medicare changes that have to do with drug coverage. These policies change frequently and previously unaffordable medications may now be much less expensive.

Learning More About Medications and Other Treatments

Where can you get more information about treatments to make good decisions about them? The internet can provide information about new treatments and be a resource for up-to-date information. But be cautious—especially when you are on sites that are selling products or services. Not every piece of information on the internet is correct or even safe. Seek out the most reliable sources. You can do this by noting the site's authors or sponsors and the site's internet address (also called its URL). Addresses ending in .edu, .org, and .gov are generally more objective (less biased) and reliable. These URLs are from universities, nonprofit organizations, and governmental agencies, respectively. They are not selling products. Some .com sites can also be good, but because they are maintained by commercial or for-profit organizations, the information on a .com site may be biased in favor of their own products.

Consulting Dr. Google

At one time or another, most of us have gone to Google or another search engine to look up symptoms or medication. There is very useful information on the internet. It was designed to give knowledge to the general public. But it is also full of misinformation. Many people use search engines to learn more about the treatments or medications that their providers prescribe. Unfortunately, what they read sometimes frightens them or they come away feeling that their provider did not do what was best for them. Here is an example. Eliana was prescribed a *short* course of steroids for a severely inflamed sinus. She googled steroids and found that there were many side effects with *long-term use* and then decided not to take the medication. Her sinus condition became worse and she needed to return to the doctor. Search engines give general information and do not take into account all the unique situations that go into prescribing for an individual. In fact, short-term use of steroids can help or even eliminate acute inflammation in different parts of the body with few or no side effects. Searching caused Eliana to make a poor decision which led to continued sinus problems.

Your health care provider has the advantage of knowing the specifics about you and also the different ways the same medication might be used. Consider aspirin. It can be used to relieve pain, reduce inflammation, prevent blood clots, and even keep flowers fresh. The amount of aspirin and the length of time it is used are different for each of these. So, if you are concerned about taking a medication after looking it up, call or message your provider or advice nurse and share your concerns. You can also ask a pharmacist. Then you can make an informed decision based on your needs and those of your care partner.

Reliable Sources of Medical Information

So, where can you find reliable sources of information? You can search the treatment or product using a search engine and asking for reviews. The following list provides some sites to explore. You can find updated URLs for these sites at www.bullpub.com/resources under the headings "Making Treatment Decisions" and "Medications, Herbs, Supplements & Other Treatments."

- **National Center for Complementary and Integrative Health** is a government agency providing research-based information from A to Z (acupuncture to zinc), including up-to-date, reliable information about chronic pain and complementary treatments.
- **MedlinePlus.gov** is an extensive online database of drugs, herbs, supplements, medical tests, and more from the National Library of Medicine.
- **NatMed** (requires subscription) is a comprehensive database that reviews clinical data on approximately 90,000 herbal products, dietary supplements, vitamins, minerals, homeopathic products, Ayurvedic (relating to Ayurveda, a traditional Hindu system of medicine) medicines, complementary alternative medicines, integrative therapies, alternative treatments such as acupuncture, traditional Chinese medicine products, and other natural remedies. It also provides an Interaction Checker that shows how natural products interact with prescription and over-the-counter medications.
- **ConsumerLab.com** (requires subscription) provides independent testing on over 1400 nutritional products.
- **Consumer Reports** reviews and evaluates both alternative and conventional treatments and products.

Canada regulates natural health products and maintains a natural health products webpage. The government of Canada also maintains the Licensed Natural Health Products Database (LNHPD). The database contains information about natural health products that have been issued a product license by Health Canada. It also includes information on vitamin and mineral supplements, herb- and plant-based remedies, traditional Chinese medicines, Ayurvedic medicines, homeopathic medicines, and many everyday consumer products.

It is not only alternative treatments that you need to look into before adopting. Just because something is commonly done doesn't mean it is always the best thing to do. Sometimes it is wise to say no to standard medical treatments. After reviewing the medical evidence, various medical specialty organizations have recommended that many common treatments should *not* be used. They also recommend tests and treatments you *should* have but may not be getting. To learn more about this, see www.Choosingwisely.org. Canada's equivalent is choosingwiselycanada.org.

For example, you may not need X-rays for back pain, antibiotics for sinus infections, whole-body scans for early detection of illness, CT scans for uncomplicated headaches, and so on. At the same time, there may be tests that are not being offered to you that are good options for you. For example, you might benefit from lung function tests for asthma or heart and kidney protective medications for diabetes. The US Preventive Services Task Force and the Canadian Task Force on Preventive Health Care provide evidence-based, critical reviews of various screening tests and medical treatments for both providers and consumers.

If your care partner has dementia or another progressive chronic condition, recommended preventive tests and treatments may be different. The goal in such situations may be to improve quality of life rather than to extend life. For example, having cataracts removed may be helpful to improve quality of life, while a colonoscopy to detect colon cancer may not be necessary.

Making decisions about new treatments for yourself or your care partner can be difficult. You don't have to research all options on your own. Review Chapter 7, Getting Help, for suggested resources and organizations in your community. A good self-manager uses the questions presented in this chapter and the decision-making steps in Chapter 2, Becoming a Better Caregiver: The Basics, to achieve the best results. If you ask yourself all these questions and decide to try a new treatment on your own, it is very important to inform your health care provider about it so they can advise you and safely monitor your progress.

Answering Health Care Providers Questions before Tests, Treatments, or Procedures

Unfortunately, two-way communication between patients/caregivers and doctors often does not happen. Studies show that fewer than 5 percent of patients getting new prescriptions ask any questions. Health care providers tend to think that if their patients are silent, it means they understand and will take the medications properly. Problems often result when patients do not get enough information about medications or do not understand how to take them. In addition, people often do not follow instructions. Safe, effective drug use depends equally on your provider's expertise and on your understanding of when and how to take the drug or give the drug to your care partner. You must ask questions to get the information you need. (See "Communicating with Members of Your Health Care Team" in Chapter 6, Communicating Effectively.)

Some people are afraid to ask questions of a health care provider. They are afraid that they will seem foolish or stupid or that the doctor will think they are difficult. Asking questions is a necessary part of a healthy provider-patient relationship. It is also a very important part of the caregiver role.

The goal of treatment is to get the most benefits with the fewest risks. This means taking the fewest medications, in the lowest effective doses, for the shortest period. (Note that some medications need to be taken for life.) Whether the medications for you or your care partner are helpful or harmful often depends on how much you know about the medications, how well you communicate with the providers, and if you or your care partner are taking the medications as directed.

Communication is key. You need to know the answers to these questions before each appointment so you can share the answers with your health care providers. Your health care provider needs to know the answer to the following questions even if they don't ask them.

What medications or supplements are you or your care partner taking?

Report to your or your care partner's health care provider (including the dentist) all the prescription and nonprescription medications you or your care partner are taking. Include vitamins, aspirin, antacids, laxatives, alcohol, supplements, and herbal remedies. An easy way to do this is to carry a list of all medications and the amounts you take (dosage). Many electronic medical records (EMRs) have a complete list of the medications that have been prescribed for each patient that you can download or copy. You can also ask a primary care provider for a list of all the medications they have in your electronic record. The patient record may include medications that you or your care partner are no longer taking. If it does, let the provider know. The important thing is that you and your health care teams have current, accurate information about what you and your care partner are taking. If you don't have a list and cannot put one together, gather together all the medications and take them to medical appointments. Saying that you or your care partner are taking "the little green pills" isn't very helpful.

If you or your care partner are seeing more than one health care provider, each one may not know what the others have prescribed. This is especially true if they are in different health care systems. Unless you know that all your providers use the same medical record, always bring a list of medications and supplements. It is necessary for correct diagnosis and treatment. For example, if your care partner has symptoms such as nausea or diarrhea, sleeplessness or drowsiness, dizziness or memory loss, or impotence or fatigue, it may be a drug side effect rather than a symptom of an illness or ailment. If your health care providers do not know all the medications, they cannot protect you and your care partner from drug interactions.

Have you or your care partner had allergic or unusual reactions to any medications?

Describe any symptoms or unusual reactions caused by medications, anesthetics, or X-ray contrast materials. Be specific: Describe the medication and the exact reaction. A rash, fever, or wheezing that develops after starting a medication may be a true allergic reaction. If any of these develop, call your health care provider at once. Symptoms such as nausea, diarrhea, ringing in the ears, light-headedness, sleeplessness, and frequent urination are likely to be side effects rather than true drug allergies.

What chronic illnesses and other medical conditions do you or your care partner have?

Some illnesses can make a drug less effective or increase the risks of side effects. The kidneys or liver can control how the body uses and breaks down a drug. The doctor may recommend avoiding certain medications if you or your care partner have ever had high blood pressure, peptic ulcer disease, asthma, heart disease, diabetes, or prostate problems. Be sure to let your doctor know if there is a history of bleeding or if you or your care partner are possibly pregnant or are breastfeeding. Many drugs are not safe in those situations.

What medications or treatments were tried in the past for this illness?

It is a good idea to keep your own records. What medications or treatments were used in the past and what were the effects? You can also usually find some of this information online in the electronic medical records (EMRs). But be sure to also keep a personal record of self-care, self-prescribed, over-the-counter, and alternative treatments, herbs, and supplements. Knowing what has been tried and how you or your care partner reacted informs the recommendation of any new medications or treatments. *Note that just because a medication did not work in the past does not necessarily mean that it can't be tried again.* Diseases change, and a medication that did not work the first time may work the second time.

Asking Questions before Tests, Treatments, Procedures, or New Medications

Ideally, you should ask the following questions before any test, treatment, or surgical procedure or before you or your care partner take a new medication. As time is often limited, you may only be able to ask these questions before more significant or risky interventions. Except for in extreme emergencies, when a health care provider orders something, this order is really just a recommendation for you. *You* make the final decisions.

Is this test, treatment, procedure, or medication really needed?

Some doctors prescribe medications or order tests not because the tests are necessary but because they think patients want and expect them to do so. Doctors often feel pressure to do *something* for the patient, so they prescribe a new drug. Don't pressure your doctor. Many new medications are heavily advertised. Some are later found to be so hazardous that they are withdrawn from the market. So, be cautious about requesting the newest medications. If your doctor doesn't prescribe a medication, consider that good news.

Instead of asking for new medications, ask about nondrug alternatives focusing on lifestyle changes, such as exercise, diet, and stress management. When any treatment is recommended, ask what may happen if you postpone treatment. Would your condition likely get worse or perhaps better with time? Sometimes the best medicine is *no medicine*. Sometimes the best option is taking a powerful medication early to avoid permanent damage or complications.

When it comes to medical tests, ask, "What happens if the result is not normal?" and "What happens if the result is normal?" If the answers are the same, then you or your care partner probably do not need the test. If the patient has already had a similar test or medication, gathering that information again can sometimes prevent unnecessary care and risk. If a test result is not normal, sometimes the follow-up test or treatment may not be something you want your care partner to undergo. In this case, there may not be a need for the test in the first place.

What are the risks and benefits of this test, treatment, procedure, or medication?

Each test, treatment, and procedure has a risk. Weighing the possible risks and benefits can be difficult, but it is very important. You and your care partner are the ones who will live with the results. Side effects and complications may range from minor, common, and reversible to major, rare, and permanent. Reading about all the possible side effects on patient information inserts can be scary. Talk with the doctor or pharmacist to help sort out the risks. *There are also risks associated with not taking a medication that is necessary and helpful.*

The doctor may prescribe several medications before finding the one that is best. You need to know what symptoms to look for in yourself or your care partner and what action to take if they develop. Should you seek immediate medical care, discontinue the medication, or call the doctor? Though the doctor cannot be expected to tell you every possible side effect, the most common and important ones should be discussed. Unfortunately, a recent survey showed that 70 percent of people starting a new medication did not recall being told by their physicians or pharmacists about precautions and possible side effects.

Medical tests carry a risk of inaccuracies or errors. A false positive result incorrectly says you are sick. A false negative result fails to identify you are sick. Such inaccuracies can lead to anxiety, delayed diagnosis, and further risky testing. However, sometimes repeating a test is necessary.

When it comes to surgery, the skill and experience of the surgeon and surgical team can make a significant difference in successful outcomes and risk of complications. While you do not always need the "best" surgeon, if possible, seek out a surgeon that has done the same surgery many times.

Being aware of and avoiding unnecessary risks is important, but there is another side to this story. Some tests, such as mammograms, vaginal exams, prostate exams, and colonoscopies (examination of the rectum and colon) are somewhat unpleasant and can be embarrassing. Some medications, such as chemotherapy, have side effects. However, these are not reasons to avoid these tests or medications. These tests, treatments, and medications can be lifesaving. As a self-manager and caregiver, you must weigh the risks and benefits. These can be different for you and your care partner. Health care providers are there to help.

What can I or my care partner expect from this test, treatment, procedure, or medication?

If you or your care partner are prescribed a new medication, you should know its name, how much to take, how you should take it, and for how long. You should also know some other facts. Is the medication intended to prolong life, completely or partially relieve symptoms, or help with better function? Some medications help prevent problems in the future and other medications treat acute problems today. For example, if your care partner is prescribed a medication for high blood pressure, the medication is usually given to prevent later complications, such as stroke or heart disease. On the other hand, if your health care provider recommends a pain reliever such as ibuprofen (or Motrin or Advil), the purpose is to help ease a headache.

You should also know how soon to expect results. Drugs that treat infections or inflammation may take several days to a week to show improvement. Antidepressant medications and some arthritis drugs typically take several weeks or even months to start providing relief.

Taking medication properly is vital. Yet nearly 40 percent of people report that their doctors failed to tell them how to take the medication or how much to take. If you are not sure about how to take the prescription medications you and your care partner have, contact your health care providers or pharmacist. Even if you get your drugs by mail order or online, you can still contact your local pharmacist with questions. For example, does "every 6 hours" mean every 6 hours while awake or every 6 hours around the clock? Should the medication be taken before meals, with meals, or between meals? What should you do if you accidentally miss a dose? Should you or your care partner skip the does entirely, take a double dose next time, or take the regular dose as soon as you remember? Should you refill and continue the medication until there are fewer symptoms or until the current medication is finished?

Some medications are prescribed on an as-needed (PRN) basis. Others need to be taken regularly. Having food in your stomach may help protect the stomach from irritation when taking some medications, but a full stomach can make other drugs ineffective. Some medications might make the patient more sensitive to the sun, putting them at increased risk for sunburn. Ask whether the medication prescribed will interfere with driving safely. Other drugs, even over-the-counter drugs, and alcohol can amplify or lessen the effects of the prescribed medication. Taking aspirin along with an anticoagulant medication, for example, can possibly result in bleeding. Some medications need lab tests to check for side effects. If you or your care partner are taking one of these medications, work with your doctor to make sure you are getting the necessary lab tests.

If a surgical procedure is recommended, it is important that you discuss the options for anesthesia and how to prepare for the operation. For example, should the patient continue taking medications? Stop eating and drinking? When? Can the patient drive to the procedure? Discuss how long recovery is likely to take and when the surgical patient can resume normal activities. After surgery, patients are sometimes given medications to relieve pain, but also ask about some of the nondrug stress management tools discussed in in Chapter 5, Using Your Mind to Manage Stress.

How much does this test, treatment, procedure, or medication cost?

Ask for an estimate in advance of the cost for tests, procedures, and medications. Ask if there are less expensive tests, treatments, or procedures that your insurance may cover. Is there a less expensive alternative or generic medication?

When a drug company develops a new drug in the United States, it is granted exclusive rights to produce that drug for 17 years. In Canada, patent terms are currently 20 years. After this 17-year period, other companies may market chemically identical versions of that brand-name drug, referred to as generic versions. Every drug has at least two names: a generic name and a brand name. The generic name is the medication's scientific name. The brand name is the name given to the drug by its developer. Generic medications are generally considered as safe and effective as the original brand-name drug but often cost much less. In rare cases, your health care provider may have a special reason for preferring a brand name instead of a generic version. Even so, if cost is a concern, ask your provider if a less expensive but equally effective medication is available.

You may also be able to save money by knowing how to best use your insurance. For example, your copayment may be less if you get your medications from a company designated by your insurer or if you order refills online and receive them by mail. Also, many national pharmacies have discount programs for seniors and individuals with low income. It pays to ask and then ask again. And it is wise to shop around. Even in the same town, different stores sell the same medication at different prices. Big box stores with pharmacies often offer lower price options.

Buying medications online is an option for saving money on prescriptions. You can safely buy medication online if you use online pharmacies recommended by the National Association of Boards of Pharmacy. This organization verifies internet drugstores throughout the United States and most Canadian provinces. You can visit the National Association of Boards of Pharmacy website (https://safe.pharmacy/buy-safely/) to find out which online drugstores are recommended and which aren't.

Don't trust an online drugstore if:

- The website doesn't ask you for a prescription.
- The drugstore isn't a licensed pharmacy. In the US and Canada, pharmacies are licensed by state or provincial governments.
- The online drugstore doesn't have a licensed pharmacist available to answer your questions.
- The website isn't secure. This means that any information you type in—your address, your credit card number—could be used by anyone who comes across it. See the box below

Prescription drugs are painfully expensive in the US. People in the US pay up to 10 times more for prescription drugs compared to residents of other countries of similar size and wealth. To save money on out-of-pocket drug costs, some people choose to order medications online through companies in foreign countries.

Medication that you buy online from sources that are not regulated can be either too strong or

How to Tell If a Website Is Secure

- Look at the URL (address line). It should start with "https." The "s" stands for secure. If it is missing, be careful.
- In the same line, look for a padlock icon. This indicates a secure site, but only in some browsers.
- Check for spelling and typos in the URL. For example, "Amazon" may be "Anozon," or "Creek" may be "Creak."

too weak or even fake. Fake medication can be expertly packaged. They look like the real thing, but they may contain ingredients like chalk, sugar, and flour instead of the medication you need. In the worst cases, a fake pill may contain drugs or chemicals that could be harmful.

Under the Canada Health Act, prescription drugs administered in Canadian hospitals are provided at no cost to the patient. Outside of the hospital setting, provincial and territorial governments are responsible for the administration of their own publicly funded drug plans. The public drug plans determine what prescription drugs are listed and under what conditions for eligible recipients. Most Canadians have some access to insurance coverage for prescription drugs through a patchwork of public and private insurance plans. The federal, provincial, and territorial governments offer varying levels of coverage and decide who is covered and what each plan pays. The publicly funded drug programs generally provide drug plan coverage for those most in need based on age, income, and medical condition. Many Canadians and their family members have drug coverage linked to employment, and some Canadians may have no effective drug coverage and pay the full cost of prescription drugs.

Where can I find written or online information about the test, treatment, procedure, or medication?

Your health care provider may not have time to answer all your questions. You may not remember everything you heard. Fortunately, there are many other good sources of information. Your pharmacist is an expert on medications and can answer questions in person, over the phone, via email, or through a secure web portal. In addition, many hospitals, medical schools, and schools of pharmacy have medication information services that you can call to ask questions. As a self-manager, you can also consult nurses, package inserts, pamphlets, books, and websites. Review Chapter 7, Getting Help, and for a complete list of suggested further readings, useful websites, and other helpful resources, please see www.bullpub.com/resources under the topic heading "Medications, Herbs, Supplements & Other Treatments."

Managing Medications

Whether you are taking medications for yourself or giving them to your care partner, understanding how to manage medications is an important job. Working closely with your doctor and your care partner's medical team is critical for the safe and effective use of medications. The suggestions offered in this chapter can be useful in managing your medications as well as the medications you are giving to your care partner.

Understanding Medications

Medications are heavily advertised. These ads are aimed at making you believe that if you just use this pill, your symptoms will be cured, and life will be better. It seems like there is a pill for every ill.

But your body is often its own healer, and given time, many common symptoms and conditions will improve. The prescriptions filled by the body's own "internal pharmacy" are frequently the safest and most effective treatments. Patience, careful self-observation, and monitoring are often excellent choices.

It is also true that medications can be a very important part of managing a chronic illness. Although most medications do not cure chronic illnesses, they can:

- **Relieve symptoms.** For example, an inhaler delivers medications that help expand the bronchial tubes and make it easier to breathe. A nitroglycerin tablet expands the blood vessels to relieve chest pain. Acetaminophen (or Tylenol) may relieve pain.
- **Prevent further problems.** For example, medications that thin the blood help prevent blood clots, which cause strokes and heart and lung problems.
- **Improve or slow the progress of the disease.** For example, nonsteroidal anti-inflammatory drugs can quiet the inflammatory process of arthritis. Antihypertensive medications can lower blood pressure. Sometimes even if medications do not stop symptoms, they slow the underlying condition or illness.
- **Replace substances that the body is no longer producing adequately.** This is why people with diabetes take insulin and why thyroid medication is prescribed for underactive thyroid.

As these examples show, most medications for chronic conditions lessen the consequences of illness or slow the disease. When you take medications like these, you may not feel anything. You may think that the drug isn't working. But the medication may be preventing complications or keeping you from getting worse. For this reason, it is important to continue taking your medications and discuss medication use with your doctor when you have questions.

Medications can be very helpful. But humans pay a price for having such powerful tools. Besides being helpful, all medications have undesirable side effects. Some of these effects are predictable and minor, and some are unexpected and life threatening. As many as 5 to 10 percent of all hospital admissions are due to drug reactions. Even herbs and supplements can cause harm. Each year, many thousands of people die from overdoses of prescription opioids and other prescription drugs. At the same time, *not taking medications as prescribed* can be dangerous. Consider the drugs for high blood pressure. Not taking them as prescribed can be a major cause of stroke, heart attacks, and hospitalization.

Using Mind Power: Expecting the Best

Medication affects the body in two ways. The first is determined by the chemical nature of the medication. The second is triggered by your beliefs and expectations. Your beliefs can change your body chemistry and your symptoms. Your beliefs can enhance how *any* medication or treatment works. You may have heard of placebos. A placebo is a treatment or substance that looks real but has no active ingredient meant to affect health. The placebo effect refers to what happens when people take so-called "sugar pills" and their symptoms improve. This effect is an example of how closely the mind and body are connected.

Many studies have shown the power of the placebo—the power of mind over body. When people are given a placebo, some of them improve anyway. Every time you take a medication, you are swallowing your expectations and beliefs as well as the pill. You can learn to take advantage of your powerful internal pharmacy along with taking medications. *Expect the best!*
Consider the following ways to do that:

- **Examine your beliefs about the treatment.** If you tell yourself, "I'm not a pill taker," or "Medications always give me bad side effects," how do you think your body is likely to respond? If you don't think the prescribed treatment is likely to help your symptoms or condition, your negative beliefs will undermine the ability of the pill to help you. You can change these negative images into more positive ones. (Review the discussion of positive [helpful] thinking and self-talk in Chapter 5, Using Your Mind to Manage Stress.)
- **Think of your medications the way you think of vitamins.** Many people associate healthful images with vitamins—more so than with medications. Taking a vitamin may make you think that you are doing something positive to prevent disease and promote health. If you regard your medications as health restoring and health promoting, like vitamins, you may get more benefits.
- **Imagine how the medication is helping you.** Develop a mental image of how the medication is doing its job inside of you. For example, think of taking thyroid hormone replacement as filling a missing link in your body's chemical chains to help balance and regulate your metabolism. Or think of an antibiotic as a broom sweeping germs out of your body. For some people, forming such a vivid mental image is helpful. Don't worry if your image of what's happening chemically inside of you is not medically accurate. Your belief in a clear, positive image is what counts.
- **Keep in mind why you are taking the medication.** You are not taking your medication just because your health care provider told you to. You are taking your medication to help you live your life and manage your health. It is important to understand and remind yourself how the medication is helping you. You can use this information to help the medication do its job. For example, suppose a woman with cancer is given chemotherapy. She has been told that it will make her feel like she has the flu, she will vomit, and her hair will fall out. This knowledge may worsen her side effects. But suppose she is also told that the symptoms will last only a few days and that her hair falling out is a good sign because it means that cells that grow fast (cancer cells and hair cells) are being destroyed. Her hair will recover but not the cancer cells. *The presence of side effects can sometimes be a positive signal that the medication is working.*
- **Present the positive.** Your positive (or negative) attitude about medication can be contagious! As a caregiver you have a lot of influence with your care partner. Even

if your care partner has major cognitive (thinking) problems, your feelings about medication sway the way your care partner acts when given medications. If you are positive and calmly persistent, your care partner might be more likely to take the medication.

Taking Multiple Medications

People with several conditions often take many medications. For example, a person may take a medication for dementia, a medication to lower blood pressure, an anti-inflammatory drug for arthritis, a pill for angina, a bronchodilator for asthma, an antacid for heartburn, plus a handful of over-the-counter remedies and herbs. The more medications you and your care partner are taking, the greater the risk of side effects. Not all drugs play well together. When they are taken together, they sometimes cause problems. Fortunately, it is often possible to take fewer medications and lower the risks. However, you should not change the medications you take without the help of your doctor. Most people would not change the ingredients in a recipe or throw out a few parts when fixing a car. If you want the best and safest results, you need expert help.

How you and your care partner respond to any medication depends on age, daily activity, the ups and downs of symptoms, chronic conditions, genetics, and frame of mind. To get the most from medications, your doctor depends on you. You have to observe yourself and your care partner closely to determine these. Report what effect, if any, the drugs you or your care partner take have on symptoms and any side effects. Based on this information, medication may be continued, increased, discontinued, or otherwise changed. In a good provider-patient partnership, continuing information flows in *both* directions.

Taking Medications

A medication doesn't work if you don't take it! Yet nearly half of all medications are not taken as prescribed. Some people refer to this as "the other drug problem." There are many reasons why people don't take their prescribed medication: forgetfulness, lack of clear instructions, complicated dosing schedules, side effects, and cost. Whatever the reason, if you or your care partner are having trouble taking medications as prescribed, discuss this issue with your health care provider. Often simple changes can make it easier. For example, if you or your care partner are taking many different medications, sometimes one or more can be stopped. If one medication needs to be taken three times a day and another four times a day, the doctor may be able to prescribe medications that only need to be taken once or twice a day.

If you or your care partner are having trouble taking your medications, read the following questions and discuss the answers that concern you with your doctor or pharmacist.

- Do you tend to be forgetful?
- Are you confused about the instructions for how and when to use the medications?

- Is the schedule for taking medications too complicated?
- Do the medications have bothersome side effects?
- Is the medication too expensive?
- Do you feel that the condition or disease is not serious enough to need regular medications? (With some diseases such as high blood pressure, high cholesterol, or early diabetes, there may not be any symptoms.)
- Do you feel that the treatment is unlikely to help?
- Are you denying that you or your care partner has a condition or disease that needs treatment?
- Have you had a bad experience with the medicine or another medication?
- Do you know someone who had a bad experience with the medication, and are you afraid that something similar will happen to you or your care partner?
- Are you afraid of the medication's effects or that you or your partner will become addicted to it?
- Are you embarrassed about taking the medication? Do you view taking it as a sign of weakness or failure, or do you fear you'll be judged negatively if people know about it?
- Do you need to review the benefits of the medication when taken as prescribed?

Reading Prescription Labels

Prescription labels can be a great source of information. They list patient name, dose, appearance, how to take the medication, precautions, and more. Figure 12.1 gives tips on how to read the labels on your prescriptions.

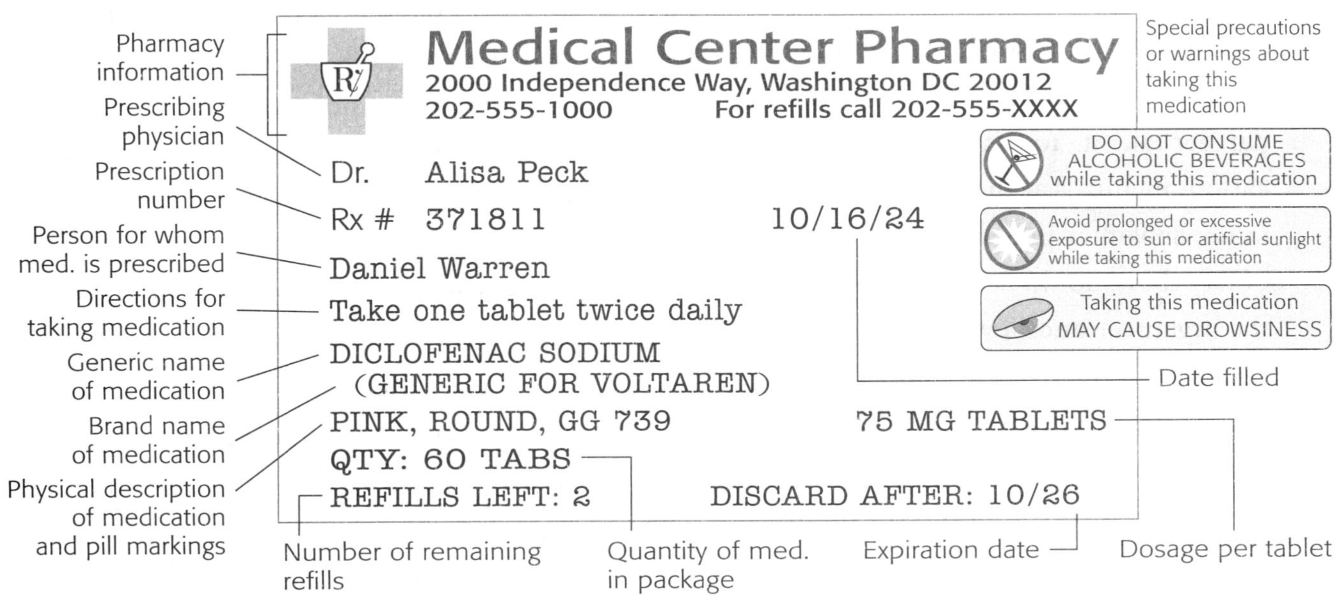

Figure 12.1 **How to Read a Prescription Label**

Remembering to Take Medications

If forgetting to take medications is a problem in your household, here are some suggestions to help:

- **Make it obvious.** Place the medication or a reminder next to your toothbrushes, on the breakfast table, in a lunch box, or some other place where you're likely to notice or stumble over it. Be careful where you put the medication if children are around. Or put a reminder note on the bathroom mirror, toothbrush, refrigerator door, coffee maker, television, or some other obvious place. If you link taking the medication or giving it to your care partner with some well-established habit such as mealtimes, brushing your teeth, or watching a television show, you'll be more likely to remember.
- **Use a checklist or an organizer.** Make a medication chart listing each medication you and your care partner are taking and the time when you take it. Check off each medication on a calendar as you or your care partner take it. You might also buy a medication organizer at the drugstore. This container separates pills according to the time of day they should be taken. You can fill the organizer once a week so that all your pills or your care partner's pills are ready to take at the proper time. A quick glance at the organizer lets you know if anyone has missed any doses and prevents double dosing. You and your care partner should have clearly labeled organizers that are different colors so that there is less chance of mixing them up. Some pharmacy services are now able to sort and prepackage medications for each day in blister packs. Each packet has the date, time, and description of the medications and nutritional supplements. Ask your pharmacist about this option. There are also websites and apps that have charts you can print to help you track your medications.
- **Use an electronic reminder.** Get a watch or cell phone that you can set to beep at pill-taking time. There are also electronic medication containers that beep at preset times. If you have a smartphone, you can download apps that remind you when you or your care partner need to take medication.
- **Have others remind you.** Ask members of your household to remind you to take your medications or give medications to your care partner at the right times.
- **Don't run out.** Don't let yourself run out of medication. When you get prescriptions filled, add a reminder to your calendar on the date one week before the medications will run out or 2 weeks if you get your medications by mail. This will remind you to get your next refill. Don't wait until the last pill is taken to order more. Most mail-order pharmacies offer automatic refills so medications arrive when you need them.
- **Plan before you travel.** If you plan to travel, put a note on your luggage reminding you to pack medications for you and your care partner. Always pack them in carry-on luggage. Don't put medications in checked

bags. Also, bring a copy of prescriptions in your carry-on bag in case you lose medications. You might even pack two sets of medications and keep them in different pieces of luggage in case one set gets lost or left behind.

Getting Your Care Partner to Take Medications

Sometimes it is difficult to get care partners to take medication. The following are some tips to try:

- Your care partner might resist taking the medication because of side effects such as nausea. Your care partner may not be able to tell you this, so look for signs of side effects. If you think you are noticing side effects, talk to the doctor about options.
- Your care partner might want to take more control. Put the pill and glass of water near your partner, but let them take their own medication. Help only as needed.
- If pills are hard for your care partner to swallow, ask about liquid medication or if pills can be crushed. Not all pills are crushable and some may be dangerous if you do crush them. Sometimes pills and liquid medications can be hidden in or combined with foods or beverages.
- Ask a health care provider if the medication is really necessary.
- Be a good role model and take your pills at the same time as your care partner.
- Use short sentences. Do not explain or reason. Stay calm and try again in 15 or 20 minutes.
- Find the best time of day (as long as medications do not have to be given at certain times). Care partners with Alzheimer's often are more cooperative in the morning than in the afternoon or evening.
- Try to stick to a daily routine, but be flexible if needed.
- Reward good behavior. Try giving a treat once the medications are taken.

Using Medications Safely

Whether you or your care partner are taking prescribed medications or using over-the-counter medications or herbs, here are some helpful suggestions:

- **Never take a drug from an unlabeled container or a container that has a label you cannot read.** Keep medications in their original labeled containers or transfer them to a labeled medication organizer or pill dispenser. Do not mix different medications in the same bottle. Mistakes also occur when people try to take medicines in the dark and pick up the wrong medication. Turn on the light!

- **Do not take medications yourself or give medications to your care partner that were prescribed for someone else,** even if you have similar symptoms.
- **Do not share medications.** The largest source of prescription opioid misuse is drugs that are borrowed or stolen from family or friends.
- **Make sure you or your care partner drink at least a half glass of liquid with pills and** remain standing or sitting upright for a short while after swallowing. This can prevent the pills from getting stuck.
- **Store medications where children or young adults cannot find them.** Poisoning from medications is a common and preventable problem. The main sources of recreational drugs used by teens and young adults are the prescription medications of relatives or the relatives of friends. Despite its name, the bathroom medicine cabinet is not usually an appropriate place to store medications. A locked kitchen cabinet or toolbox with a lock is far safer.

Medications and other treatments can help or harm. What makes the difference is your knowledge about medications and treatment, the care you take when using medications, and clear two-way communication with your health care team about medications and treatment for you and your care partner.

Using Alcohol and Recreational Drugs

The use of alcohol and recreational drugs (illegal or prescription medications used for nonmedicinal purposes) has increased in recent years, particularly among people over the age of 60. These drugs, whether legal or illegal, can cause problems. Alcohol and recreational drugs can interact with both prescription and over-the-counter medications, making them less effective or even causing harm. They can also fog judgment and cause problems with balance. This can, in turn, cause accidents and result in injury to you and others. In some cases, alcohol or recreational drugs can make existing long-term conditions worse. Alcohol use is associated with higher risk of hypertension, diabetes, gastrointestinal bleeding, sleep disorders, depression, erectile dysfunction, breast and other cancers, and injury.

If you or your care partner are drinking an at-risk amount of alcohol or are regularly using recreational drugs, consider reducing or stopping. Talk to your doctor or other health care provider about use of these drugs. Doctors are often hesitant to raise the issue because they don't want to embarrass you. So, it is up to you to bring up the subject. Doctors will be very willing to talk about it. They have heard it all, and they will not think less of you or your care partner. An honest conversation may save your life or your care partner's life.

Limiting Alcohol

At-risk alcohol use for women is drinking more than seven drinks per week or more than three drinks per day. For men, at-risk alcohol use is drinking more than 14 drinks per week or more than four drinks in a day. Women of any age and anyone over age 65 should average no more than one drink per day, and men under 65 should have no more than two drinks per day on average. Canada's Guidance on Alcohol and Health states that research shows that no amount or kind of alcohol is good for your health. It doesn't matter what kind of alcohol it is—wine, beer, cider, or spirits. Drinking alcohol, even a small amount, is damaging to everyone, regardless of age, sex, gender, ethnicity, tolerance for alcohol, or lifestyle. That's why if you drink, it's better to drink less. If you are going to drink, don't exceed two drinks on any day.

One alcoholic drink equivalent contains 0.6 fluid ounces (17 g) of pure alcohol, which is equivalent to 12 fluid ounces (355 mL) of regular beer (5 percent alcohol), 5 fluid ounces (148 mL) of wine (12 percent alcohol), or 1.5 fluid ounces (44 mL) of 80 proof distilled spirits (40 percent alcohol). Note that these guidelines may change with new evidence.

Avoiding alcohol altogether may be best depending upon the medical conditions and history of you and your care partner. It is also important how you react to alcohol.

Using Medical Marijuana

Some US state governments have approved the use of marijuana (also known as cannabis or pot) for medical use. The US federal government continues to classify marijuana as a Schedule I controlled substance. This technically makes it illegal to possess and limits medical research into the potential benefits of cannabis.

Many people believe that cannabis will lessen their pain. They may also believe that cannabis will reduce their reliance on opioids. Some people may believe both. The current evidence on how cannabis affects pain and opioid use is uncertain. A recent large review of studies found there are few, if any, studies on cannabis use that meet the standards for good research. The good news is that researchers are beginning to conduct high-quality studies and should have the answers in a few years.

Research is also progressing on isolating the individual compounds in cannabis. For example, you may have heard of cannabidiol (CBD), which is one of the individual compounds found in cannabis. Products such as CBD oils, topical pain-relief treatments, edibles, and other nonsmoking applications are now available. When isolated, some of these compounds may be found to be valid medical treatment options that do not produce the high that the compound commonly known as THC produces.

Some evidence suggests there are benefits of cannabis use for nausea and vomiting associated with cancer chemotherapy. Cannabis may also help with muscle spasms in multiple sclerosis, epilepsy symptoms, appetite stimulation, anxiety and stress reduction, and possibly the management of certain types of chronic pain. Some experts are concerned about negative effects of marijuana on memory and mental ability, increased incidence of accidents, and damage to the lungs from smoking it. Before using cannabis products in any form, have a thorough discussion with your health care provider.

Since 2001, medical cannabis has been a legal treatment option in Canada for certain health conditions. Medical cannabis is not a Health Canada-approved treatment. Talk to your health care provider about the benefits and risks of using medical cannabis. They can help you decide if medical cannabis is an option. Your health care provider will give you instructions on what type of medical cannabis to try, how much to use, how to take it, and how often to take it. In Canada, it is a good idea to become a registered user for medical cannabis to make sure you get the right dosage, you are protected as an employee, the cannabis can be claimed as a medical expense, and that you are purchasing products that are government regulated for safety and consistency standards. If you registered with Health Canada, you can grow your own cannabis for medical purposes or designate someone to do this for you. If you have side effects or think you have a problem with cannabis use, contact your health provider.

For a complete list of suggested further readings, useful websites, and other helpful resources, please see: www.bullpub.com/resources.

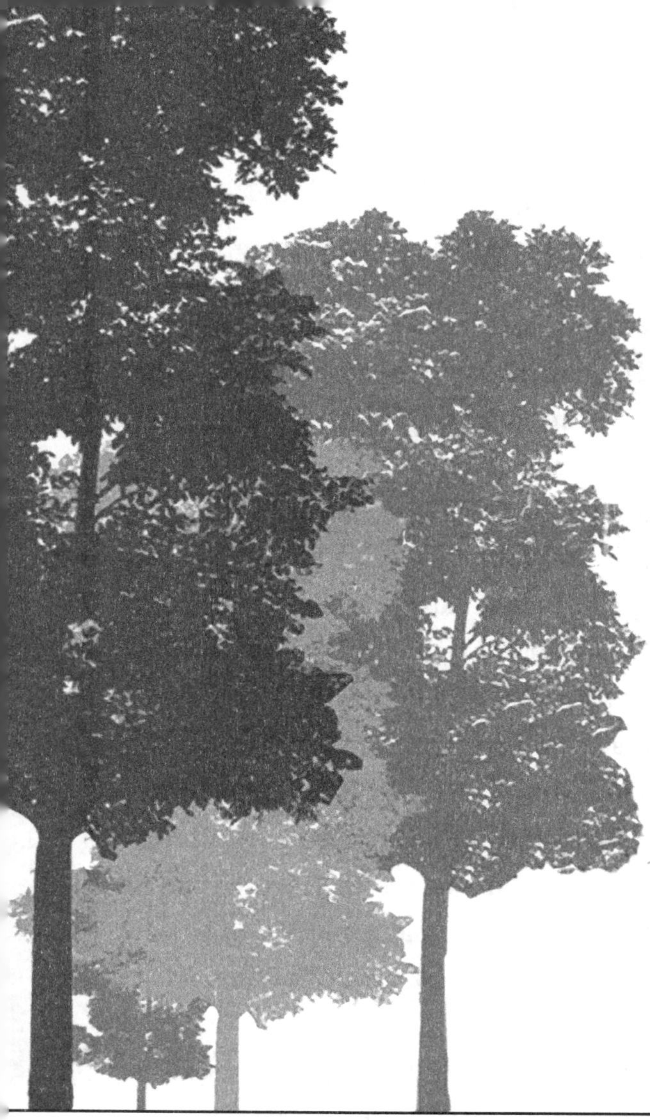

Chapter 13

Planning for the Future: Fears and Reality

Caregivers often worry about what will happen next. In fact, as a caregiver, you have double the worries. What will happen to your care partner over time and what will happen if you can no longer be a caregiver? One way to deal with these fears about the future is to take control and plan. You may never need to put the plans into effect, but there is reassurance in knowing that you have plans in place if the events you fear come to pass. Because of the special relationship between caregivers and care partners, you may be responsible for both planning your own future and your care partner's future at the same time. Although the future can involve difficult events and topics to discuss and plan for, you are in a unique position. You are likely best suited to help your care partner better prepare for the future. This chapter examines the most common concerns people have about the future and offers some suggestions.

What If I Can't Take Care of Myself or My Care Partner Anymore?

Regardless of how healthy they are, most people fear becoming helpless and dependent. This fear is even greater among caregivers. Caregivers not only need to make choices for their own future care but also for their care partner. Their fears involve the management not only of physical challenges, but also of financial, social, and emotional ones.

Addressing Physical Day-to-Day Living Needs

As your own health condition changes, you may need to consider changing how and where you and your care partner live. This could involve hiring someone to help you in your home or moving to a place where more help is provided. How you make this decision depends on your needs and how they can best be met. Most people think only about their physical needs, but we also have social and emotional needs. It is best to consider these as well.

Start by evaluating what you can do for yourself and for your care partner. In this book, we are most concerned about you and your health as the caregiver. What caregiving tasks are a problem for you and affecting your own health? Which of your own activities of daily living (ADLs) will you need help with? ADLs are everyday tasks including getting out of bed, bathing, dressing, preparing and eating meals, cleaning house, shopping, and paying bills. Most people can do these things, even though they may have to do them slowly with some adjustments or with some help from assistive devices. However, when you are responsible for doing these things for your care partner as well as yourself, you need to evaluate which of these tasks you can continue to do, and which may be too difficult for you.

Some people eventually find that they can no longer do one or more of these tasks without help. For example, you might still be able to fix meals but are no longer able to do the shopping. Or if you have problems with balance and coordination or mobility, or have bouts of dizziness, you might need someone around all the time to help. You may also find that some activities you enjoyed in the past, such as gardening, are no longer pleasurable.

Use the problem-solving steps discussed in Chapter 2, Becoming a Better Caregiver: The Basics, to evaluate and make a list of the potential problems. (This is Step 1: Identify the problem. Review the problem-solving steps on page 12.) Once you have this list, you can solve the problems one at a time. Begin by first writing down every possible solution you can think of. (This is Step 2: List ideas to solve the problem.) These examples are problems followed by possible solutions:

Can't go shopping.

- Find a volunteer shopping service.
- Shop at a store that delivers.
- Ask another family member to shop for me.

- Ask a neighbor to shop for me.
- Shop on the internet and have groceries delivered to me.
- Get home-delivered meals or meal kits.

Can't be by myself or can't leave my care partner alone.

- Hire in-home care.
- Move in with a relative.
- Get a Lifeline Emergency Response system.
- Move to a skilled nursing or assisted-living facility.

When you have listed your problems and the possible solutions, choose one solution to try that seems the most workable, acceptable, and within your financial means. (This is Step 3 of problem solving: Choose an idea to try.) Your choice will depend on financial, family, and other resources available, as well as on how well you think each potential solution will solve your problem.

Sometimes a single solution might be the answer to several problems. For instance, if you can't shop and can't be alone, and housekeeping chores require help, you might consider a retirement community that offers meals, regular housecleaning, and transportation for errands and medical appointments. Even if you are not of retirement age, some facilities accept younger people. Some facilities for the retired people accept residents who are 50 or younger. If you are a younger person, the local center for people with disabilities or independent living center may be able to direct you to an out-of-home care facility.

When looking for a retirement community, consider the levels of care offered. These usually include:

- **Independent living**, where you have your own apartment or small house.
- **Assisted living**, where you get some help with daily living activities, such as with taking medications, chores, and errands.
- **Skilled nursing**, which includes help with daily activities and some medical care.

  Often there is also a specialized memory care unit.

As you begin to make changes in your life and that of your care partner, go slowly, one step at a time. You don't need to change your whole life to solve one problem. Remember that you can always change your mind. Be careful not to make major changes in your lives that you cannot reverse. For example, if you are thinking of moving out of your own place to another location (a relative's, an assisted-living home, or elsewhere) don't give up your present home until you and your care partner are sure you want to stay in your new home. Here we would like to mention that the solution might not be the same for you and your care partner. For example, it may be that you go to live with a relative and your care partner goes to live in a nearby skilled-nursing facility or assisted-living facility.

If you think you need help, hiring someone to help you at home might be a less drastic solution than moving. Or, if your care partner can't be alone and you have no other family or friends who could stay with your care partner when you need to be away, you might also look into finding an adult or senior day care center to keep your care partner safe, comfortable, and maybe entertained while you run your errands or take a respite.

Reaching out to Family for Help

When you know you cannot do something yourself, consider reaching out to family and friends. Sometimes, people fear rejection, so they never ask for help. Other people try to hide their need for fear their loved ones will withdraw from them. Families often complain, "If we'd only known . . ." when they find out that a family member or friend has needs that were unmet. Just as you can feel scared and embarrassed of becoming physically dependent, you may also be fearful of being abandoned by family members. Tales of being dumped in a nursing home by children who never come to visit haunt many people. They worry that this may happen to them. Your care partner might have these same fears. A more common situation is that people who you thought would help don't help. Sometimes this is because they don't know how. Don't expect that people should know what to do. Often, they do not and they too are overwhelmed by the situation. Remember from Chapter 6, Communicating Effectively, that you cannot change how others communicate, but you can change how you communicate to be sure you are better understood.

When talking with family members or friends, be as open and reasonable as possible. At the same time, try to make them understand that you are the one who decides to accept or not accept help. To gain their cooperation, use "I" messages. For example, "Yes, I do need some help with , but I still want to do myself." There is more information about communicating with "I" messages and tips on asking for help in Chapter 6, Communicating Effectively, and Chapter 7, Getting Help.

Asking for help does not mean giving up your right to choose and decide about issues relating to you and your care partner's lives. Insist on being asked about all the important decisions that affect both you and your care partner. Early on, lay the ground rules with your advisors. Ask to be presented with options when it is time to make choices about what is best for you and your care partner. Try hard to weigh good suggestions, and do not dismiss every option that isn't your own idea. If you learn to be a good decision maker, people will see that you can make reasonable decisions and will continue to give you the opportunity to do so.

Be appreciative. Recognize the goodwill and efforts of people who want to help you and your care partner. Even when you need help, you maintain your dignity by gracefully accepting help. Getting assistance might feel embarrassing, but in the long run, getting help can allow you to maintain independence. If you believe that you are being offered help that you don't need, decline it with tact and appreciation. For example, "I appreciate your offer to have Thanksgiving at your house, but I'd like to continue having it here. I could really use some help though. I would like to roast the turkey, but could the rest of you bring the other food and clean up after dinner?"

If you are unable to come to terms with your increasing needs for help from others, talk with a professional counselor. Find a counselor who has experience with the emotional and social issues of people with disabling health problems and the challenges of caregiving. Your local agency providing services to caregivers, seniors, or the disabled can refer you to the right kind of counselor. The Area Agency on Aging or online resources, such as the Canadian Seniors Directory, may also provide referrals.

Getting Professional Help with Decision Making

If you cannot turn to close family or friends because they are unable or unwilling to become involved, turn to helpful agencies. It may help to discuss your wishes, abilities, and limitations with a trusted friend or professional. Sometimes another person can identify things you have overlooked or would like to ignore. Seeking ideas from others and using other resources are important parts of becoming better caregivers. (This is Step 6: Use other resources.)

Case managers can make it easier to get help. They assess your needs and then work with you to organize community services to meet those needs. There are at least two situations where case managers might be helpful: when you cannot rely on family or friends for help or when you are trying to help someone who refuses help. You can find case managers through your local social services department's adult protective services program or Family Services Association. Religious service organizations, such as Jewish Family Services or Catholic Charities, also have case managers. In Canada, publicly subsidized home and community care is available through the provincial/territorial governments. The social services department in your local hospital can also put you in touch with the right agency.

Organizations serving people with a specific health condition can also direct you to support groups and classes. (In the United States, these include organizations such as the Alzheimer's Association, Parkinson's Association, American Cancer Society, American Lung Association, American Heart Association, and American Diabetes Association.) In addition, Veterans Affairs (VA) can also direct you to support groups and classes. You can locate the agency you need through the internet.

In Canada, organizations include Alzheimer Society Canada, Parkinson Canada, the Canadian Cancer Society, Canadian Lung Association, Heart and Stroke Foundation of Canada, and Diabetes Canada.

A social worker at your local senior center, center for people with disabilities, or hospital social services department can help by providing information about resources in your community. This person can also give you some ideas about how to deal with your partner's care needs. There are several kinds of professionals who can help.

Social workers are good for helping you decide how to solve financial and living arrangement problems and to locate appropriate community resources. Some social workers are also trained in counseling people with disabilities and the elderly. They can help you deal with emotional and relationship problems that could be associated with the health problems of you and/or your care partner.

Another helpful professional is an occupational therapist (OT). An occupational therapist can assess the daily needs of both you and your care partner. If needed, they can suggest assistive devices or changes to make your home life easier. (Chapter 8, Preventing Injuries, also has ideas for you to look at about these kinds of things.) OTs can also help you find ways to keep doing the activities you and your care partner enjoy.

If you or your care partner have been hospitalized, you can use the hospital's resource center for help. Most hospitals have a discharge planner on staff. This person—usually a nurse or social worker—will see you or your care partner before you go home and check that you and/or family members know what to do and how to do it. If necessary, they will help find resources so that when you leave the hospital you and/or your care partner are safe and continue to heal. It is very important that you are honest with this person. If you have concerns about your ability to care for your care partner or yourself, say so. Solutions are usually available. However, the planner can help only if you share your concerns. Many hospitals also have chaplains who can be helpful. They might know about resources within your own religious or spiritual community.

Financial planners and attorneys are also very useful resources. Financial planners not only provide advice about investing and managing your money, they also can help you plan for your retirement and discuss your options, including the need for types of insurance such as disability or long-term care. If you use a financial planner, be sure that their compensation is not tied to investing your money. Look for certified financial planners, who are formally recognized as experts in their field.

Attorneys, especially those specializing in elder law, should be on your list of resources. They can help you set your financial affairs in order. Attorneys can help you protect your assets, prepare a proper will, and execute a durable power of attorney (DPA) for both health care and financial management. (A general durable power of attorney deals with financial matters, while a durable power of attorney for health care, which is discussed on pages 264 and 266-272, is for health care decisions only.)

To find an attorney, you can contact your local bar association. They can provide you with a list of attorneys experienced in this area. These attorneys are generally familiar with the laws applying to younger persons with disabilities as well. If you are living with a disability, even if you are not a senior, your legal needs are much the same as those of the older person. If budget is a concern, ask your local senior center for the names of attorneys and financial advisers who offer free or low-cost services to seniors. AARP (formerly known as the American Association of Retired Persons) and CARP (formerly known as the Canadian Association for Retired Persons) are other important resources for finding this advice. The sooner you can plan for these in the present, the better prepared and more in control you will feel about the future.

Will I Have Enough Money to Pay for Care?

Many people are scared of not having enough money to pay for their own and their care partner's needs. Managing chronic health problems often requires expensive care and treatment. If you are not able to work due to your own illness or disability or because you are a full-time caregiver, the loss of income, and especially the loss of your health insurance coverage, might present an overwhelming financial problem. You can, however, avoid some of these risks by planning and knowing your resources.

In the United States, health insurance and Medicare may meet only a part of your care costs. The days of covered skilled nursing, if needed, are limited. Medicare does not cover everything, and most private "Medigap" insurance policies only pick up the 20 percent out-of-pocket expenses that Medicare does not cover. Medigap plans usually do not cover any procedure or treatment that is not also covered by Medicare. However, some Medigap plans may pay for certain health services outside the United States that are not otherwise covered by Medicare.

In addition to Medigap policies, there are other types of supplemental insurance policies that may pay for care not covered by Medicare and Medigap insurance. These supplemental policies may be available as a benefit from your employer, or you can purchase a policy directly from an insurance company. Examples of supplemental insurance include long-term care, critical illness, hospital indemnity, and accidental death insurance. If you plan to buy such insurance for yourself and/or your care partner, carefully read the whole plan, especially the sections on benefits, limitations, and exclusions. For example, a supplemental policy may not cover all the expected expenses. It may require waiting periods before payments start. Or it may have limits based on how much you paid for the policy and how long you have had the policy. Be sure the policy covers nursing home care at a daily rate that is realistic for your community. Make sure you know how long they will pay for care. There is usually a cap of around three months for skilled nursing or rehabilitation facilities, less if you or your care partner are judged to be "not getting better" and in need of custodial care.

Governmental health care reforms continue to bring many changes in Medicare, Medicaid, and private insurance in the United States. Changes can be difficult to understand. Your local senior center, Area Agency on Aging, or disability organization can refer you to trustworthy sources of information.

If you or your care partner are too sick to work—either permanently or for some extended period—you may be entitled to Social Security based on disability. If you or your care partner have dependent children, they could also receive benefits. As of this writing, if you or your care partner have been disabled for two years, you may be entitled to Medicare coverage for medical treatment needs. Disability payments are based only on disability, not on need. If Social Security benefits are not available or not enough, the Supplemental Security Income (SSI) program is available to individuals who meet the eligibility criteria for Medicaid.

If you or your care partner have minimal savings and little or no income, the federal Medicaid program may pay for medical treatment and long-term skilled or custodial care. The eligibility rules on assets and income differ from state to state. Consult your local social services department to see if you are entitled to benefits. An attorney specializing in elder care may also be able to help.

If you or your care partner have been hospitalized, the social services department in the hospital where you or your care partner have been treated can advise you about your situation and the probability of your being eligible for these programs. The local agency serving the disabled also usually has advisers who can refer you to programs and resources for which you or your care partner may be eligible. Senior centers often have counselors knowledgeable about health care insurance.

If you or your care partner are a United States military veteran, check with your nearest Veterans Affairs (VA) facility or the VA website about services. You may be eligible for a range of services at very low or no cost. In Canada, Employment Insurance Caregiving Benefits provide financial assistance while a person is away from work to care for or support a critically ill or injured person or someone needing end-of-life care. The three benefits are family caregiver benefit for children (a critically ill or injured person under 18), family caregiver benefit for adults (a critically ill or injured person 18 or over), and compassionate care benefits (for caring for a person of any age who requires end-of-life care).

Veterans Affairs Canada has the Caregiver Recognition Benefit (CRB), a monthly, tax-free payment of $1,000 (indexed annually by the Consumer Price Index) paid directly to informal caregivers to recognize the contribution they make to the health and well-being of disabled veterans.

If you or your care partner own a home, you might be able to get a reverse mortgage. If a person takes out a reverse mortgage, the bank pays a monthly amount based on the value of the home. The nice thing about a reverse mortgage is that no matter how long you live, you can never be thrown out of your home. It is usually better to take out a reverse mortgage than to borrow against the assets you have in your house. Be sure to talk to a good financial planner who is knowledgeable about health- and aging-related issues before making any decisions. There are both risks and benefits to reverse mortgages.

It is never too soon or too late to start financial planning for expected and unexpected future events. Even when the idea of discussing the future makes you and your family feel uncomfortable or uneasy, the sooner you begin this process, the better off and more secure you will all feel knowing there is a plan in place. You and your care partner will also be better prepared if something happens.

In Canada, the Canada Health Act covers in-hospital and physician services, but other services may not be covered by the public system. It is up to you to find out which health benefits are or are not covered. In some cases, a person may qualify for more than one disability benefit. In Canada, private insurance such as disability, long-term care, and critical illness is available. Employers may offer short-term and long-term disability benefits. Provincial disability income programs may supplement Canada Pension Plan (CPP) disability benefits. Eligibility depends on the medical condition and financial criteria. CPP provides disability benefits (disability pension and post-retirement disability benefit) to people who have made enough contributions to CPP and who are disabled and cannot work at any job on a regular basis. Provinces have their own disability income programs for people who are eligible and do not qualify for other disability income programs. Publicly subsidized home and community care is also available through the provincial/territorial governments.

Can I Get Paid for Being a Caregiver?

There are some programs that pay caregivers for their work. While not everyone qualifies for these programs, you may be able to benefit.

Medicaid Programs

If your care partner is receiving Medicaid because of a disability, your state may have programs for a family member or friend to become a paid caregiver. This differs by state. To find out more, contact your state's Medicaid office.

Veterans Affairs Programs

There are programs for veterans enrolled in the VA system. Even if your care partner is not enrolled in the VA, they may be eligible. It is worth contacting the VA to find out.

The first is the veteran-directed home and community-based services program. This is open to all veterans enrolled in the Veterans Affairs who are eligible for community care and meet some specific clinical criteria. To find out more, talk with a social worker at the VA where the veteran receives care. The purpose of this program is to help veterans stay in their homes.

The VA also has aid and attendance benefits. These are for veterans who receive a VA pension and spend most of their time at home because of a permanent disability. You can find out more from the nearest VA regional office.

The Program of Comprehensive Assistance for Family Caregivers (PCAFC) offers enhanced clinical support to family caregivers of eligible veterans. Benefits may include a monthly stipend paid directly to the family caregiver. To find out more, contact your local VA Caregiver Support Program coordinator at your local VA.

In some cases, the VA also supplies respite care. Respite care is temporary care for a person who is unable to care for themselves, allowing their primary caregiver to take a break.

US State Programs

Some states have special programs to pay family caregivers. To learn more, your Area Agency on Aging is the place to start.

Long-Term Care Insurance

Some long-term care insurance policies allow for the payment of family or friends as caregivers. If you have one of these, check your policy or call your insurance agent.

I Need Help but Don't Want Help—Now What?

In addition to practical and financial concerns, there are emotional aspects of needing help. Most people leave childhood wanting and reaching for independence—the driver's license, the first job, the first credit card, the first time you go out and don't have to tell anybody where you are going, and so on. In these and many other ways, you demonstrate to yourself as well as to others that you are "grown up"—in charge of your life and able to take care of yourself.

If you realize that you can no longer manage your own needs or those of your care partner, it may feel like a return to childhood. It may seem like a loss of independence. You and/or your care partner again find yourselves with somebody else in charge of parts of your lives. This can be very painful and embarrassing for both you and your care partner.

Some people faced with this situation become depressed and no longer find any joy in life. Others deny their need for help. They may even place themselves and their care partners in danger, making life difficult for those who want to be helpful. Still others give up and expect others to take care of them completely. They may demand attention and help from their children or other family members. If you are having one or more of these reactions, you can help yourself feel better and develop a more positive response.

The idea of "changing the things you can change, accepting the things you cannot change, and knowing the difference" is key to staying in charge of your life and your care partner's life. Take a hard and realistic look at your situation. Identify the activities that require help, such as going shopping or cleaning house, and those that you can still do yourself, such as getting dressed, paying bills, and cooking light meals. Another way to look at this is to ask for help from others for the things you least like to do. If you get help with the tasks you dislike, you will have the time and energy to do the things you like.

Figuring out what kind of help you need means making decisions. And if you are making the decisions, you are in charge. It is important to make decisions and take action while you are still able to do so. Don't let events force someone else to make decisions for you and your care partner. Be realistic and honest with yourself. Use the decision-making tools on pages 12–14 in Chapter 2, Becoming a Better Caregiver: The Basics.

Even though you are the decision-maker and caregiver, you don't need to figure everything out alone. Some people find that talking with a sympathetic listener, either a professional counselor or a sensible close friend or family member, is comforting and helpful. As noted earlier in the chapter, a thoughtful listener can often point out options you may have overlooked. You may see things in a new light.

Review the content earlier in the chapter on reaching out to family and getting help with decision-making on pages 254–256 to get some ideas on people you can seek out for information and help. Choose your advisers carefully and be cautious when you take advice. Don't take advice from somebody who is selling something.

There are many people whose solution to your problem is whatever they are selling—this can include things like health or burial insurance policies, annuities, special and expensive furniture, "sunshine cruises," special magazines, or health foods.

Grieving: A Normal Reaction to Bad News

When people experience any kind of a loss—small losses, such as losing a special keepsake, or big ones, such as seeing their care partner's condition worsen with no hope for improvement or finally losing their loved one—they go through an emotional process called grieving. This is natural. It helps people come to terms with the loss.

Caregivers experience a variety of losses. These include loss of companionship, loss of confidence, loss of self-esteem, loss of independence, loss of the lifestyle you knew and cherished, and perhaps the most painful of all, loss of a positive self-image. Many caregivers tell us that no matter what they do, they feel they do not do enough. Many report feeling they are not good enough and are failing as caregivers.

Elizabeth Kübler-Ross, a psychiatrist who wrote extensively about this process, describes the stages of grief:

- **Shock**, when you feel both a mental and a physical reaction to the initial recognition of the loss.
- **Denial**, when you think, "No, it can't be true," and proceed to act for a time as if it were not true.
- **Anger**, when you ask, "Why me?" and search for someone or something to blame (if only the doctor had diagnosed it earlier, it's the care partner's fault because they refused to change their unhealthy habits, and so on).
- **Bargaining**, when you promise, "I'll never smoke again," or "I'll follow my treatment regimen absolutely to the letter," or "I'll go to church every Sunday, if only I can get over this."
- **Depression**, when awareness sets in, you confront the truth about the situation, and experience deep feelings of sadness and hopelessness.
- **Acceptance**, when you recognize that you must deal with what has happened and make up your mind to do what you must do to move forward.

People do not necessarily pass through these stages one after the other. You are more apt to flip-flop between them. So, don't be surprised or discouraged if you find yourself angry or depressed again when you thought you had reached acceptance.

If you find yourself experiencing any, some, or all of the stages of grieving, first know that this is normal. The grief is real but need not be overwhelming. Reaching out to others—friends, family, or professionals—can often help with the pain of grieving. Review the content in this chapter about reaching out to family for help and getting professional help with decision-making on pages 254–256 as well as Chapter 4, Dealing with Difficult Emotions, and Chapter 5, Using Your Mind to Manage Stress. The important thing is that you are not alone.

Making End-of-Life Decisions

Decisions about the end of life can be very difficult. It means dealing with the idea of your own mortality. For caregivers, it also means dealing with your care partner's end of life. As you age and as your care partner's condition worsens, you may begin to have fears about death. This is especially true when something happens to bring you face-to-face with the possibility or your own death. Losing a friend, surviving an accident, or learning you have a health condition that may shorten your life can cause you to think about your own passing. It may also force you to think about your care partner's condition and who will take care of them if something happens to you.

Attitudes about death are shaped by core attitudes about life. These attitudes are the product of your culture, your family, perhaps your religion, and certainly your life experiences. You might pray or wish that you or your care partner be released form suffering, feel guilty about these wishes, or fear dying. Sometimes you may have all these feelings. If this is how you feel, you are not alone. Many people try to avoid these feelings. They do not want to face the future because they are afraid to think about death.

If you are ready to think about your own and your care partner's future—about the near or distant prospect that your lives will most certainly end—then the information that follows will be useful to you. If you are not ready to think about this just yet, put this reading aside and come back to it when you are ready.

Taking positive steps to prepare for death is often healthful. This means putting things in order and attending to all the necessary details, large and small. It also means gathering information about what to expect and what is possible. If you avoid dealing with these details, you create problems for yourself and for those who love and care about you. You may also lose your ability to stay in control and make these important decisions for yourself and your care partner.

Whatever you decide about your future and the future of your care partner, it is important to tell others. What are your wishes about how and where you want your care partner to be during those last days? Do you want the same thing for yourself? Does your care partner want to be in a hospital or at home? What do you want for yourself? When do you want procedures to prolong life stopped for your care partner and yourself? At what point do you want to let nature take its course? Who should be with your care partner or you—only the few people who are nearest and dearest, or all the people you care about and want to see one last time? What will happen if you can no longer provide care to your care partner? What will happen if your care partner cannot manage their affairs? What do you want to happen at the end of your or your care partner's life? Most people have very definite ideas of what they would like. Share both your ideas and wishes as well as those of your care partner with others.

This kind of end-of-life planning is hard and sometimes frightening. People do not like thinking about all the what-ifs. Nevertheless, such planning is necessary for both you and your care partner. Good planning protects both of you and ensures that your wishes are understood and carried out.

If your plans are not written down and recorded in legal documents, your wishes or those of your care partner might not be followed. In the following content, we discuss the types of legal documents you should have in place. If you are not sure what you have, or you do not have any of these, consult a lawyer. This is not something you can do yourself. Many people worry that going to a lawyer will be very expensive, but many lawyers will allow a free meeting or consultation where you discuss your needs. Law offices can give you the price of each service during a consultation. Also, lawyers' fees do vary. Shop around to find one whose fees fit best with what you can afford to pay. Preparing the two documents that we discuss, the power of attorney and the advance directive for health care, should not be too expensive and are essential for ensuring that you and your care partner's wishes are respected.

Legal Planning

Preparing legal documents should be done now, not later. This is especially true if your health is worsening and/or your care partner's mental abilities are declining. Attorneys who are consulted about legal end-of-life planning are required by law to determine that a person is "of sound mind" and able to make these decisions for themselves. Therefore, it is best not to wait.

First, a disclaimer: The following discussion is not complete. Also, the laws are different for each state, province, and country. For more complete details, seek legal counsel. These are just the basics to prepare you for a deeper discussion with your care partner, family, and legal counsel. It should also be noted that both you and your care partner need these documents. One last note: Even if you have these documents, check that they are up to date. In some places, documents must be reviewed and updated every so many years. In other cases, your or your care partner's life circumstances may have changed but not be noted in the documents.

Power of Attorney

A general power of attorney (POA) is a legal document that gives a person that you appoint the power to make financial or business decisions for you when you are not mentally or physically able to represent yourself. You can set a POA to take effect immediately or to take effect when or if there is some future event that will leave you unable to act on your own behalf because you are mentally incapacitated or have a physical disability. For caregivers, it is recommended to have a POA in place and ready for when your care partner is no longer able to make these types of decisions on their own.

If you do not have a POA in place and you need to pay for care, then you, your family, friends, or even sometimes the state, will need to go to court to pay those bills. A POA can avoid the need to file for conservatorship which involves a court hearing where one person, the conservatee (care partner), is found to be unable to handle their own affairs, and another person, the conservator (caregiver or some other person), is appointed to handle these affairs. This is expensive and usually means going to court many times. Talk to a lawyer about the advantages and disadvantages of a POA for you and your care partner.

Advance Directives for Health Care

Advance directives are written instructions that tell your medical professionals what kind of care you would like to receive when you or your care partner are not able to make medical decisions for yourselves (for example, if you are unconscious, in a coma, or mentally incompetent). Usually, an advance directive describes both the types of treatments you want and those you do not want.

Everyone faces death, but how each of us dies, like other aspects of our lives, is something we can help manage. You, along with your care partner, can have input and make decisions that will affect the quality of your or your care partner's final days. Planning and proper management can lessen the negative impact of death on our family and friends. An advance health care directive can help you manage some of the medical and legal issues concerning death as well as help you plan for both expected and unexpected end-of-life situations. You and your care partner, if they are able, should put an advance health care directive in place as early as possible. This is important even for people who do not have any chronic health conditions. Without this directive, your wishes or those of your care partner may not be followed. Even as the caregiver, your partner's wishes may not be followed without an advance directive unless you have conservatorship.

There are different types of advance directives. The most common types are described in the following list:

- **Living will.** A living will is a document that states what kind of medical or life-sustaining treatments you or your care partner would want if seriously or terminally ill. A living will, however, does not let you legally appoint someone to make those decisions for you. It expresses your or your care partner's desires, but it is not a legally binding document.
- **Durable power of attorney (DPA) for health care.** A durable power of attorney (DPA) for health care (or more simply a power of attorney for health care) allows you or your care partner to name someone to act as your agent. It also gives your agent guidelines about your health care wishes. If you want, you can let your agent make the decisions without your guidance. Many people, however, prefer to give guidance to their agent. This guidance can indicate almost anything you want done for your and your care partner's care. The guidance may range from wanting the use of aggressive life-sustaining measures to not wanting these measures. Whereas a living will applies only if you or your care partner have an illness that will end life, a DPA for health care can be used anytime you are unconscious or unable to make decisions due to any illness, accident, or injury.

In Canada, terms used for a DPA for health care include substitute decision maker, proxy, mandatary (Quebec), agent, or power of attorney for health or for personal care. We refer to DPA for health care for the rest of this section, but the discussion applies equally to Canada. (Note that a general DPA deals with financial matters, whereas a DPA for health care is for health care decisions only.)

It is important to understand that a DPA allows you to appoint someone else to act as your agent for *only* your health care. It does not give this person the right to act on your behalf in other ways, such as in handling your financial matters. In general, a DPA for health care is more useful than a living will because it allows you to appoint someone to make decisions for you. It can be used anytime that you are unable to make health care decisions. The only time a DPA for health care may not be the best choice is if there is no one you trust to act on your behalf. The next section of this chapter on pages 266–269 contains more detailed information on preparing a DPA for health care. In most states, you do not need a lawyer to prepare this document.

- **Do not resuscitate (DNR) order.** A DNR is a request that a person not be given cardiopulmonary resuscitation (CPR) if their heart stops or if they stop breathing. **A DNR can be included as part of a living will or durable power of attorney (DPA) for health care**. However, you do not need to have a living will or a DPA for health care to have a DNR order. Your doctor can put a DNR in your medical chart so that it may guide the actions of the hospital and any health care provider. You can also put a DNR on your refrigerator or somewhere else in your home so that emergency personnel will know your wishes. Without a DNR order, hospital or emergency personnel will make every effort to resuscitate you. DNR orders are accepted in all states in the United States.
- **Advance directive for mental health care.** Although advance directives for health care are generally used for end-of-life situations, they may also be prepared to direct the type of mental health treatment given in the event a person with dementia or mental illness becomes incapacitated due to that illness. Under US federal law, most states may combine advance directives for health care and mental health care in one document and allow you to appoint an agent to act on your behalf for both health and mental health issues. Some states, however, require separate documents, which also allow you to choose different agents, one for health care and another for mental health care. For more information on mental health advance directives and the specific practices in your state, visit the website of the National Resource Center on Psychiatric Advance Directives (www.nrc-pad.org).
- **Physician Orders for Life-Sustaining Treatment (POLST).** Another advance directive form that is becoming more common is the POLST. Doctors introduce this form (which is usually pink) to their patients during an appointment. A POLST is part of your medical record, but it does not appoint someone to act on your behalf, so a DPA for health care is still important.

In Canada, the terms for advance directives vary across the country. An advance directive may be called a personal directive, health care directive, advanced care plan, protection mandate (previously known as a "mandate in case of incapacity"). The term "living will" originated in the United States and has no legal status in the US or Canada. In Canada, a health care directive can be created without the assistance of a lawyer. Most provinces and territories in Canada have their own DNR forms for residents to use. The names of these forms and when they can be used may differ. In Canada, practices on mental health care directives differ by province. For more information, check with your local health authority or hospital, or contact your local branch of the Canadian Mental Health Association (cmha.ca). In Canada, POLST is referred to as "Goals of Care" while the province of BC uses MOST (Medical Orders for Scope of Treatment).

Preparing a Durable Power of Attorney (DPA) for Health Care

All adults (anyone age 18 or older) should have a durable power of attorney (DPA) for health care. Unexpected events can happen to anyone at any age. Although each state has different regulations and forms for advance directives, this information is useful wherever you live.

Many states recognize durable powers of attorney for health care that are created in another state. However, this is not always the case. To be on the safe side, if you move or spend a lot of time in another state, it is best to check with a lawyer in that state to see if your document is legally binding there.

Make sure your doctor has a copy of your DPA for health care, and when you go to the hospital, be sure the hospital also has a copy. If you cannot bring your DPA yourself, be sure your agent knows to give a copy to the hospital. This is important because your doctor may not oversee your care in the hospital. Do not put your only copy of your DPA for health care in your safe deposit box. It needs to be easily accessible when it is needed.

Choosing Your Agent

The first step in preparing a DPA for health care is to choose your agent. An agent can be a friend or family member, but it cannot be any of the providers who give you care. Your agent should probably live in your area. If the agent is not available on short notice to make decisions for you, the agent will not be much help. Just to be safe, name a backup or secondary agent who will act for you if your primary agent is not available. Some documents ask for three names.

Be sure that your agent thinks like you or at least is willing to carry out your wishes. You must be able to trust that this person has your interests at heart and truly understands and will respect and carry out your wishes. Your agent should be mature, composed, and comfortable with your decisions. Sometimes a spouse or child is not the best agent because this person is too close emotionally. This can be the case if that spouse or child is also the caregiver. For example, if you or your care partner wishes not to be resuscitated in the case of a severe heart attack or other illness, the agent must be able to tell the doctor not to resuscitate. This could be very difficult or impossible for a caregiver or family member to do. Be sure the person you choose as your or your care partner's agent is up to this task and would not say "do everything you can" at this critical time if this is not something you want. You want the agent to be someone who will not find this job too much of an emotional burden.

In review, look for the following characteristics in an agent:

- Someone who is likely to be available should they need to act for you
- Someone who understands your wishes and is willing and able to carry them out
- Someone who is emotionally prepared and will not feel burdened by doing so

Finding the right agent is a significant task. This may mean talking to several people. These might be the most important interviews that you will ever conduct. We talk more about discussing your wishes with your family, friends, and doctor later in this chapter.

Expressing Your Choices

Once you have chosen your agent, spend some time with your care partner to think about your choices and determine what you want for yourselves. In other words, what are the directions you will give your agent? What you want is guided by your beliefs and values. Some DPA forms give several general statements of desires concerning medical treatment. These can help you decide what you want. The following are some examples of general statements:

If my primary physician finds that I cannot make my own health care decisions, I grant my agent full power and authority to make those decisions for me, subject to any health care instructions set forth below. My agent will have the right to:

a. Consent, refuse consent, or withdraw consent to any medical care or services, such as tests, drugs, surgery, or consultations for any physical or mental condition. This includes the provision, withholding, or withdrawal of artificial nutrition and hydration (feeding by tube or vein) and all other forms of health care, including cardiopulmonary resuscitation (CPR).
b. Choose or reject my physician, other health care professionals, or health care facilities.
c. Receive and consent to the release of medication information.
d. Donate organs or tissue, authorize an autopsy, and dispose of my body, unless I have said something different in a contract with a funeral home, in my will, or by some other written method.
e. Prolong my life to the greatest extent possible without regard to my condition, the chances I have for recovery, or the cost of the procedures.

If you use a form containing suggested general statements such as these, all you need to do is initial the statements that apply to you.

Other forms include a "general statement of granted authority," in which you give your agent the power to make decisions. In this case, you do not write out the details of what these decisions should be. Instead, you trust that your agent will follow your wishes. Since these wishes are not explicitly expressed in written form, you must discuss them in detail with your agent.

All forms also have a space in which you can write out any specific wishes. You are not required to give specific details, but you may wish to do so. Knowing what details to write is a little complicated. None of us can predict the future or knows the exact circumstances in which the agent will have to act. You can get some idea by asking your doctor what the most likely developments are for someone with your or your care partner's condition. Then you can direct your agent on how to act. Your directions can include outcomes, specific circumstances, or both. If you specify outcomes, the statement should focus on which types of outcomes would be acceptable and which would not (for example, "resuscitate if I can continue to fully function mentally").

The following is information about specific conditions:

- **You or your care partner have been diagnosed with Alzheimer's disease and/or other neurological problems that may eventually leave you with little or no mental function.** These conditions generally are not life-threatening, at least not for many years. However, other things can happen, too, that can be life-threatening, such as pneumonia, a stroke or heart attack. Therefore, you and your care partner need to decide how much treatment you want. For example, do you want antibiotics if you get pneumonia? Do you want to be resuscitated if your heart stops? Do you want a feeding tube if you are unable to feed yourself? Remember, it is your choice as to how you answer each of these questions. You may not want to be resuscitated but may want a feeding tube. If you want aggressive treatment, you might want to use all means possible to sustain life. On the other hand, you might not want any special means to be used to sustain life. For example, you may want to be fed but may not want to be placed on life-support equipment.
- **You or your care partner have very bad lung function that will not improve.** If you or your care partner become unable to breathe on your own, do you want to be placed in an intensive care unit on a mechanical ventilator (a breathing machine)? Remember, in this case, you will not improve. To say that you never want ventilation is very different from saying that you don't want it if it is used to sustain life when no improvement is likely. For example, mechanical ventilation can be lifesaving in cases such as a severe asthma attack when it is used for a short time until the body can regain its normal function. In this case, the issue is not whether or not to ever to use mechanical ventilation but rather when you want to use it.
- **You or your care partner have a heart condition that cannot be improved with surgery.** Imagine you are in the cardiac intensive care unit. If your heart stops functioning, do you want to be resuscitated? As with artificial ventilation, the question is not, "Do you ever want to be resuscitated?" but rather, "Under what conditions do you want resuscitation?"

From these examples, you can begin to identify some of the directions that you might want to give in the advance directive or durable power of attorney for health care for you and/or your care partner. Remember that in order to understand these possible situations better and to make them more personal to you or your care partner, it is important to speak with your health care providers about what the common problems and decisions are for people with your conditions.

In summary, there are several questions to answer before directing your agent on how to act in your behalf:

- Generally, how much treatment do you want? This can range from the very aggressive—doing many things to sustain life—to the very conservative, which is doing almost nothing to sustain life, except to keep you or your care partner clean and comfortable.
- Given the types of life-threatening events that are likely to happen to people with your or your care partner's condition, what sorts of treatment do you want under what conditions?
- If you or your care partner become mentally incapacitated, what sorts of treatment do you want for other illnesses, such as pneumonia?

In this section, we have focused not only what kinds of decisions you want yourself should something happen to you as the caregiver, but also what you should think about the different scenarios that might happen with your care partner. If your care partner's wishes are recorded in a document, you can prepare yourself emotionally for the time you will need to act on those decisions. Asking your care partner's health care provider about the usual things that can happen with your care partner's condition can help you think about how you would react if and when these things happen. You will be better able to effectively direct the health care team if you have prepared yourself emotionally. When your care partner is near the end of life because of their illness or some other life-threatening event, it is best to change the focus of your caregiving efforts. Rather than seeking treatment to extend your care partner's life, you can ask their health care team to provide care to make them as comfortable as possible so that you can make the most of the time you have left together.

Check out our resource page at www.bullpub.com/resources under the heading "Planning for the Future." Some of the websites have downloadable forms for durable power of attorney (DPA) for health care.

Sharing Your Wishes about End-of-Life Issues with Family and Friends

Recording your and/or your health care partner's wishes and having your advance directive for health care, including the DPA for health care, in place is not the end of your work. If you want your wishes and those of your care partner carried out, these need to be shared fully with your agent, family, maybe friends, and the health care team. This is often not an easy task.

Before you can have this conversation, everyone involved needs to have copies of your and/or your care partner's DPA for health care. Once you have completed these documents, have them witnessed and signed. In some places, you can have your DPA for health care notarized instead of having it witnessed. Make several copies. You will need copies for your agents, family members, and health care providers. Also, give one to your lawyer if you have one. Sometimes these are also placed in your electronic medical record such as MyHealth or MyChart.

Now you are ready to talk about your wishes and those of your care partner. People don't like to discuss their own death or that of a loved one. Therefore, it should not surprise you that when you bring up this subject, the response is often, "Oh, don't think about that," or "That's a long time off," or "Don't be so morbid; you're not that sick." Unfortunately, this is usually enough to end the conversation. Your job is to keep the conversation open. There are several ways to do this. First, plan on how you will have this discussion. Here are some suggestions:

- As noted earlier, prepare your and/or your care partner's DPA for health care and give copies to the appropriate family members or friends. Ask them to read it and then set a specific time to discuss it. If they give you one of the avoidance responses, explain that you understand that this is a difficult topic but that you must discuss it with them. This is a good time to practice the "I" messages discussed in Chapter 6, Communicating Effectively. For example, say, "I understand that death is a difficult thing to talk about. However, it is very important to me that we have this talk."
- Another strategy is to get blank copies of DPA for health care forms for all your family members and suggest that everyone fill one out and share them. This could even be part of a family get-together. Present this as an important part of being mature adults and family members. Making this a family project involving everyone may make it easier to discuss. Besides, it will help clarify everyone's values about death and dying. Even teens can be a part of this discussion.
- If these two suggestions seem too difficult or for some reason are impossible to carry out, try writing a letter or e-mail or prepare a video to send to family members. Talk about why you feel your and/or your care partner's death is an important topic to discuss and that you want them to know your wishes. Then state your wishes. Give the reasons for your choices. At the same time, send them a copy of your and/or your care partner's DPA for health care. Ask that they respond in some way or that you set aside some time to talk in person or on the phone.

As mentioned before, when deciding on an agent, it is key that you choose someone with whom you can talk freely and exchange ideas. If your chosen agent is not willing to or is unable to talk to you about your wishes, you have probably chosen the wrong person. Remember, the fact that someone is very close to you does not mean that that person understands your wishes or would be able to carry them out. This topic should not be left to an unspoken understanding unless you don't mind if your agent goes against your wishes. For this reason, you may want to choose someone who is not very emotionally close to you and/or your care partner. If you do choose someone outside of close family members, make sure your family knows who you have appointed and why.

Talking About End-of-Life Issues with Your and Your Care Partner's Doctor

In our research, we have learned that people often have a more difficult time talking with their doctors about their wishes than they do talking with their families about end-of-life issues. In fact, only a very small percentage of people who have written DPAs for health care or other advance directives ever share these with their physician.

Even though it is difficult, you should talk with both your doctor and your care partner's doctor. You need to be sure that your doctors' values are like yours. If you and your doctors do not have the same values, it may be difficult for them to carry out your wishes. Second, your doctors need to know what you want. This allows them to take appropriate actions such as writing orders to resuscitate or not to use mechanical resuscitation. Third, your doctors need to know who your agent is and how to contact this person. If an important decision must be made and your wishes are to be followed, the doctor must talk with your agent. Sometimes your wishes for yourself and what your care partner wants or what you want for your care partner, might not be the same. This is OK, but the doctors giving care for each person must know each person's wishes and have those wishes in writing.

Be sure to give your doctor a copy of your DPA for health care so that it can become a permanent part of your medical record. The same is true for the doctor of your care partner. As mentioned earlier, there is another advance directive form, the POLST (Physician Orders for Life-Sustaining Treatment) form used for people in the final year of life or who have an advanced-stage terminal illness or an illness from which they are not expected to recover. Many doctors complete this form with their patients during an appointment. This gives both you and the physician an opportunity to discuss what could happen and what you want when it does. A POLST is part of your medical record but it does not appoint someone to act on your behalf, so it is still important to have a DPA for health care.

As surprising as it may seem, many physicians find it hard to talk to their patients about their end-of-life wishes. Doctors are in the business of keeping people alive and well. They don't like to think about their patients dying. On the other hand, most doctors want their patients to have durable powers of attorney for health care (and sometimes a POLST). These documents can prevent added stress and worry for both you and your doctor.

Plan a time with your doctor when you can discuss your wishes. This should not be a side conversation at the end of a regular visit. Rather, start a visit by saying, "I want to discuss my wishes in the event of a serious problem or impending death." When put this way, most doctors will make time to talk with you. If the doctor says that there is not enough time to talk with you about this topic, ask when you can make another appointment. This is a situation where you might need to be a little assertive. Sometimes a doctor, like your family members or friends, might say, "Oh, you don't have to worry about that; let me do it," or

"We'll worry about that when the time comes." Again, you must take the initiative, using an "I" message to communicate that this is important to you and that you do not want to put off the discussion.

Sometimes doctors do not want to worry you. They think they are doing you a favor by not describing all the unpleasant things that might happen to you in case of serious problems. You can help your doctor by telling them that having control and making some decisions about your future will ease your mind. Not knowing or not being clear about what may happen is more worrisome than being faced with the facts, unpleasant as they may be, and dealing with them.

Even if you know all this information, it is still sometimes hard to talk with your doctor. It might be helpful to bring your agent with you for this discussion. The agent can facilitate the discussion and at the same time meet your doctor. This gives everyone a chance to clarify any misunderstandings. It opens the lines of communication so that if your agent and physician must act to carry out your wishes, they can do so with few problems. If you cannot have this conversation with your doctor, your doctor should still receive a copy of your DPA for health care for your medical record.

When you or your care partner go the hospital, be sure to take a copy of your DPA for health care with you. If you do not take it, be sure your agent knows to give a copy to the hospital. If you or your care partner do not have a DPA prepared and available, the hospital will ask you to fill out the advance directive form for the institution that is treating you. This is important so the doctors who oversee your care in the hospital know your wishes.

Again, do *not* put a durable power of attorney in a safe deposit box—no one will be able to get it when it is needed. And remember, you do not need to see a lawyer to draw up a durable power of attorney. You can do this by yourself with no legal assistance. If you are writing a DPA for your care partner, however, you may want legal advice.

Preparing Yourself and Others

Now that you have done all the important things, much of the hard work is over. And it is important to remember that you can change your mind at any time. Your agent may no longer be available, or your wishes or your care partner's might change. Be sure to keep your DPA for health care updated. Like most legal documents, the DPA for health care can be revoked or changed at any time. The decisions you make today do not have to be forever.

Sharing wishes about how you and your care partner want to be treated in case of a serious or life-threatening illness is one of the most important tasks for managing your own health as a caregiver and that of your care partner.

Here are some other steps to help reduce the emotional burden to your care partner, family, and friends:

- **Make a will for both you and your care partner**. Even if your estate is a small one and your belongings are few, you may have ideas about who should inherit what. If you have a large estate, the tax implications could be significant. A will ensures that your belongings go where you would like them to go. Without a will, some distant or long-lost relative could end up with your estate. You might also want to consider a trust. Your will should include information about what you want done with your financial accounts and give directions about who can access them and how. Do not put passwords to your accounts in a will. Talk with your lawyer about these options of will and/or trust. Be sure to review this every few years to be sure it is up to date.

- **Plan your funeral and that of your care partner.** Write down your wishes or arrange for the funeral and burial. You and/or your grieving family will be very relieved not to have to decide what you would want and how much to spend. Prepaid funeral plans are available. You can purchase a burial space in the location you prefer. Be sure that the people you want to handle things after your death are aware of all they need to know about your wishes. This includes your plans and arrangements, and the location of necessary documents. Talk to them or at least prepare a detailed letter of instructions. Give the letter to someone trusted to deliver it to the right person at the right time.
- **Organize all important documents and papers.** You can purchase (at any well-stocked stationery store or online) a kit in which you place a copy of your will, your durable powers of attorney (for health care and for financial and legal matters), important papers, and information about the financial and personal affairs of you and/or your care partner. Another useful source to help organize this information is My Life in a Box, which is listed in the resources at www.bullpub.com/resources under the heading "Planning for the Future." It includes forms to fill out about bank and charge accounts, insurance policies, the location of important documents, passwords to online accounts, where your safe deposit box and its key are kept, and other related information. This is a handy, concise way of getting everything together that anyone might need to know about. If you keep these documents on your computer, be sure others can find the passwords to access the information.
- **Wrap up your dealings with the world around you.** Mend your relationships. Pay your debts, both financial and personal. Say what needs to be said to those who need to hear it. Do what needs to be done. Forgive yourself. Forgive others. (This is a good idea at any time, not just at the end of life.)
- **Talk about your feelings about death.** Most family and close friends are reluctant to start this conversation but will probably appreciate it if you bring it up. You may find that there is much to say to and to hear from your loved ones. If you find that they are unwilling to listen to you talk about death and the feelings that you have, find someone who will be comfortable and understanding in listening to you. Most hospitals and hospice services have chaplains who have these types of conversations daily. You

may find it helpful to talk to a person with this experience and training. Your family and friends might be able to listen to you later. Just as you may have to go through the stages of grieving, people who love you go through the stages of grieving.

A large part of the fear of death is fear of the unknown: "What will it be like?" "Will it be painful?" "What will happen to me after I die?" Most people who die from a chronic or terminal illness are ready to die when the time comes. Painkillers and the disease process weaken body and mind. The awareness of self diminishes without the realization that this is happening. Most people just slip away, with the transition between the state of living and that of no longer living hardly noticeable, like how a river meets the ocean. Reports from people who have been brought back to life after being in a state of clinical death say that they experienced a sense of peacefulness and clarity and were not frightened.

People who are dying sometimes feel lonely and abandoned. Many people cannot deal with their own emotions when they are around a person who is dying. They avoid the dying person's company, or they may engage in superficial chitchat, broken by long, awkward silences. This is often puzzling and hurtful to the person dying. If your care partner is dying, this avoidance can be difficult for you, the caregiver, as you are seeking companionship and solace from the people you count on.

You can help by telling your family and friends what you want and need from them—attention, entertainment, comfort, music, practical help, and so on. A person who has something positive to do is more able to cope with difficult emotions. If you can engage your family and loved ones in specific activities, they can feel needed and can relate to you around the activity. This will give you something to talk about, and it will occupy everyone's time in a beneficial way. It helps to define the situation for them and for you.

Considering Palliative Care and Hospice Care

Both palliative care and hospice care are available in most parts of the world. The goal of both palliative care and hospice care is to provide comfort. The word *palliative* refers to relieving symptoms such as pain associated with a serious illness and improving quality of life. The word *hospice* refers to care provided for the terminally ill at home or in the community rather than a hospital. Palliative care can begin at diagnosis and occur at the same time as treatment. Hospice care begins after treatment of an illness is stopped, when it is clear the illness will probably end in death. The primary aim of hospice is to make the patient more comfortable, but hospice professionals also help the family prepare for death with dignity. They help the surviving family members with emotional and support services during the dying process. This help often continues after the loved one's death.

In everyone's life, there comes a time when regular medical care is no longer helpful, and it is time to prepare for death. Today, people

In June 2016, the Parliament of Canada passed federal legislation—Medical Assistance in Dying (MAID) —that allows eligible Canadian adults to request medical assistance in dying. Health Canada encourages patients to contact their physician or nurse practitioner (if applicable) for questions about access. Patients may also wish to contact the resources set up within their province or territory to get information on medical assistance in dying and other end-of-life care options.

often have several weeks or months, and sometimes years, to make these preparations. This is when hospice care is so very useful. In hospice, medical and other care is aimed at making the patient as comfortable as possible and providing a good quality of life. Studies have shown that—at least for some illnesses—people who receive hospice care live longer than those who receive more aggressive treatment. Most hospices only accept people who are expected to die within six months. Rest assured, however, that this does not mean that you or your care partner will have this care taken away if you live longer.

Most hospices are in-home programs. This means that patients stay in their own homes and the services come to them. In some places, there are also residential hospices where people can go for their last days. Skilled nursing facilities often bring in hospice care as well, and they oversee the comfort for the last days, for both the person and the family.

One of the problems with hospice care is that people often wait until the last few days before death to ask for this care. They somehow see asking for hospice care as giving up. By refusing hospice care, they often put an unnecessary burden on themselves, friends, and family. Or the reverse occurs, and the caregiver and family might say they can cope without help. Although this may be true, the care partner's life and dying may be much better if hospice cares for all the medical things so that the caregiver, family, and friends are free to give love and emotional support to the dying person.

If your care partner, you, a family member, or a friend is at the end stage of illness, we encourage you to find and make use of your local hospice. It is a wonderful final gift. Hospice workers are very special people who are kind, thoughtful, and supportive. An added benefit is that many hospice care services are covered by Medicare, Medicaid, and regular private insurance policies, as well as the Veterans Affairs (VA).

In Canada, hospice palliative care is paid for in diverse ways across the country. Who pays often depends on whether care is provided at home, in the hospital, in a hospice residence, or other situation.

At home, the provincial health plan may pay. After the hours are used up, people need to look for other ways to pay for these services. People may use private insurance or their own money to pay for palliative care services at home. Some may receive assistance from social agencies, service clubs, local cancer societies, and other similar organizations.

In the hospital, care is paid for by provincial health plans. These plans usually cover most care including drugs, medical supplies, and equipment while the person is in the hospital. In long-term care facilities, residents are usually required to pay for some of their care. Costs vary among facilities.

In hospice residences, there is usually no charge as they are partially covered by provincial health plans and the rest is raised through donations and community support.

Bereavement support is often provided as part of hospice palliative care services offered in hospitals or by nonprofit or volunteer organizations in the community.

In closing, we would like to thank you for choosing to be a caregiver. Throughout this book, we have tried to give tips and tools to make this role easier for you and to encourage you to take care of yourself so that you stay healthy and live a more satisfying life as a caregiver.

For a complete list of suggested readings, useful websites, and other helpful resources, please see: www.bullpub.com/resources

Index

Note: Page numbers followed by *f* or *t* indicate a figure or table